STILL
AWAKE

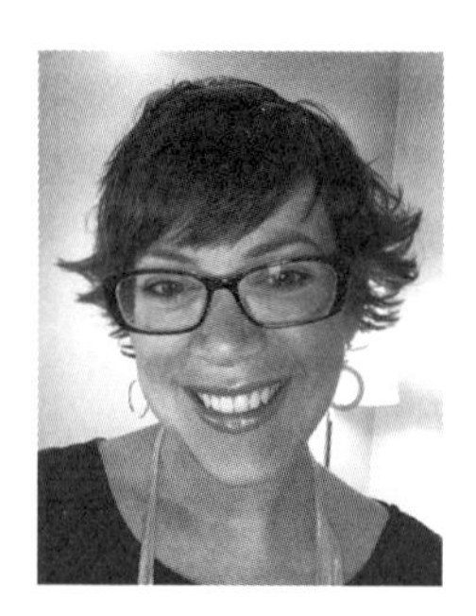

About the author

Lyndsey Hookway is a London-trained paediatric nurse, health visitor, IBCLC, holistic sleep coach, independent lecturer and international speaker. She has an international private practice supporting families with sleep, breastfeeding, bottle-feeding and responsive, gentle parenting, and has supported thousands of families with early parenting over the last 15 years.

Lyndsey runs a successful online sleep programme which promotes responsive parenting and family-centred care and is particularly known for her creative sleep solutions for toddlers and preschoolers.

She is the author of *Holistic Sleep Coaching* (2018), *Let's talk about your new family's sleep* (2020), and *Still Awake* (2021).

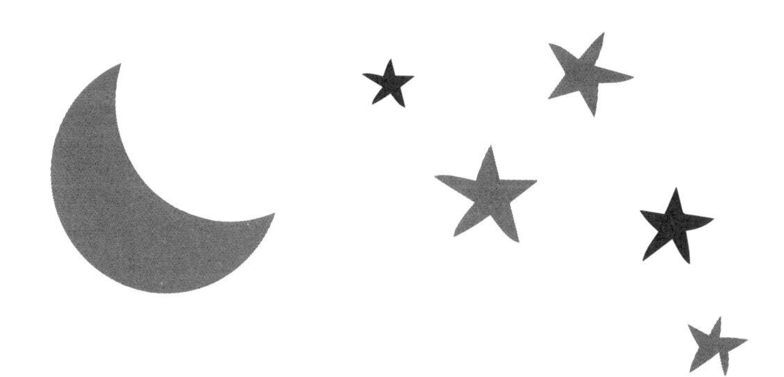

STILL AWAKE

RESPONSIVE SLEEP TOOLS FOR TODDLERS TO TWEENS

LYNDSEY HOOKWAY

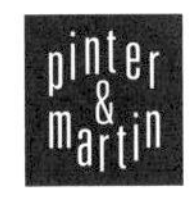

Still Awake: Responsive sleep tools for toddlers to tweens

First published in the UK by Pinter & Martin Ltd 2021

ISBN 978-1-78066-730-0

Also available as an ebook

Index by Helen Bilton

British Library Cataloguing-in-Publication Data
A catalogue record for this book is available from the British Library

Printed in the EU by Hussar

This book has been printed on paper that is sourced and harvested from sustainable forests and is FSC accredited

Pinter & Martin Ltd
6 Effra Parade
London SW2 1PS

pinterandmartin.com

CONTENTS

INTRODUCTION

WELCOME TO THE TODDLER (AND BEYOND) CLUB!

You did it – you raised your child beyond infancy. You navigated the sleep deprivation of the early weeks, teething, the inevitable poo-up-the-back-in-public situation, learning to crawl, and the 'firsts' – first birthday, first meeting of Great Aunt Aggie, first holiday.

You've done the hard part haven't you? Toddlerdom and raising a preschooler should be a piece of cake. Once they start school your work is pretty much done, right? After all – they'll sleep now, won't they? Fatigue should be a thing of the past...

Except that sometimes the answer is, not so much. If yours is one of the millions of families whose two-year-old, four-year-old, or even nine-year-old still thinks sleep is for the weak, then trust me, you're in good company. In fact, I'm going to go out on a limb here in assuming that since you're reading this, you have a child who finds it hard to fall asleep, stay asleep, or sleep where you want them to sleep (maybe even all three).

I managed to give birth to two sleep-allergic children, both with their fair share of sleep dramas, so please know that you have my virtual empathy. I really do know what it is like to have years, not months, of sleep deprivation. To know what it feels like, physically and emotionally, to be chronically sleep deprived. To know what it is to wonder if you can die from lack of sleep. To feel like your eyes are on fire, your fuse is non-existent, and you're sick of not being able to finish your sentence because you are *that tired*.

My eldest daughter woke frequently until she was three. One day,

she had finished her bedtime feed, had a story and a cuddle, and she just *went to sleep*. It was like some kind of magic. That's not to say that sleep was a breeze from that moment on – we continued to have various sleep dramas for many years, but the acute horror story of the two-hour bedtime and multiple night wakes was finally over.

Our second daughter was the polar opposite. She slept beautifully from birth. I had to wake her to feed her, and she slept 8–10 hour stretches from about two months. I felt that the universe had repaid my patience with my eldest. But it didn't last. Our youngest soon started waking frequently, and this lasted for many more years in the end than her sister. She became very ill with cancer, which really messed up her sleep, and it was only once she was fully recovered, aged six, that her sleep became predictably solid. So I've clocked nine years of pretty shoddy sleep. I really do get it.

Right at the outset of this book, I also want to offer you hope. Almost all children's sleep eventually gets better. Those who continue to struggle usually have an underlying problem or condition. I'm not here to sell you a dream, offer false promises, or provide unsubstantiated quick-fix tricks. I'm not going to recommend a programme that will have your child sleeping a certain number of hours per night, in a certain number of days. I have no magic, but a lot of experience and, most of all, a lot of love for children. In fact, if I'm going to be honest with you, although most people who talk about sleep write about babies, I've always been drawn to working with toddlers and older children.

I love working with older children because it's more interesting to me. The areas that you as a parent can work on to improve sleep are immensely rewarding. The tools we can use are more creative. We can involve children in the plan. And while I'm a big fan of no crying at any age, with toddlers and older children it's very likely that there will be minimal and usually no crying when using the suggestions. You do not need to put a stairgate on your child's room, ignore them, or leave them alone. You just don't. Stick with me – I promise I have solutions other than 'live with it', or 'they'll grow out of it'.

I truly believe that most sleep education is out of date. A large proportion of it assumes that behavioural approaches to sleep will work for most problems. This is the idea that most children do something because their behaviour is reinforced by our actions. In doing whatever

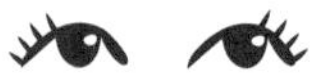

it is we do to help, we reinforce the behaviour. The problem is that this is an outdated theory, and even if some sleep problems *are* behavioural, firstly, there are more constructive and creative ways to work on them, and secondly, not all problems *are* behavioural in origin. We do children a huge disservice to distil their sleeping patterns down to a simplistic behavioural cause. I need to be careful not to have a rant here! I am tired of hearing of parents who have been told to ignore their child, put up a stairgate, teach them who is 'boss' or only reward and acknowledge 'good' behaviour. There is so much more to it. That is not to say that I'm trying to make something more complicated than it needs to be, but that children *are* more complicated than this narrow vision. Treating their complexity with a one-size-fits-all behavioural approach serves nobody.

Thank you for trusting me with your family's sleep. Together, we will explore sleep in a meaningful way, and you will find plenty of strategies to try right away, which will not conflict with your gentle parenting ethos.

How your child slept as a baby

Maybe your little one has always been an 'interesting' sleeper. Maybe they used to sleep well, and things have gone belly-up recently. Perhaps it was a big change, or an event that sparked a deterioration in sleeping behaviours. Or maybe their sleep has undergone peaks and troughs, but, basically, it's never covered itself in glory.

Wherever you position yourself and your child's sleep, I assure you that all this is a common story to me. It is certainly true that some children seem to struggle with sleep from the beginning. Sometimes there is a theme – the child who has always had tummy trouble, or the child who has always needed parental presence and reassurance.

You may hear sleep described as a developmental milestone. Well, it is and it isn't. Sleep is not a learned skill, and nor is it something that children acquire competence with at certain ages. But on the other hand, some of the aspects of a child's development, such as their emotional maturity, comfort, self-confidence, and ability to comprehend simple instructions, can all facilitate an easier transition to sleep. This is why sleep does get better with increasing age, though of course all children may struggle with their sleep because of different factors.

But if there is one thing I hear every week, it is the agonised groan of a parent of a toddler or older child who is worried that something they did or didn't do when their child was a baby is why they are in the position they are today.

You need to know that whatever parenting support you offered your baby is *not* why your child struggles with sleep. In fact, it probably needs to be categorised under 'normal parenting'. Your child may be sensitive, and they may have struggled with sleep whatever you did. Perhaps your child had specific needs as a baby, which you met. Can the way in which you met their needs become a habit? Yes, of course – but does this make it a mistake? No way. If your little one would only settle with breastfeeding, you were just meeting their need. If your baby only slept while being held upright in the baby carrier, you were meeting their need.

Whatever it was that you did for your baby to keep them happy and comfortable, and support their sleep, was entirely appropriate. The fact that this has now become unsustainable, or they still don't sleep without your help, is not some kind of proof that you did the wrong thing. All of us as parents do our best at the time. There is no place for guilt, blame or shame here.

One last thing while we're on this subject. If some wise guy is trying to tell you that you should have tackled your child's sleep ages ago and not left it till now, I'm here to tell you that they are wrong. All families are different, and you will need to do whatever is best for you and your family.

Why toddlers and older children are different

This may sound like an obvious point, but there are many differences between the ways in which babies, toddlers and older children sleep.

Older children are different first of all because the amount and distribution of sleep that they need is different. The total amount of sleep that children need reduces as they get older.[1] Again, this is stating the obvious, but most books seem to assume that all children under five will sleep from 7pm–7am. I hate to break it to you, but not all children sleep like this. It's also a culturally incompetent idea to assume that all children (or adults for that matter) work steadily towards monophasic sleep – which is one long chunk of sleep overnight, followed by being awake all day. In many cultures, biphasic sleep is prevalent. This is where people take a long nap in the afternoon, and it's common in parts of southern Europe and the Caribbean. In other parts of the world, such as Asia and Africa, polyphasic sleep (multiple naps throughout the day) is

common. With both biphasic and polyphasic sleep, there will be a shorter nighttime sleep duration.[2] So it is absolutely wrong on a number of levels to assume that children will achieve a solid unbroken stretch of sleep overnight. Not only does this assume a relatively high total sleep duration over 24 hours, but it also assumes the predominantly post-Industrial Revolution Western pattern of monophasic sleep.

A recent study found that the *function* of sleep dramatically changes just before a child reaches 2.5 years old. Scientists have discovered that the primary function of sleep before this age is to grow the brain. Young infants, and especially premature infants, spend a much higher percentage of time in REM sleep, and this seems to organise the brain. After this age, sleep seems to facilitate repair and maintenance of the brain.[3] In essence, while your 2.5 year old is sleeping, their brain is taking out the rubbish bins. (It's pretty awesome really...)

Another difference is that the reasons for night waking change as children get older. In infancy, sleep may be fragmented due to night feeding, reflux, teething, and the excitement of learning to crawl. Older children may wake up for entirely different reasons – wet beds, nightmares, lost teddies, sadness over a nursery friend leaving, school playground spats... you name it.

Infants and older children have different types of interactions with their parents. Young infants have limited mobility and need their parent physically more. Older children have more interactive and complicated conversations and communication with their parents, and have different needs.

Infants and children also have different abilities to understand instructions and requests. As their language acquisition and cognitive understanding grows, they are able to comprehend more complex instructions. But they are also able to negotiate, procrastinate, ignore instructions and push limits.

Finally, the tools that may work for infants and children of different ages are different. So often, people apply tools that might work for some infants to toddlers or preschoolers, only to find that they are inappropriate. If the tools someone has are limited to only what works with infants, and also what works with a really simple sleep situation, or a compliant infant, then it is doubly or triply doomed.

Toddlers and older children need different approaches because they are different developmentally, socially, emotionally, cognitively, physically, behaviourally and in terms of their growth and nutritional needs. If you're feeling frustrated because the solutions you've read in a generic sleep blog or book don't work – take heart. You're not applying the tool wrongly, and your child is not broken. It's probably just a poor fit for their situation, age or developmental stage.

How you may be feeling

Many parents of older children fully anticipated that their baby would wake in the night and need their help. But in our culture we are led to believe that this is a problem of relatively short duration. We psyche ourselves up for perhaps 4–6 months of sleep deprivation. But then six months pass, and the universe seems to laugh at our naïve expectation that sleep would be better by now. Eight months rolls into a year... Surely they will sleep after their first birthday?

Before you know it, you are the proud parent of an amazing, talented, brilliant, resourceful, funny, loving and sleep-avoidant toddler. Or preschooler. Or school-aged child.

And here you are. Yet none of this is your fault.

But for the record, it's not your child's fault either. In fact, let's just bin the word 'fault' shall we? The truth is, some children sleep brilliantly from the word go. Others sleep like babies, but their sleep gradually consolidates and the night-wakings reduce gradually over the first year. Other children seem to have missed the memo on how to sleep, and seem to struggle with it for longer.

Friends, family, and society at large don't help do they?

'Is he still waking at night?'

'You're not still struggling with bedtime are you – you poor thing!'

'I never had this problem with my kids – have you tried x/y/z?'

'You pander to her too much'

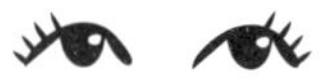

Whether friends and family are smug, condescending, horrified, or pitying, none of that makes you as a parent feel any better about the situation. You may feel even more alone, blamed, wretched or hopeless than you did before. None of these comments are empowering or helpful, and they tend to close down conversation. You're not likely to seek support from someone whose only suggestions are either something that is not acceptable to you, or patronising ideas that have not worked for you in the past. In this way, not only can you end up feeling worse about your sleep situation, but you can also end up feeling lonely, misunderstood, and foolish. These comments seem to assume that you have rather stupidly let this situation happen, have encouraged it, or have not tried anything to improve it. The reality could not be further from the truth. When I speak to parents of toddlers, they are always intelligent, insightful people who have tried a great many ideas or tricks.

You may also hear this rhetoric from health professionals, books, articles and social media. Because our culture is so set up for unrealistic expectations, it's like a whole conversation about toddler and child sleep has gone underground. There seems to be a total lack of widespread information about how to support children with sleep beyond babyhood. Pithy suggestions like trying a bedtime routine (as if you haven't!), an earlier bedtime, sticker chart, or giving a child a comforter seem to be the limit of the suggestions offered to help older children with sleep.

I'm not suggesting that we need to scare parents by saying that 2–3 years of fragmented sleep is to be expected, but in many ways, this is a more realistic perspective. Many research studies find that children continue to wake in the night into their second and third years and beyond,[4] and there are many reasons for persistent night waking that affect children older than this.

"Whether friends and family are smug, condescending, horrified, or pitying, none of that makes you as a parent feel any better about the situation. You may feel even more alone, blamed, wretched or hopeless than you did before."

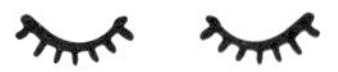

Whenever I talk to parents of toddlers and older children, they always describe a range of big emotions – resentment, anger, frustration, embarrassment, confusion and sadness, as well as exhaustion. You are of course allowed to feel whatever you feel. Your feelings and emotions are valid. But my hope is that you will feel a sense of solidarity by imagining all the people reading this book. The people, like you, who parented their children in the way that felt right, and for whom sleep has reached a point where it is becoming unsustainable, either for you, your child or your family.

Start with your own sleep

It might sound strange to leap straight to *your* sleep, in a book about children's sleep. After all, you wouldn't be tired if it wasn't for your child waking in the night, right? Well, perhaps you would. Fatigue can be caused by many things, as well as sleep deprivation. Without wanting to sound dismissive – parenting is tiring. Heck, *adulting* is tiring. I don't want to patronise you – of course if you had a full night's sleep you'd probably feel less tired. I just mean that there is more to fatigue than just sleep.

We recently brought home our new puppy, who is currently waking me up 2–4 times per night between 11pm and 6am. It's pretty brutal, especially having been sleep deprived for years with my girls. I'm definitely tired because I'm having to take the pup for a middle-of-the-night bladder break. But am I *only* tired because of that? No way. I've been tired for years, and it's not just about sleep deprivation and sleep fragmentation.

The pragmatic reason for exploring your own fatigue is that it is a whole lot easier to work on *your* sleep, lifestyle, habits and behaviours than it is to adjust your child's. An obvious point perhaps, but if you're looking for a way to feel better quickly, you might have more success with adjusting your own habits first. I'm not suggesting that will solve all your problems, but it might at least make life a bit more manageable.

Some areas you could consider:

- Your own self-care: looking after yourself isn't just a 'good idea', it's essential. This includes prioritising your obvious basic needs (eating, drinking, washing, going to the toilet) but also the needs that you

might have shelved as less important – such as laughing, talking to people who 'get it', your own need for touch and intimacy, learning ways to manage stress, alone time, having some privacy, headspace, and time to devote to your own interests.

- Managing any mental health concerns: if you've been parking your anxiety, depression, insomnia, phobia or trauma because you haven't the time to deal with it, then you definitely need to make time. Mental health problems and sleep problems/fatigue go hand in hand and are bidirectional. That is to say that having anxiety or depression can worsen your sleep, and sleep problems can worsen mental health problems.[5,6] Sometimes, addressing just *one* of these will make the other problem better too.
- Addressing any physical health needs: if you are suffering from chronic pain, an inflammatory condition, thyroid dysfunction, vitamin deficiency or some other health problem, this will make you feel worse. Please get help if you are suffering, and don't forget to take a multivitamin, including vitamin D.[7]
- Your support networks: friends, family and community are essential. Now, not everyone is on the same page, so you may need to be selective about who you ask to help you, or who you offload on. But one thing is for sure – you need friends and support.
- The people you talk to about sleep: you can choose to unfollow unhelpful accounts, seek out like-minded people, and to only share details of your sleep story with those who truly are on the same page.
- Your relationship with your partner: if you have a partner, then working on your relationship, the way you function as a team, and the way you communicate your appreciation for the respective roles you have can have a positive impact on your general stress levels, coping and fatigue.
- Your own sleep hygiene: these are the habits and behaviours you have around going to sleep. Optimising your own sleep through keeping a regular bedtime and wake up time, having a cool, dark, uncluttered bedroom, and avoiding caffeine and screens in the 1–2 hours before going to sleep can make a big difference.
- Lifestyle: I know you've heard it before, but eating well, having plenty of time outdoors, taking regular exercise and both managing and avoiding too much stress will improve the quality of your sleep, and make you feel better.

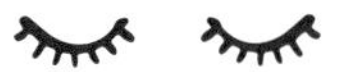

I'm not saying your problems will all be solved, but the point is that these are changes you can make that depend on nobody but yourself. Even if all this does is slightly reduce your fatigue to the point where you can think a little more clearly, it's worth it. You may find that improving your own sleep, health and wellbeing increases your tolerance for your child's nighttime shenanigans. Finally, there is something about trying and implementing a change and seeing a positive outcome that makes us feel buoyed up and more confident about implementing changes elsewhere. You can use this increase in positivity as a springboard to make changes in other areas.

You're not alone

You really are in good company. You are not the only parent whose child is still waking in the night. You didn't screw up. You haven't missed your opportunity to make sleep better. You haven't broken your child.

You may feel like you're the only one of your circle of friends dealing with a middle of the night party, or the only parent at school whose child still needs them to hold their hand while they fall asleep. But I assure you, you're not. Fragmented childhood sleep is normal and common. It's also hard, and you're allowed to complain about it. You deserve to be listened to without someone suggesting that the only solution is to leave your child to cry, while you sob next door. There are better ways to handle this.

We also need to get the balance right in how we think about childhood sleep. It's very easy for a conversation about sleeping children to descend into defining their sleep as a 'problem' that needs 'fixing'.

I do not want anyone to feel that if they do not 'sort out' their child's sleep now, that they will still be sleeping this way in several years' time. I also want to provide a safe space for those who are sick of being told to sleep train, or that their child will not develop properly if they don't learn to fall asleep by themselves. If you're here for reassurance, stick around: there's plenty of that. If, however, you are in need of creative, respectful, gentle and kind solutions to support your child to sleep as well as they can – you're also in the right place.

Most children's sleep is totally normal. In saying that, I do not mean to diminish how hard it is to be woken in the night, or have a three-hour bedtime every day. But at the same time we do not want to pathologise the fact that many children need parental support to go to sleep.

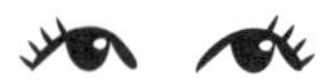

All that said, it's also okay if you have reached the end of your tether, and cannot keep going the way you are. While most sleep situations are normal and will resolve spontaneously with time, I do not know your specific situation. Every individual has a different threshold for what they can cope with. If your situation is unsustainable, then it is absolutely appropriate for you to reach out for some help.

You'll find no non-responsive, archaic, draconian or authoritarian parenting and sleep tools in this book. Rest assured, everything I suggest will fit well with your responsive parenting style. Through learning more about sleep, and supporting your child in a number of different ways, I aim to help parents feel calmer, more confident and more connected to their child, and support biologically normal, age and developmentally appropriate and attachment-promoting sleep strategies.

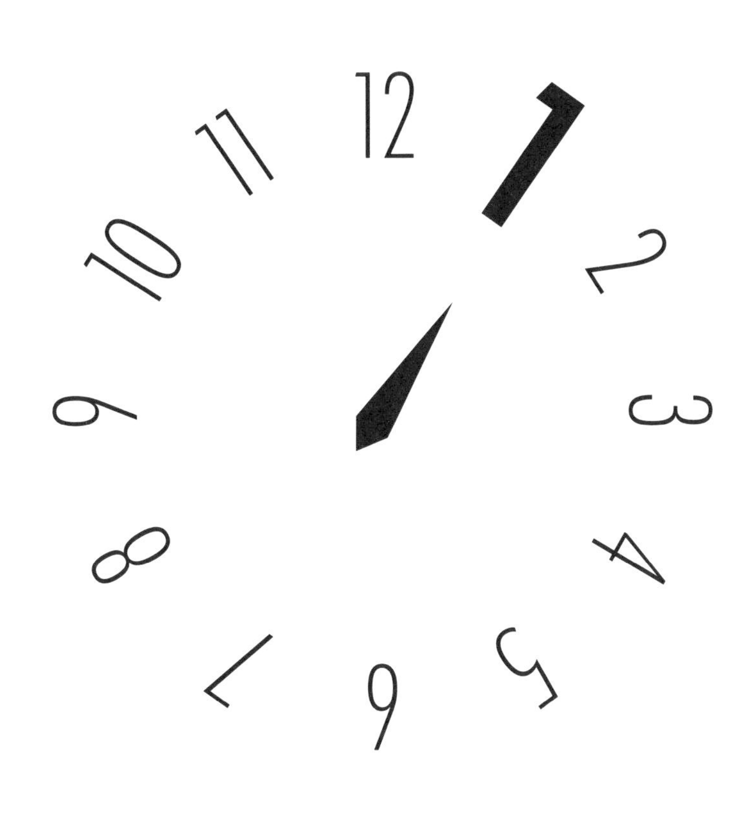

CHAPTER ONE

HOW SLEEP WORKS

This is not intended to be a clunky academic sleep textbook. However, to unpick toddler and older children's sleep, it can be useful to understand normal sleep. Children, just like babies, (and adults for that matter) do not need to be taught how to sleep. Sleep is a normal bodily function. But different children sleep differently. Some children wake more often, or seem to need a lot more support to fall asleep and stay asleep than others. Toddlers, preschoolers and older children often have different worries that keep them awake and different things that wake them up in the night. They also have different sleep needs.

The way we sleep is controlled by two separate mechanisms: circadian rhythm (body clock) and sleep pressure.

Sleep pressure

Sleep pressure builds throughout the time we spend awake. Obviously, the amount of time we can tolerate being awake varies – both according to age, and also between individuals. When sleep pressure builds enough, the drive to fall asleep becomes overwhelming, driven by a hormone called adenosine, which makes us feel sleepy.[1] Have you ever nodded off during a class, or in front of the TV? Has your toddler ever fallen asleep without you doing anything (for example when you didn't want them to)? That's sleep pressure!

Sleep pressure builds at different rates for different people. That's why some children can last longer between a nap and bedtime than others.

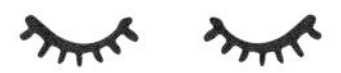

When sleep pressure builds up a lot, children sometimes get a little fussy or cranky.

You can resist sleep pressure for a while – those heavy lids may droop on a long and boring car journey, but you open the window, crank the music up and blink furiously to stay awake don't you? Eventually though, sleep pressure becomes impossible to hold back.

Ideally, when we're thinking about children's sleep, we want sleep pressure to be high before they have a nap (if they still need one) and before bedtime. It's less useful to have high sleep pressure when you ideally need to be awake, or at 6pm on those dreaded car trips which then make for a bedtime write-off... (I have absolutely been there).

All this sounds pretty obvious really, but it's important, because it really is very difficult to fall asleep with low sleep pressure, just as it's hard to remain awake with high sleep pressure. You would be amazed at how often a solution to a sleep problem is to work *with* rather than against sleep pressure.

If sleep only relied on sleep pressure, it might actually be a little simpler to understand. But the plot thickens, my friends. This is where we need to consider the role of the circadian rhythm.

Circadian rhythm

Circadian rhythmicity is not present from birth but by toddlerhood should largely be well-established, though some circadian-linked body functions, like urine production, are still immature.

The body clock is in charge of lots of different body functions that are related to time, such as blood pressure, hormone release, alertness, temperature and other bodily functions.[2] It's amazing really that we don't have to think about any of this – our bodies just get on with it. Your child's body clock can be influenced by exposure to natural daylight, timing of eating and normal activity levels.[3] Importantly, the body clock keeps ticking no matter what time of day it is, and no matter whether we are asleep or awake.[4]

This means that provided you have a relatively regular wake up and bedtime, your body clock pretty much runs on autopilot, controlling all those many body functions that are time-critical. So far, so wonderful. The body clock can get out of rhythm though, like a clock that loses time. Have you ever gone to bed really late and found that you woke up at your

usual time anyway? Or have you ever tried to nap in the day because you know you're about to go on to a night shift, and found it really hard? Or have you gone on holiday and forced yourself to stay up late to try to get into the local time zone, only to wake up alert and ready to go at 3am because back home, it's actually 9am?

This is why jet lag is so grim – your body clock will tell you it's time to wake up at your *usual* wake up time, so even if the local time is 3am, your darling body clock is releasing wake-up hormones and saying it's time to get up. This signal is even stronger than sleep pressure in most cases, which is why, even if you force yourself to stay up later to go to bed at the locally normal time, you will *still* wake up early until your body clock catches up. This can take a few days. The best way to organise your body clock is to wake up and go to bed at about the same time every day, expose yourself to bright natural daylight in the day, and keep the lights off at night.

The body clock releases alerting hormones (cortisol) and sleepy hormones (melatonin) according to the time of day. Cortisol begins to rise in the early hours of the morning, and this helps us to be alert and get ready to wake up. Melatonin begins to rise in the evening, about two hours before the usual bedtime, under the influence of decreasing light levels. Trying to fall asleep when your body clock is telling you to get up is really hard.

With a well-established body clock, it becomes more important to have a consistent bedtime. One reason for this is that about 1–2 hours before the *habitual* bedtime, the body clock is actually signalling wakefulness. This is called the wake maintenance zone (WMZ) and it is extremely hard to fall asleep during this window.[5]

Many a time I have worked with parents who describe a two-hour bedtime, lots of frustration and a really wide-awake child. This wakefulness is sometimes blamed on 'overtiredness', and a common idea is to make the bedtime even earlier. What you will instantly realise, having read the information above, is that bringing the bedtime earlier still will drag out this process even further, because even if sleep pressure is pretty high, it will be hard to fall asleep against the will of the body clock.

That 1–2 hours of wake maintenance zone before the usual bedtime is not spent with your body doing nothing. In the background, changes are occurring to get you ready to fall asleep. Melatonin is released after about

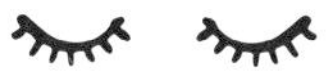

1–2 hours of consistent dimming of light in the evening. That's why it helps to turn the lights down, avoid screens and close the curtains/blinds, to allow your brain to register the dimming of light. Even though it's not quite sleep time yet, if we are exposed to bright light when we would usually be getting sleepy, this can make it harder to fall asleep. Melatonin does not actually *make* you fall asleep, like a magic pill, but it *does* make you feel sleepy.

The easy zone...

The easiest time to fall asleep, therefore, is when sleep pressure is high, and the circadian rhythm is sending all the right signals to fall asleep, like this:

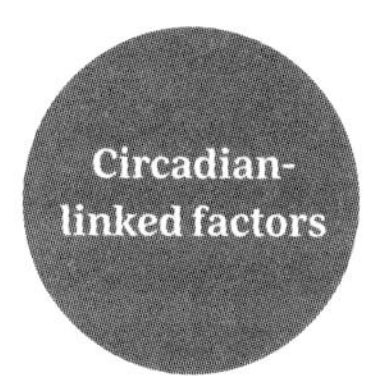

Melatonin levels rising +
Dim lights +
Cortisol levels low +
Body temperature falling

AND

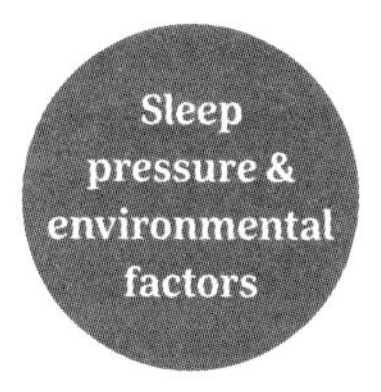

High sleep pressure (adenosine) +
Outside of the wake maintenance zone +
Free from discomforts +
Feeling calm and relaxed

If you put a child to bed when all these conditions are present, you are setting yourself up for the easiest possible bedtime.

Body clock and sleep pressure mismatch

Many bedtime problems are caused by a mismatch between the sleep pressure and the body clock. This is why it is so important to understand the science behind what is going on. So often I hear parents becoming frustrated and confused. You may have become baffled by why your apparently exhausted five-year-old is appearing to 'resist' sleep. Understanding what is going on may demystify this situation, reduce the irritation factor and also make for a more successful bedtime experience.

Let's imagine that your child usually goes to bed at 8pm. That means that from 6–7.30pm (approximately) your child's body clock is signalling wakefulness. It will be extremely hard to get them to bed at this time, even if they are unusually tired and cranky.

For instance, if your child's sleep pressure is high (perhaps because they woke up early, or had a disrupted night), then their sleep pressure may be very high at let's say 6pm. You might start bedtime early, thinking that what they need is an early night. Then what happens is that your child messes about, can't fall asleep, and needs you more. This can be bewildering – after all, your child *seemed tired!* Lots of parents doubt themselves at this point, because they thought they were observing that their child was tired – so this behaviour leads many parents to feel that either they are getting it all wrong, or their child is unusual, hard to read, or broken in some way. It only makes sense when you understand that there is another process as well as sleep pressure affecting your child's ability to fall asleep. If this has ever happened to you – you were absolutely right. You *were* correctly observing fatigue. The problem is that you were seeing sleep pressure, but the sleep pressure didn't match the circadian rhythm. They may not be 'messing about' at all, but just experiencing a biological process that they can do nothing about.

If you try to put your preschooler to bed when they are not ready, it is much harder, because their body clock is telling them that it's wake-up time. You've probably experienced the frustration of your preschooler bouncing around their room when you thought it was bedtime! There may be a reason behind the apparent madness.

If this is becoming problematic, then you may need to think about:

Is there a reason for your child getting so tired at that awkwardly early time? If your child still naps, then could you make the nap later? This may mean that they can last a little longer in the evening so their sleep pressure peaks closer to the usual falling asleep time.

Is this a tricky phase because they are learning a lot, attending school or have a lot going on in their world? If so, you may need to just accept this for a while.

If you're consistently having a two-hour frustrating bedtime, then just start bedtime later, and aim to get your child to go to sleep within one hour of starting the routine. Take the stress out of bedtime first, before adjusting the timing.

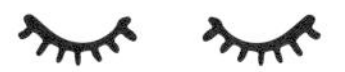

Sometimes children draw out bedtime because they have a need to connect. Make sure you've built in plenty of time to connect throughout the day. If they are at school or nursery, or you're at work, then try some highly focused one-to-one play when you get back together again. It doesn't have to be hours – just 10–20 minutes can be enough to fill your child's love tank up and stop their need to connect from derailing bedtime (more on this in on pages 125–7).

If you're concerned that bedtime has crept really late, then focus on making bedtime nice and succinct first, and then bring bedtime forward in 15-minute increments every few days.

Sleep needs

Sleep needs are also different for different people. There are many charts or tables, apps and downloadable resources suggesting how much sleep your child should achieve at certain ages. There's nothing wrong with these: they are based on large research studies and can give you an idea of how much sleep is realistic. But do remember that all children are different. In my experience, if you are the parent of a child who is at the low end of the sleep need spectrum, then looking at charts which tend to display the average amounts of sleep can be disheartening. Some of us just need more sleep than others. Do you know anyone who can cope well on only five hours' sleep per night? And do you also know people who absolutely *have* to have 9–10 hours' sleep to feel well-rested? That's due to individual sleep needs. Your child may fall outside of the normal sleep ranges illustrated by popular books and charts.

The average amount of sleep your 2–5 year old child needs is about 10–13 hours of sleep in total. This may include a nap (more on naps in chapter 9). So, for example, if your four-year-old still needs a one-hour nap, this may mean that they only achieve nine hours of nighttime sleep if they are at the lower end of the sleep need spectrum.

By the age of six, all the way through to the teenage years, your child's sleep needs will change again, reducing to about 9–11 hours of sleep in total, with no nap.

So, all these sleep amounts are within the normal range:

- A two-year-old sleeping from 8pm–6am
- A three-year-old sleeping from 9pm–7am

- A four-year-old having a 30-minute nap after nursery and then sleeping 8pm–7am
- A five-year-old sleeping from 8pm–6am
- A six-year-old sleeping from 7pm–5am
- A seven-year-old sleeping from 7pm–4am
- An eight-year-old sleeping from 10pm–7am

As you will notice, these amounts are variable, and may be less than you thought. This may be the first place that you need to start with your child's sleep. What is realistic? What is within your control? Are there areas to improve, or do you need to accept that your child is getting enough sleep? Perhaps the total number of hours seems okay, but the timing is not working: for example, with our example of a seven-year-old sleeping from 7pm–4am, clearly 4am is an ungodly hour to be waking up. But my point is that if your child only needs nine hours' sleep, then it may simply be unrealistic to put them to bed at 7pm and have them sleep until 6am. You may need to adjust their bedtime, rather than try to prolong their sleep duration.

Knowing the total amount of sleep your child needs is important, because it helps to ensure that our expectations are realistic. If your child only needs 10 hours' sleep in 24 hours, and your main problem is their early rising, then it could be that the only solution is a later bedtime.

Sleep cycles

During sleep, we all move between different stages of sleep. We shift from awake, to light sleep, to deep sleep, to dreaming sleep, then we wake up again. Most of the deep sleep is in the first half of the night, and most of our dreaming sleep is towards the morning. The sleep cycle doesn't always look the same: sometimes we spend a little more time in one sleep stage than another, but you don't need to get hung up on that. Your child's brain actually takes care of this by itself. We don't need to micromanage it.

Your child's sleep cycles are a little longer now than they were as an infant, but may not be fully mature yet. For some children, the sleep cycle does not lengthen to the classic 90–120-minute mature sleep cycle until they are 3–4 years old, but sleep cycle maturation is also linked to pubertal stage and other developmental factors.[6]

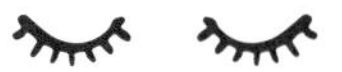

Night waking

Now you have an idea about how sleep works, why some children wake more often, and what makes us sleep in the first place. You might also have some questions about how much sleep toddlers need at different ages, and how to organise this and manage naps.

I have a love-hate relationship with sleep charts, because the last thing I want to do is cause people anxiety. But on the other hand, it's sometimes useful to have a rough idea of what to expect. So, please know that your toddler may fall outside of these average ranges. That may be fine. It may be due to their genetics, or their temperament, or something else.

I am often asked if toddlers will be sleep deprived if they wake up frequently at night. It sounds logical, doesn't it? After all, if someone wakes *us* up 4–10 times per night, we feel very tired the next day. But is it the same for our little ones? Well – it depends.

Remember that we all wake after every sleep cycle. If your child wakes and needs something from you to go back to sleep, then as long as they get what they need promptly and return to sleep, no – they are not sleep deprived. So, if they fall asleep at 8pm and wake up at 7am, they had 11 hours of decent sleep (*even if* they woke up six times in between, needing your help to fall asleep again). You can probably tell this yourself because your toddler will be happy during the day, have plenty of energy, and want to play and have fun with you.

On the other hand, if they wake up and are unsettled in the night, or they wake up because they're uncomfortable or ill, then this may make them wakeful for more than just a brief moment. This may mean that they lose out on some overnight sleep. This is often particularly noticeable when toddlers are unwell with a cough or cold. They are often very miserable and wakeful at night, and then may need to sleep more in the day to compensate. But it is pretty obvious when a little one is genuinely tired in the day. If your toddler is happy, they're probably *not* significantly sleep deprived.

In my experience, we often assume our little ones are tired or even exhausted, because *we are*. We sometimes assume our toddlers need an early night or a longer nap because *we need those things*. But remember that fragmented sleep is not the same as sleep deprivation. I'm not saying that *you* aren't tired. Of course you are! But hopefully some small comfort is that your toddler is likely to be just fine.

Sadly, one of the things that some parents are told is that if they don't sleep train their toddler, they will not develop properly, will struggle to learn in school, put on weight, or their brain will not grow. This is simply not true. Many people talk about the public health outcomes of inadequate sleep, but this needs a bit of unpacking.

We need to remember four things about the research that examines the correlation between obesity,[7] poor memory,[8] behaviour problems[9] and learning difficulties and sleep.[10] There are many studies that have looked at these, and they are really important areas to consider. But we do need to be very careful about how we apply research to different age groups. So consider:

1. The studies were generally looking at school-aged children (not infants and toddlers)
2. The studies were not looking at fragmented sleep (lots of wake-ups at night) but at total sleep time. So the children who had a higher risk of the negative outcomes they mention genuinely weren't getting enough sleep – in one stretch or in chunks. The children were achieving fewer than the 9–11 hours in total that is usually needed at this age.
3. If children are achieving fewer hours of sleep than they physically need, then an important question is why? Are they being prevented from getting the hours of sleep they need due to a chaotic lifestyle? Are there inappropriate boundaries present? Is there too much screen time? What are the environmental and parenting factors that led to the late bedtime? It's important to separate out the reasons that are parent-related, and the reasons that are child-related.
4. Many studies do not separate out the children who had a genuine sleep pathology – such as sleep apnoea. This is a big problem, because if this is the case, the sleep disorder is causing the nighttime awakening, rather than the child just having a late bedtime.

Some people equate those brief awakenings at night (which are normal) with significant sleep deprivation. I can assure you that if your toddler seems fine in the day, then they probably are.

With all this said then, here is a chart of average sleep needs, including naps. Please bear in mind that although this is based on data

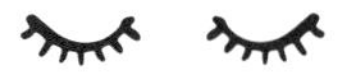

from large studies, there is considerable variability between children, especially in terms of daytime napping. So if your child is getting enough sleep in 24 hours but their naps don't look anything like this – don't worry. You're in good company I assure you!

Age	Number of naps	Total daytime sleep (hours)	Total nighttime sleep (hours)	Total sleep in 24 hours
0–3 months	evenly spread	varies	varies	14–17
3–6 months	4	3–5	9–10	13–15
6–9 months	3	2–4	10–11	12–15
9–16 months	2	2–3	10–11	11–14
16–24 months	1	max 2–3	10–11	11–14
2–2.5 years	1	up to 2	10–12	10–13
2.5–5 years	0–1	0–2	10–13	10–13
6–13 years	–	–	9–11	9–11
14–17 years	–	–	8–10	8–10
18–64 years	–	–	7–9	7–9
65 years +	varies	varies	7–9	7–8

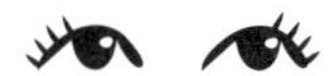

Using the chart on the previous page, you can work out your child's needs and compare it with their actual sleep here:

My child needs	*My child's actual total is*
approximately ______ hours of sleep in 24 hours.	*approximately ______ hours of sleep in 24 hours.*
This is made up of approximately ______ hours of daytime sleep, including ______ naps,	*This is made up of approximately ______ hours of daytime sleep, including ______ naps,*
and approximately ______ hours of nighttime sleep.	*and approximately ______ hours of nighttime sleep.*

In terms of the amount of total sleep (forgetting the number of wake-ups) my child's nights are:

less than average	*about right*	*more than average*

In terms of naps, when I count up all my child's naps combined, my child's daytime sleep is:

less than average	*about right*	*more than average*

My child's sleep is:

on the low side	*completely normal*	*more than average*

When you go through this, you'll be able to see if there are any areas of difference where you might be able to make some changes. For example, if naps are great, but nights are difficult, and your child's total sleep time is normal, then it may be that you have to shorten some naps in order to improve your nights. If your nights are good, and naps are short, then the tradeoff for decent nights may be short naps.

Having realistic expectations will help you know whether there is anything that you might be able to adjust.

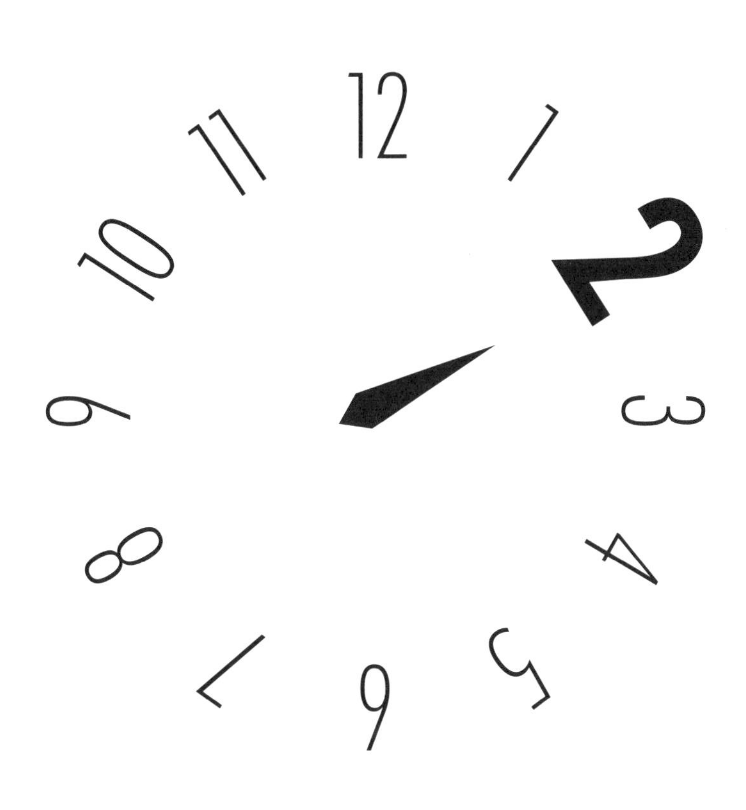

CHAPTER TWO

SELF-SOOTHING

You're probably sick of hearing from others that you need to let your toddler or older child learn to self-soothe (don't worry – I won't tell you this!). But what *is* self-soothing? Well, there are lots of ways that people interpret this term.

Some people interpret it as the ability to become calm once you feel stressed. This is actually quite an advanced skill, and certainly not something we can expect of toddlers and young children. Toddlers will have a few more self-regulatory abilities now that they are getting older, but these are still quite basic. If you are the parent of an older child, they gradually acquire more ability to become calm, but this is still a work in progress.

Other people say that you can teach a child to self-soothe by leaving them to cry, and eventually they will fall asleep. This isn't really self-soothing though. All children learn is that when they cry, nobody comes, so they eventually stop crying, or become tired out, and fall asleep.

Some people interpret self-soothing as a child's ability to fall asleep by themselves, without help from a parent. I'm going to focus on this interpretation in this chapter, as this is what I have found most people get confused about.

Self-regulation

Imagine a really stressful piece of news. Imagine the excitement you feel before you go on holiday. Imagine the rush you feel after you walk away having ridden a rollercoaster. Your autonomic nervous system is an incredibly efficient machine, ready to go at the drop of a hat. Your stress response and alerting mechanisms are automatic – which is a good thing. It wouldn't be very useful if you had to rationally think through the steps right before you need to run to try to board a train that is about to leave. Your body does the work for you, without you needing to think about it. Lots of people talk about a stress response, but it's also important to mention that your body's alerting mechanisms get all fired up with exciting events, as well as stressful ones. To me, this is really important to state explicitly, because a whole range of human emotions is perfectly normal, for both adults and children. Children can become dysregulated because they are really excited, as well as when they are nervous or worried. Whether your child is positively or negatively experiencing a heightened state of arousal, they may lack the ability to self-regulate.

This stress response is present from infancy, but the ability to rationally process stress, problem-solve, think creatively and talk ourselves down from that heightened state of arousal is one that develops gradually. This is why young children have more meltdowns than adults, and gradually this improves with age and developmental and emotional maturity. Self-regulation skills are a learned coping mechanism for when we are dysregulated – either by excitement or stress. This is not a switch that is pressed when your child reaches a certain age – self-regulation builds over time.

There are two things that you can do to help your child develop self-regulation. Firstly, children need to see self-regulatory behaviours modelled by you. If you think about it, children learn so many skills and behaviours by copying. If you regularly demonstrate how *you* deal with something super stressful or exciting, your children will subliminally copy what you do. It helps to be quite intentional about this. I know that as adults we often keep our thoughts to ourselves, quietly coping with life's stresses and irritations, but if you can sometimes remember to articulate this out loud, it will normalise the fact that everyone gets stressed sometimes and needs a tool up their sleeve to help them calm down.

I'm not saying we need to over-share, or wear our hearts on our sleeves. Our children don't need to know everything that bugs us, but try to show a little of your vulnerable side from time to time. For example:

'I'm feeling a little stressed – will you help me take some deep breaths?'

'Yikes, we're going to be late. But you know, there's nothing we can do

about it, so shall we sing a song to take our minds off it?'

The other part of helping our children deal with dysregulation, until they can spontaneously do this for themselves, is to co-regulate them.

Co-regulation

We are social beings aren't we? We just can't do this life alone. Sometimes, we all need a little bit of help to calm down when we are overwhelmed, overstimulated, overloaded or just over it. Little people particularly need help to calm down when they are dysregulated. Remember that your stress response works from infancy, but the ability to calm it down develops over time. Full maturity in this area is not reached until adulthood, but major changes occur in adolescence.[1] So it's perfectly normal that your child of two, five, or nine years old needs help sometimes. What this means in practice is that if your child gets upset about something, if they are uncomfortable, if they miss you, or if they are frustrated, they will probably need you more both day and night.

I've found that people sometimes separate daytime and nighttime behaviour, as well as the response to that behaviour. For example, most people completely understand that a toddler may cry and need comfort if a balloon bursts near their face. Most people appreciate that a six-year-old who is sad because their best friend wanted to play with someone else needs some reassurance. But sometimes I run into the idea that children somehow don't need this sort of comfort overnight. I know it's an obvious point, but daytime and nighttime parenting is the same, it's just that one is more fatiguing and less convenient than the other! Another obvious but important point is that children have no more ability to self-regulate at night than they do in the day. If your child needs support in the night do not panic – they are entirely normal, and responding to them is the right thing to do. You see, we learn independence and self-sufficiency over time, and through having those needs initially met by a warm, responsive, attuned caregiver. You have not 'created a monster', or made a 'rod for your back'. Instead of thinking 'my child is this way because I have taught them to need me', think 'my child is this way, and I have responded accordingly'. The way your child needs you is just who they are. It's not the result of you failing to teach them to not need you. Some little people just need more co-regulation than others, particularly if they are more sensitive. They will gradually develop the ability to calm down more independently with age and maturity. Don't forget, too, that two-year-olds have two-year-old sized problems. They may seem trivial to us, but two-year-olds do not have the life experience yet to understand that their two-year-old problem is not really a problem in the grand scheme of things. To them, it's a problem, and so we must take it seriously.

Essentially, with co-regulation you are providing a bridge back to calmness for your dysregulated child through your regulated presence and behaviour. Let's say your three-year-old's stress response is triggered by something. It could be a dog that barked loudly, a friend who took their toy, or a broken banana. Whatever it is, their heart may race, they may get sweaty, shouty, and start hitting or crying. Because they don't have the developmental maturity or cognitive ability to problem-solve, rationalise, or logically reason, they need you, with all your regulating prowess, to come along and bridge them back to calm. You do this already I'm sure: you hug, rock, sing, rub their back, use soothing words, and hold space for those feelings. That's co-regulation. You're nailing it. The tricky part about co-regulation, however, is that you need to be regulated and calm yourself, in order to calm someone else. My husband and I used to say that as a couple, there was only room for one of us at a time to have a meltdown. If we were both stressed and upset about something, neither of us were any good to the other. That's where you either need the self-awareness to realise what is going on, and take some steps to become regulated yourself, or you need someone else in the picture.

I'm mindful that as you read that paragraph, you may feel stressed about being stressed, or anxious about being anxious. I would hate anyone to think that they must remain calm and in control at all times for the sake of their child. Firstly, that's not real life. And secondly, it's normal to find bedtime, or your child having a tantrum in the supermarket, stressful. I would simply urge you to be aware of your own emotional state. I often turn those negative thoughts around from 'what if me being stressed is stressing my child out', to 'what if my calm was able to calm my child'. It is true that your own emotional state may influence your child, which is why it's important to acknowledge the normalcy of certain behaviours or situations being stressful or triggering, and then manage that. If you're able to, take a moment, pause, and collect yourself before attending to your child. You will probably find that calming them is easier if you take one minute to calm yourself first. Think of your calm as being contagious!

Soothing ourselves to soothe our children

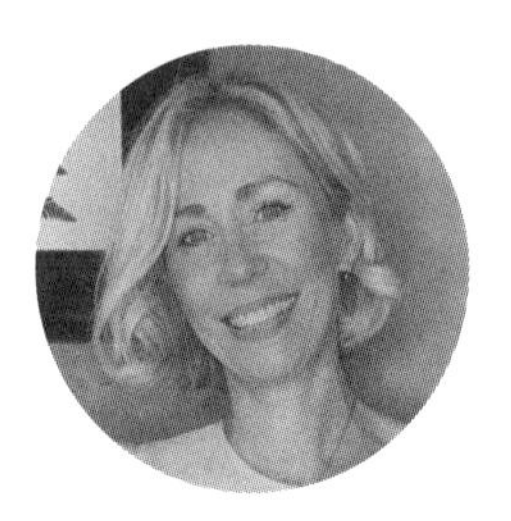

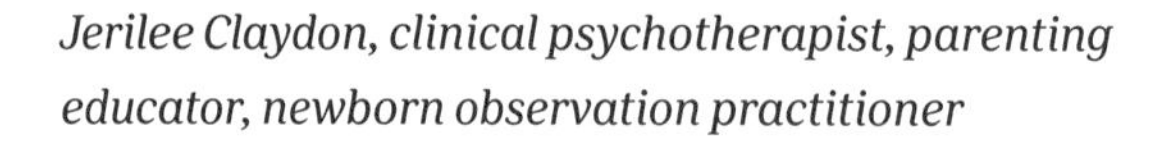

Jerilee Claydon, clinical psychotherapist, parenting educator, newborn observation practitioner

It's a life-long project to figure out who we are, but within that quest can you identify a sense of yourself along the way? Can you step back with an awareness and witness yourself moment to moment? Pausing to question – do my actions align with my values? Is that how I really wanted to respond?

Perhaps it feels like a choice to feel the way you do. According to attachment theory your relationships with yourself and others are shaped by your earliest relationship with your caregiver. The early years really are *that* important, shaping us for life and even influencing how we parent. I encourage you to become curious about yourself, especially if you feel stuck emotionally. Consider that you have a choice in each moment, and opportunities to choose how you'd like to parent. This growth mindset is crucial to our parenting journey, especially when we feel we are remiss. Our willingness to choose differently and to evolve is a pillar in our healthy loving relationships.

Why would this awareness of our self be important to the parenting journey? Because during stressful situations we can become triggered and lose sight of our intentions. In a triggered state you are no longer in the moment of reality. Instead your brain has been pulled off balance and is reminded of a past trauma. The reaction will be one of anger, yet it is often a mask for another more vulnerable emotion such as hurt.

When we become emotionally triggered, we are no longer fully present to the situation in front of us. Which means we are no longer able to parent through choice. This interferes with our capacity to regulate not only ourselves, but our children.

I personally get triggered when I'm not being listened to. It makes me feel out of control. It can be something simple like asking my five-year-old daughter to glance up while I wipe her face in the morning. After several attempts, with her looking anywhere but at me, I feel a thunderous rage within me. I feel irrationally annoyed and want to disengage.

The act of not being heard catapults me to a place of threat, so in moments like this I am no longer able to see my daughter's world view, only my distorted version.

The perceived threat my brain detected isn't a threat to me at all. I misinterpreted the situation and over-reacted. My daughter was simply distracted by all that was around her and actively engaged with her environment – which is totally normal and healthy for a five-year-old brain.

In moments like this we cannot make rational thinking decisions. We act out a younger part of the self that lacked emotional regulation at the time of our own childhood. As adults when we are triggered it is rarely the situation in the moment causing us such distress, but the childhood memories. However, for a child witnessing the distress they quickly believe it is about them.

Without having to change the past we can reform this. So what can you do?

1. Develop an awareness of yourself in heated moments. Your feelings might not be relevant to the situation. This recognition is valuable in guiding you to step back and take a breath.

2. Think about your own childhood attachments. What didn't you like and how might this trigger you today? Can you recall the feelings you had during childhood? Do you notice those feelings surface as an adult?

3. A therapeutic Cognitive behavioural therapy (CBT) approach is to let the fear run its course... so in my example; 'I am worried if I can't wipe your face you'll go to school dirty, if you are dirty your teachers and friends might judge you, if you are judged you might not get on with everyone, if you don't get along then you might be alone, if you are alone then you'll struggle socially....'. See how an initial thought can unconsciously unravel itself. In this example I know logically that some peanut butter on the face doesn't really mean she'll never have friends, but unconsciously this is where my mind would run.

4. What relationships were beneficial to you as a child? How do you remember the experience? What would you like to replicate?

How can I make myself feel better when I get it wrong?

We all get triggered, I still do! what is key is developing an awareness to minimise and manage eruptions. Not feeling good enough as a parent is painful. To remedy this, I recommend practising self-compassion, replacing any negative punishing dialogues with words of comfort. When we blanket ourselves in compassion rather than judgement we soften back into the here and now, the present moment where your child is waiting for you.

As adults we are rarely in the here and now, but rather thinking about the past or the future. Being lost to our thoughts in this way challenges our parenting rhythm. A child's demands can feel jarring, yanking us from our thoughts, yet if we are present to the moment the exchange flows, which means we respond to our children rather than react. But how can we be present to the moment? We need to self-regulate, which means checking in emotionally with ourselves.

What does this look like?

Soothing our mind and body through breathing techniques and developing an awareness of our thoughts. Simply asking yourself 'how are you doing?' is a great question to pause the moment.

A great technique to release tension is to soften the jaw and arms before holding your child. A child will always know when we are strained and can become fussy themselves.

What if my child is upset (dysregulated)?

If your child is dysregulated they won't yet have the higher brain skills (the pre-frontal cortex) to manage big uncomfortable emotions. Discovering a favourite cereal box is empty may be experienced like grief. The feelings they have are visceral – which means they can't think or make rational decisions.

When we remain calm, as the adult staying in a regulated state, we are able to re-regulate the child back into a calm state. So you are essentially *lending* them your brain to soothe them. A child will need assistance to regulate any big emotions, happy or sad. Whether over-excited or unhappy, a young child needs assistance to develop self-regulation skills. These aren't learned through demonstration, but rather through an interaction known as co-regulation.

If you have ever spent time with someone who is really down in a depressed mood, you will know that after some time you may come away feeling depressed yourself. Children are even more impacted by that type of emotional exchange than adults.

When a child is having a tough time, it's helpful as the adult to stay regulated ourselves – avoiding those triggered states – so we can step in as the co-regulator. As Dan Siegal describes it, in these moments you are playing your PART – Presence, Attunement, Resonance and Trust. This will promote connective interactions – attachments – that then become self-soothing skills. In these moments it's about having a connection where you honour differences.

When this is repeated as a parenting approach, the practice of being present rewards us with connection which means an integrated healthy developing brain in the child.

How can you co-regulate your child?

Slow your words, speak quietly, reflect.

Imagine the world from your child's point of view. Become curious about what life is like for them. What can they see? What do they feel is happening around them?

Respond with gentle movements of rocking or touch.

Provide a soothing narrative of what you see. 'You sound hungry, I'm sorry you needed me and I wasn't here, I can hear how sad you are' rather than 'You're okay! Come on don't be silly, there's no need to cry'. The second is by no means intentionally harmful, but it's dismissive of the child's experience – reflecting the carer's world view and not the child's. When it all goes wrong and we hear ourselves ROAR come back to this acronym.

- **REWIND**. What just happened?
- **OWN IT**. This is not about you, this is about me
- **APOLOGISE**. Acknowledge the hurt you've caused: 'I'm sorry for reacting like that'.
- **REFLECT** with empathy and actively listen.

If there is one thing to take away it's that there is no such thing as a perfect parent and nor are we trying to train children to self-regulate. It's about having a connection and building a trusting relationship with yourself and your children. In doing this, your child eventually develops resilience and self-soothing skills.

Recommended reading

A staple for reliable easy reading is Margot Sunderland and her book *What every parent needs to know*. Stuart Shanker writes about self-regulation if you'd like to read more on how to help your child (and you) break the stress cycle and successfully engage with life.

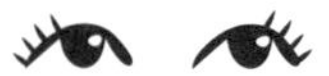

What exactly is 'self-soothing' in a sleep context?

The first thing you need to remember is that we all wake up briefly after each sleep cycle. All of us. Even you and me. We punch the pillow, inhale deeply, look around, clear our throat. Or we might get up to use the bathroom, have a drink of water, or rearrange the covers. But ultimately, we don't really remember this in the morning, and we don't involve anyone else, by and large, when we wake briefly.

Little ones generally fall in to two camps when they wake briefly: the self-soothers and the signallers.[2] You may already have a good idea based on your experience so far with your child which camp they drift towards. This is more likely to be an issue for toddlers and young preschoolers, but if you're a parent of an older child who wakes in the night, this section will be relevant for you too.

The self-soothers wake briefly, like everyone else, and provided they do not have a significant need – like fear, hunger, discomfort or pain – they might suck their fingers or thumb, wriggle around, make a noise and then go back to sleep. They don't need parental help to go back to sleep as often. These children tend to sleep for consolidated stretches when they are ready, and as babies and toddlers they are able to sleep longer between feeds. Often these children were labelled 'easy' or 'good sleepers' from an early age, but the reality is that there is probably nothing their parents did in infancy to make their child behave this way. If your toddler slept like this as an infant, but only recently started to wake more, then take heart, there is plenty of troubleshooting information later on.

The signallers, on the other hand, aren't quite so able to fall back to sleep on their own. Not only do they wake when they have a significant need, but they are much more likely to need help going back to sleep after the other sleep cycles as well. These toddlers can be slower to sleep for consolidated stretches, and find it harder to link sleep cycles. They may wake every 1–2 hours, and do this for a longer time. If this is your child, it's very likely that you might say 'they've never slept well'. People might label these children as 'difficult' or 'sensitive', or 'high need'. If you're nodding along, don't worry – plenty of ideas coming up to soothe your sensitive little one.

The reason this matters is that the strategies that might work really well for a self-soother, may not work so well for a signaller, because the signaller needs more help. For example, one common piece of advice is that if a toddler wakes in the night, you can give them just a minute to see if they settle themselves. The idea is that if you go to them immediately, you may stop them settling, and you might also create a new habit. Now, this idea will fall apart if you have a signaller. Your signaller does not have these skills, so all that will happen is their crying will escalate, they will fully awaken, and it will be harder, and take longer, for you to get them back to sleep. People sometimes become baffled when their thriving healthy toddler who eats more than they do is waking at night for a feed. 'They can't possibly be hungry!' people say in bewilderment. No, they may not be, but the signaller will wake for comfort, and feeding is their preferred way of being comforted – so guess what, they will wake and probably want a feed.

Now, the bad news is that you can't teach a toddler to be someone they're not. If your toddler is a signaller, they can't help it, and they can't help needing you more. What you *can* do is help them adjust to *other* ways of going back to sleep. You can also help them by eliminating as many possible causes of sleep disturbance as you can. Take heart – there is hope! The great news with toddlers is that there are *more* tools you can use to help them, because they are generally more verbal, have greater understanding, and there are more factors that might be disturbing their sleep – this is helpful, trust me! If there's something bugging your toddler, and you can figure out what it is, then you can probably improve their sleep.

Finally, you may feel that your child *sometimes* falls in to the self-soothing camp, whereas at other times, for seemingly inexplicable reasons, they seem to reside firmly in the signalling camp. This is also pretty common. If you think about it, it's normal that at times your child may need you more or less. These broad categories are not strictly binary, but children may drift in and out of being able to shift into another sleep cycle without your help. Part of responsive parenting is identifying and understanding that it is normal for your child to need you more during certain phases, and meet those needs without overthinking the 'why factor' too much.

Sleep-training

We can't really go much further without bringing up how sleep-training fits in to the overall picture of self-soothing, attachment and regulation. I'm acutely aware of everyone's individual journeys with their children up to this point, and of how emotive a topic sleep-training is. For this reason, while I don't want to be vague and accepting of sleep-training in a bigger context, I also don't want anyone to feel judged. My friends, this is not an easy task. After all, everyone has an opinion on sleep-training. You have firm beliefs about your child, their sleep story, and sleep approaches in general. So do I. With this section, I seek to share evidence-based information, with a healthy dose of compassion and empathy. Does that sound good? I don't know your story, or what you've tried so far. I don't know the hours you've spent in the middle of the night with your child, and I don't know who you have spoken to, which books you've read, or what your friends and family think. Please just know that wherever you sit on the sleep-training debate, if we met face-to-face, there would be no judgement.

It seems sensible to start by defining sleep-training. Sleep-training may mean different things to different people. For some, it is any active management of a child's sleep other than being entirely led by them. For others sleep-training is the term used to describe leaving a child to cry alone in order to attempt to improve sleep. In between doing nothing and leaving to cry, there are a hundred other changes that you could potentially make. Personally, I define sleep-training as non-responsive strategies that misunderstand a child's needs (emotional, social, psychological, developmental, health, nutritional or relational) and urge a child towards a pattern of behaviour or sleep that is not individually age or developmentally appropriate. The reason I don't *only* define cry-it-out, or controlled crying, as sleep-training, is that I have seen plenty of non-responsive strategies that involve a parent being in the room with their child. I honestly don't think a parent being present physically with their child is the definition of 'gentle'. I have spoken to literally hundreds of parents who were told to stay in the room but not make eye-contact, or stay in the room but not pick their child up if they cry. I just don't think it's sensible to define sleep-training by the activity you undertake – it's about the heart attitude behind it. Some little ones are quite happy for their parent to be in the room and barely looking at them. Others become hysterical while their parent rubs their back and shushes. Responsive sleep strategies, at the heart, mean that a parent aims to meet the needs of their child at the time, and is led by how well they are coping. So rather than define sleep-training by the strategy used, I prefer to define it by thinking about what is temperamentally, developmentally and age appropriate. I also believe that the way a parent and child inter-relate, the way a parent responds to and manages their child's needs, and the way a parent is able to adapt and modify what they are doing in response to how a child is coping, is paramount.

What's the premise of most non-responsive strategies?

Most behavioural sleep-training is based around the idea that if a child falls asleep with a particular sleep cue, they will learn to expect that same cue whenever they wake up. It is also based on the idea that a child comes to learn to wake up in order to receive that particular cue because it is worth waking for. The idea is that if you stop whatever it is you're doing to help your child back to sleep, they will eventually develop the skill they need alone and then not need your help. This behaviourist approach was heavily criticised even in the 1920s and has largely been refuted in recent years[3] but many people have internalised it into conventional parenting wisdom. It's not sensible if you really think about it, because how can you train a child to not need you? Does stopping whatever it is you're doing to get them to sleep help to teach them self-regulatory abilities or independence? Almost certainly not.

The truth is, if you have sat with your child, held their hand, rubbed their back, fed them to sleep, or had them in the bed with you, you may well have heard that these activities are 'sleep associations', 'props' or 'crutches'. You know what I call this? *Normal parenting.* Parents have been soothing and parenting their children to sleep for thousands of years, and will do for thousands more. It's normal, it won't last forever, and you didn't do anything wrong if this is how you have parented your child. I'm always aware though that when people read sentences like this it is easy to interpret these words as 'it's normal, therefore nothing can be done, so deal with it'. I don't mean to imply you're stuck with an unsustainable way of soothing your child in the night until they grow out of it on their own. But we have to start from the basis that this is normal parenting, and normal child behaviour.

What's the harm of sleep-training?

I get asked this question a lot. Well, we have to start by asking ourselves what is the risk in not responding to a child, or not responding in the way a child needs? Risk, of course, is relative and not absolute. So a small chance of something happening is not the same as a high chance of something happening. And not everyone is affected in the same way.

If I buy hardy flower seeds and fragile flower seeds and want to know how to raise them, I might check reputable gardening websites. I might read a book, look online, ask my mum, or talk to a gardener. Depending on who I ask, and their knowledge, training, bias and experience, I may be given good or bad advice, and depending on my patience and capacity as a gardener, I may or may not choose to act on or ignore certain advice. Let's say I decide to just plant them straight out in my garden in the winter. Will they all survive to flower? Perhaps. The hardy ones have a greater chance of making it, but that's not to say the fragile ones won't make it. Certainly the environment makes a difference. Putting all the seeds in a propagator first, watering and feeding them and keeping them warm would provide the optimum conditions. But even in those circumstances, some seeds may not flower. Of course, I could plant them all outside, but cover them with fleece. I could add fertiliser and compost, which would enhance the chances. You get the idea.

Will *all* children be harmed by sleep-training? No, I don't think this is a sensible conclusion. Might the children who were sleep-trained, like the seeds that were planted outside, thrive and flower? Of course. Some cry only momentarily, and then settle down quickly – I call these the 'rapid responders'. Others seem to have a harder time, and might cry for a longer period, or for more days – I call these children the 'slow responders'. But there are some who cry long and loudly, every night for many weeks – I call these children the 'non-responders'. I suspect that when we think about the children who seem to have a rapid response to sleep-training, in the context of an otherwise loving and responsive relationship with their parent or parents, it is unlikely that sleep-training is or was harmful. We will never know of course, whether it would have been easier for them to have not been sleep-trained. But I don't pretend to know the circumstances of all these children either. I also don't know what position the parents of those children were in at the time, or what advice they were given. I don't know how vulnerable they were, or how desperate the situation was.

The evidence we have about sleep-training isn't very good. There doesn't seem to be conclusive proof of harm, but there is not good enough proof of safety either – particularly for those children who do not have that rapid response. In the context of what we know about responsive parenting, attachment, attunement, and relationship building, as well as the uncertainty we have about individual children's responses, and their internal vulnerabilities and resilience levels, it's not something I personally am willing to take the risk with, which is why I continue to advocate for responsive sleep support.

If you tried sleep-training in the past, then I can't imagine that was easy for you to do. I know from having listened to many parents over the years, that it isn't a decision that many parents take lightly. I truly want you to know that this is not intended to shame. I imagine that if you tried sleep-training, either recently, or years ago, with the child you had in mind when you bought this book, or an older child, you would have had one of three outcomes:

1. You tried it, and it worked
2. You tried it and it didn't work
3. You tried it and it worked for a while but the improved sleep hasn't lasted

Sleep-training doesn't always work for all children and families. When you break this down, it may not work because the child did not settle, became too distressed, and the parents decided this was not the right strategy. Or it may not work because despite the parents following the strategy consistently, their child may not seem to settle and continued to cry for many weeks. For many more parents, it works for a while, or even years, and then suddenly sleep deteriorates. These parents often ask me – 'my child has been self-soothing for years, why did they forget how to do it?'. The truth is, they *hadn't* learned to self-soothe. When a child has been sleeping well for a time, and then sleep deteriorates, there are two things to bear in mind. Firstly, it is common and normal for sleep to go up and down. Secondly, for whatever reason, something has changed. Either they are developing and learning, or they are anxious about something, but for whatever reason, they can no longer just fall asleep like they've been doing up till now, and they need their parent more.

The context changed. They changed. Their sleep changed. In a way,

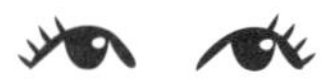

it's really simple. Of course, the reality is far from simple – it is confusing, frustrating and tiring.

But whether we are talking about a deterioration after sleep-training, or a family that has never tried sleep-training, I am firmly of the view that, with older children in particular, sleep-training is not the best approach. The main reasons are that it is likely that with a mobile, verbal child, it will be louder, more difficult and more stressful. It is also unlikely to address the root cause, and misses an opportunity to build confidence and connection, both individually, and between the child and parent.

Attachment security

Attachment patterns affect many areas of our wellbeing, functioning and psychosocial development. The very first meaningful relationship that we have is our relationship to our primary caregiver in infancy. When parents sensitively and promptly respond to their infants at times of need or distress, children are more likely to develop a secure attachment style. Secure attachment is associated with better outcomes, including good mental health, positive future relationships, better job prospects and even fewer long-term adult sleep problems.

Thinking about secure attachment can be quite triggering for many parents. I meet hundreds of parents who beat themselves up about whether they manage to fully understand their child and interpret their behaviour accurately. Some parents feel that their child is still a bit of an enigma they will never quite understand. There is so much research about attachment behaviours and patterns, and what contributes to the development of secure attachment, but much of it boils down to the fact that as parents we need to do two main things: provide safety and security, and be sensitive to our children's needs. Sensitivity is the ability of a parent to recognise, accurately interpret, and promptly respond to infant cues. This is often called attunement, and it is important as it promotes bonding, improves relationships and facilitates empathy and social awareness. Secure base provision, on the other hand, is similar to sensitivity, but is more specific to providing safety and interpreting attachment-seeking behaviours – specifically crying, preventing exposure to and supporting through frightening experiences, and picking babies up and holding them chest to chest.

Some recent research[4] suggests that while parental sensitivity and secure base provision are both important, some parents struggle with sensitivity, perhaps because they have not had a good role model, are themselves stressed, anxious or traumatised, or suffering from depression. Researchers found that it was secure base provision more than parental sensitivity that most predicted secure attachment. There seems to be a much smaller link between sensitivity and attachment than previously thought, and it is specifically those behaviours that provide safety during distress that are particularly important for secure attachment. This is actually really positive and realistic news, and while of course we should aim to understand our children as much as we can, it's reassuring that when life doesn't go quite to plan, our early experiences are far from perfect, and we are tripped up by common difficulties, that attachment won't necessarily all go to pieces.

Children don't need us to get things right all of the time. Getting it right enough of the time – which is about 50 percent – seems to be good enough. We may worry whether we have done enough. It's been my experience in general that one of the signs of having done enough is that you worry whether you have done enough. The fact that you care about it is probably indicative that you knew it was important. I'm not suggesting that we can all relax and disregard the importance of attachment, but we need to get our thoughts about it into perspective. The purpose of this section is not to make parents question whether their child is secure, but to reinforce and affirm the importance of all your hard work, and how this relates to your child's attachment behaviours *now*.

Attachment behaviours are those that a child exhibits in order to get physically close to the primary attachment figure. This is usually referred to as separation anxiety and in plain English what this means is that a baby or toddler may sometimes cry when you leave, or cling to you to try to stay near you. Later on, a child's attachment behaviours are driven by conditions that the child can't manage or struggles to cope with – such as pain, discomfort, dysregulation, tiredness, hunger, or something distressing or scary. It's also common to have a second, third or fourth wave of separation anxiety around big life changes, such as starting school, another sibling arriving on the scene, or illness. Adults display these behaviours as well, especially during stress, but they may be directed toward a partner. For example, if an adult experiences bad news, grief, or they are sick, they may desire close contact with a partner or family member.[5]

Remember that attachment behaviours, or separation anxiety, are normal,[6] and kind of a compliment. After all, it's normal to miss the people we love. If your child is sad when you say goodbye, and only calms down when you reappear, this is entirely normal. My best suggestion is to know that it is normal, will pass, and there is nothing you can really do to speed it up. However, being endlessly patient while you have a Velcro toddler is tiring and emotionally draining, so I hope you have a way of getting some space – even if it's just 15 minutes in the bath, or listening to an audiobook on your commute. We all have a limit, and need space to regroup.

Child sensitivity

Some children are more sensitive than others. You may have heard many different words to describe this – 'high need', 'fussy', 'spirited', 'emotional', and others. An emerging concept is the dandelion and orchid theory, developed by Dr W. Thomas Boyce in 2008. There may be genetic and epigenetic factors that predispose children to behave and act in certain ways. The metaphor explains why some people are more sensitive and reactive to their environment. It is probably overly simplistic to label, typecast or categorise children as either 'resilient', or 'vulnerable', because after all we all have good days and bad days, and seasons that are harder or easier. Some days your child may tolerate something, and on others may baulk and have a meltdown. However, the orchid-dandelion metaphor is helpful to understand different patterns of temperament and behaviour, and the impact that this may have on parenting confidence.

Orchid and dandelion children

When you think of a dandelion, you imagine a plant that is tough, resilient and can flower anywhere. It springs up in poor soil, between cracks in the pavement, grows back after it's been cut down, and survives poor weather conditions. The dandelion can be seen everywhere and you do more or less what you like – it will still come back and flower, whether you want it to or not. Features of dandelion children include:

- Low levels of neuroticism
- Low sensitivity to environmental stimuli
- More likely to be extroverted (feel energised by being around lots of people)

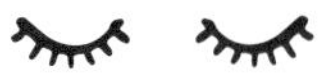

- Not easily overwhelmed
- Cope well under pressure

Dandelion children may be described as happy-go-lucky, easy-going, adaptable, sociable, or textbook children. As a parent it is perhaps easier to feel like you're 'getting it right' with a dandelion child. Dandelions can cope better with difficult circumstances, and seem to take knocks more easily. My second child is a dandelion, and has coped with very serious illness, and other problems, with cheerfulness and stoicism. The evidence suggests that while dandelion children do get affected by knocks and trials, they seem to bounce back more easily. It is probably not fair to say that they necessarily sleep better. A dandelion may still be a signaller, have low sleep needs, and feel anxious about going to sleep. But it's been my experience that their sleep struggles are generally easier to contain and deal with, and they may respond more quickly to changes, limits and boundaries that you put in place.

When you think of an orchid, you imagine a flower that needs the exact right conditions in order to thrive. They need the right soil, the right temperature, the right light aspect, and quickly droop, fail to flower or die if not provided with the right conditions. I've always loved orchids. I grew up in south-east Asia and there were orchids everywhere – truly beautiful plants. Later, as a teenager, I had an orchid that lived in my south-facing room under a sloped window. It was stunning for years, until the day I moved it so that I could redecorate. That was the end of the orchid. I tried to repot it, and put it back in the same place, but no. I had upset it by changing its environment and couldn't seem to make it happy again.

Features of orchid children include:

- Higher levels of neuroticism
- Highly sensitive to environmental stimuli
- More likely to be introverted (find being surrounded by people exhausting)
- Easily overwhelmed
- Do not cope well under pressure, particularly social pressure or feeling scrutinised

It is common to feel like parenting is harder work with an orchid child,

or that you don't quite understand your child. Parenting an orchid does not mean they will have a poor outcome – after all, orchids are intensely beautiful flowers, but the conditions they need may be more specific in order to help them grow. There is also some evidence that they respond more positively to therapeutic interventions, such as interventions to reduce depression, than dandelion children. So it is a tale of hope! My first child is an orchid, and though she is easier to predict now, she was a highly sensitive child who found change, transitions, as well as certain sensations and activities, very hard.

There is a third type of flower in the metaphor. You may wonder about the children you know who don't really fit into either of these extremes. 'Tulips' are described as having medium sensitivity. They fit somewhere in the middle of the sensitivity spectrum. Of course, these categories are not necessarily binary, but you probably have a sense that your child fits broadly into one of these types. You may also wonder where you would put yourself. All of us have tendencies towards different sorts of behaviour, sensitivity thresholds and tolerance levels. You may feel like you are a different flower to your child, which may explain why sometimes you feel like you're on a different page, and don't understand their response. Conversely you may feel like you are more in tune with your little one and can predict how they will react. This may be down to your careful, close observation over the years, your commitment to learning what makes them tick, or it may be because you instinctively feel the same way and can relate on a visceral level.

The point about understanding attachment, regulation, and sensitivity is that all this affects sleep, your child's response to sleep, and how we approach sleep. If you can get inside your child's mind and understand the world from their point of view, it will make it easier for you to meet their needs, whether asleep or awake.

"If you can get inside your child's mind and understand the world from their point of view, it will make it easier for you to meet their needs, whether asleep or awake."

Parenting orchids

Tracy Cassels, PhD, parenting and sleep consultant. Founder: Evolutionary Parenting

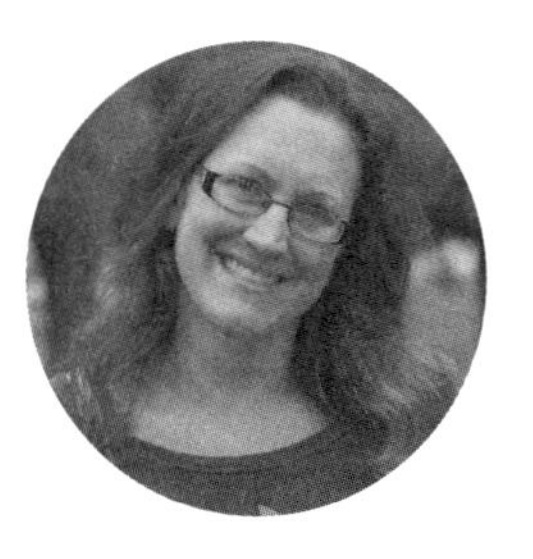

Tell me if this sounds familiar: you have a child that just doesn't seem to be like anyone else's child. Their child went through these 'independent' milestones relatively quickly and smoothly. You're already wondering if you're going to have to go off to university with your child. Their child seems to be rather even-keel. Your child seems to feel the spectrum of emotions on 11 – every time. Their child is a typical kid who forgets things and doesn't always know what's going on around them. Your child doesn't miss a thing and will remember things from ages past. If it does, congratulations: you are very likely the parent of an orchid child.

What is this 'orchid child'? These are the children who are far more in tune with and affected by their environments. They have biological differences that lead to these behaviours that parents can find so demanding – especially in our society where understanding and support are scarce. These children are also far more reactive. You know when your orchid gets upset and just loses their mind? That's thanks to the fact that their stress reactions are actually far greater than for other kids.

For parents, you may feel like you've done it wrong or that your job is to force your orchid to be like others. This isn't the case. Because orchids are so affected by their environments, we have to be very careful how we raise them. You see, unlike other kids who tend to do well as long as they have a 'good enough' environment, orchids are quite specific in what they need. If they get this environment, they thrive and will often be the adults who have *more* emotion regulation, *more* empathy, *better* health (physical and mental), and are the innovators in our society. If they don't, they wither and face a greater risk of physical illness, mental health problems, and less life success.

The problem is that what they need is *not* what our society tells us they do. Modern parenting practices – like solitary sleep, early daycare, early independence – are the opposite of what orchids need to thrive. Thanks to their stress reactivity, they need a lot of social buffering in the form of physical contact with an attached caregiver. This means things like co-sleeping, babywearing, and being responded to (and often held) at all times. It puts a lot of pressure on you – the parent – that can be difficult.

Parents of orchids often feel more run down, more stressed, and face more struggles because of the intensity of the needs of their child. If you aren't supported by others, you can feel done with parenting. If you are being blamed by others, you can feel like a failure. If you're an orchid yourself (there is a genetic component after all), you may feel completely overwhelmed and triggered, especially if you didn't have the type of upbringing that would have allowed you to thrive.

It's okay to feel all these things. I always want parents of orchids to know that although our children need this specific environment, they do not need us to be perfect. As long as we are open to apologising and modelling forgiveness to ourselves, our orchids will likely thrive even through our mistakes.

What they really need is us. This means you need to focus on getting your needs met too. This is so hard for many, but is essential if you're going to survive this ride of a lifetime. Some parents get help in whatever form they can – with housework, caring for other kids – and some just take more time to do something that brings them peace and allows them the space to be just focused on them. It can also help to find other parents of orchids to realise how much it's not you doing it wrong. Support and understanding are crucial and other families can offer that. I personally try to educate as many people as I can about orchids through talks, videos, courses, and articles and you can see these at Evolutionary Parenting.

I promise you though, these hard times are worth it. As our orchids get older, you get to see their brilliance shine through and you may even heal a bit of yourself in the process.

Website: evolutionaryparenting.com
Email: tracy@evolutionaryparenting.com

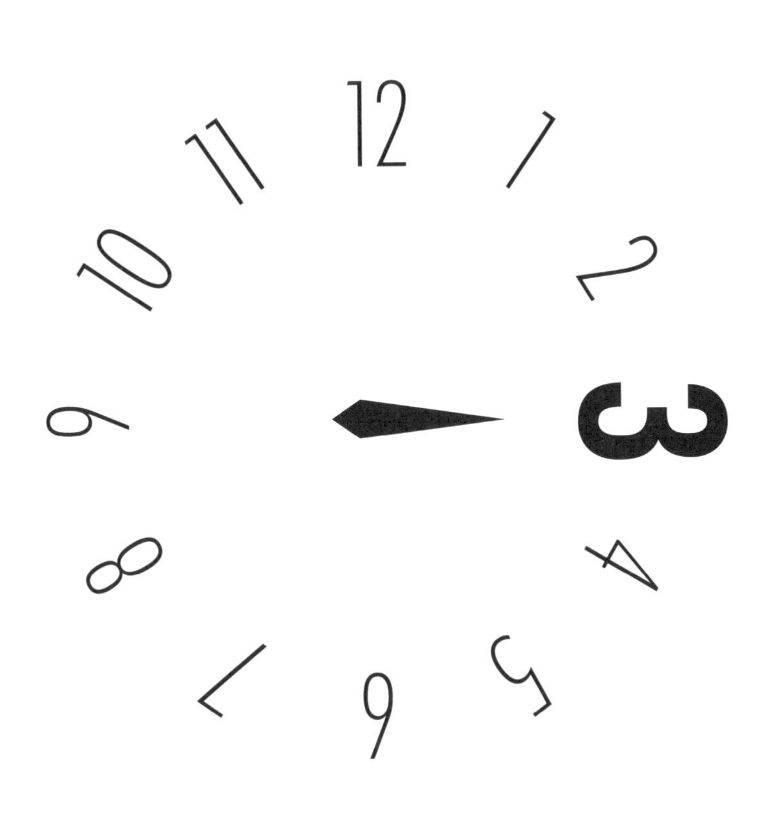

CHAPTER THREE

SUPPORTING SLEEP WITHOUT SLEEP-TRAINING

There are lots of things you can do to support your toddler to sleep as well as possible. One idea is to work with your child's circadian rhythm, understand sleep timings and biology, and how to calm your child for bed. None of these ideas will be stressful or difficult, and I often recommend starting with these easy fixes. Every child is different, and they change rapidly as they grow, which means you have a constant dance of adaptation to the ever-changing needs of your child. Their sleep needs may also be changing or reducing, and some aspects of their daily routine may need adjusting.

- **Exposure to sunlight** – this is one of the best ways to make your child's body clock more robust. It can also help if they tend to get sleepy later in the day and you can't avoid that late nap that is a disaster for bedtime! Exposure to sunlight also helps with early rising.
- **Nap time** – toddlers often need a longer stretch of awake time between their nap and bedtime. I often suggest having a good look at their nap. If it's too long, you may pay for this at night. If it's too early, they may not be able to last till bedtime, and then you can end up in a cycle of early rising and early bedtimes. If it's too late, you may not get your toddler down till much later than you'd like. While every child is different, as a loose rule of thumb, aim for a nap right in the middle of the awake time. So if they wake at 6am and go to bed at 8pm, aim for a nap at around 12.30/1pm, for 1–2 hours. More on naps later!

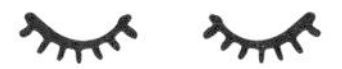

- **Predictable wake up time** – try if you can to start your day at the same time every day. If you have a partner who can take the toddler for an hour or two, while you catch up on some sleep, then all the better! Just because the toddler's day has to start, doesn't mean you can't catch a break.

Your toddler's natural bedtime is likely to get later as they get older. It may fluctuate when they drop their nap or naps, and at these times, when they are between one and two naps, or about to drop their only nap, they may need a temporarily earlier bedtime as they adjust.

Right before your toddler's natural bedtime, there is a time of wakefulness and alertness.[1] This often lasts about 1–2 hours, and as you might remember from chapter 1, is called the 'wake maintenance zone' (WMZ). You may notice that your toddler is super playful, active or even hyper in this time. This behaviour is often mistaken for 'overtiredness'. While some children anecdotally do get a little wired if they are very tired, overtiredness is very over-diagnosed. This period before the usual circadian-linked bedtime is a natural time of alertness and it will be very difficult to fall asleep during this time. You're better off waiting for this naturally wakeful time to pass and then try bedtime when they're calmer.

Sleep hygiene

There is no one right way to make a comforting, sleep-inducing space for your child, but here are some principles of good sleep hygiene that you can treat as a checklist:

- Regular bedtime
- Simple, soothing bedtime routine
- Cool room temperature (16–18°C is ideal)
- Breathable cotton clothing
- A comfort object or toy if your child finds this soothing. Not all children attach themselves to one toy. If your little one is in this camp, then you could ask your child which toy they would like to take to bed with them tonight – it may be different every day.
- Drink of water in case they are thirsty in the night

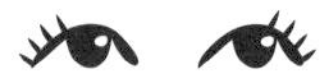

- Consider how you separate the functions of your child's bedroom. If they play there, are you able to tidy the toys away so there is a distinct shift in the room's purpose, from playtime to sleep time?
- Never send your child to their room when you are angry – this can create an association of stress with a space that needs to be peaceful (more on behaviour and limits in chapter 5).
- Are there stickers, suspended items or objects that could be casting scary shadows?
- Is the room cluttered and crowded? This can sometimes be distracting.
- If your child shares their room with a sibling, do they each have a separate space to call their own?

The take-home message with sleep hygiene is that the bedtime routine, being in the bedroom, being in bed, and the falling asleep process should be associated with calm, peace, and a rapid onset of sleep.

Sleep occurs in the rest/digest state, not the fight/flight state. I often explain this to people by saying *you can't sleep with your foot on the gas pedal*. Essentially, our autonomic nervous system responds to our environment and situation. We don't just have a simple stop/go system though – it's a little more sophisticated than that. If your nervous system needs to be still, calm and conserve energy then it will. If it needs to be alert and ready, it will be and, conversely, if there is an acute threat, it will kick into action. You can't really micromanage what your nervous system is doing, though increasingly, as we discussed with self-regulation and co-regulation in chapter 2, you can learn tools and techniques to try to calm down.

During the resting state, our bodies have lower heart and breathing rates, and energy is diverted to our gut for digestion. In the alert/aroused state, the heart and breathing rates increase, and more energy is diverted to large muscles. If levels of alertness rise further then the stress response is activated. Many people split up autonomic states into zones or stages.

One way to think about it is the way Brazelton breaks down the stages of regulation:[2]

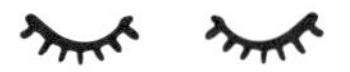

1. Deep sleep
2. Light sleep
3. Drowsy
4. Quiet alert
5. Active alert
6. Crying/dysregulated

Another simpler way to think about it is Leah Kuyper's[3] zones of regulation:

1. **Blue zone**: running slow
2. **Green zone**: good to go
3. **Yellow zone**: becoming unsettled or dysregulated
4. **Red zone**: dysregulated, disorganised or distressed

If you think about it, the only zone that sleep can easily occur in is the blue state. Green states are great to be in if you need to learn, play, communicate or work. Yellow states are shifted into when we become unsettled, uneasy, excited or stressed. There's nothing 'wrong' with being in the yellow zone, but the key is to understand why a child is yellow, and how to manage this. Ultimately, when we think about good sleep hygiene, we want the bedroom and bedtime routine, and falling asleep, to be a calm and relaxed process with a child in the blue zone. If they are bouncing around the room in the yellow zone, then sleep will be harder, and you may need to take some steps to shift the zone.

What does this have to do with sleep hygiene? Well – if your child is overthinking their day at nursery or school they may be dysregulated and find sleep harder. If your child had a late nap and is still full of energy in the green zone, they will simply not be tired, and sleep will be harder. If they have come to associate their room with a place of isolation, stress or homework anxiety – you guessed it, sleep will be harder.

The longer and more consistently your child has a long, stressful or frustrating bedtime, the more it becomes associated with wakefulness and alertness, rather than a rapid onset of sleep. And that, my friends, is not what we want. So, when you're overhauling your child, their bedtime routine, the timing of bedtime, their sleep space and the

associations with their bedroom environment, ask yourself:

- Is my child's bedtime conducive to sleep?
- Is my child ready for sleep when we start bedtime?
- What zone are they in?
- What has bedtime become associated with?

You may feel that bedtime has become associated with frustration, negotiation, playtime, tension, anxiety, hyperactivity, or something else. Whatever it is, start with that. Work out why this is happening. Is it the activities your child uses their room for? Is it the relational interplay at bedtime? Is it unrealistic expectations? Are the timings off? Is your child simply not ready for sleep?

Sleep hygiene and the environment for sleep are crucial. It all starts with this. You will probably find that no matter how clever the ideas we could discuss for managing the middle of the night antics, they will not work without also addressing this piece of the puzzle.

Essential oils

Now, essential oils aren't everyone's thing. That's okay. I'm not going to suggest that they offer some kind of miracle cure. But if you happen to like them, and you are relaxed by pleasant smells, this seems like a no-brainer. Most people consider lavender essential oil to be a bit of a cliché, and in fact, if I'm honest, it isn't my favourite essential oil for sleep and calming. But there are a number of essential oils that may help with sleep. If nothing else, your home will smell even better!

It must be said that most research on essential oils seems to be specific to either young or older people who are unwell, or healthy adults. There is a big gap in research that has explored the effects of essential oils on healthy children. We must therefore a) use common sense, b) exercise caution with interpretation, and c) keep an open mind.

Essential oils are extracted from different parts of plants – for example the flowers, bark or roots. They have been used in many different cultures around the world, for thousands of years, and many people use them either in massage, mixed with a carrier oil, in the bath, or added to water in a diffuser. I have deep respect for plants and the

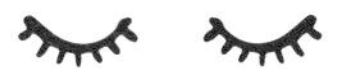

power that they have – after all, many of our medicines are derived from plants. It is not ludicrous to me, to think that they have anti-anxiety and sleep-inducing properties.

One recent small study from Iran[4] found that children with sleep disorders who inhaled rose essential oil dropped on to a cotton ball had less trouble falling asleep, staying asleep, and had fewer nightmares. A systematic review found that lavender, rose and orange essential oils were effective at improving the quality of sleep, including the sleep of children with leukaemia.[5] Another study found some possible positive effects of using neroli and lavender for sleep.[6] Finally, one study found that orange essential oil positively reduced anxiety and therefore improved sleep in children with diabetes.[7]

With so little data, and so few essential oils studied, relative to the bewilderingly vast array of oils anecdotally reported to have benefit, it is hard to form a solid conclusion about whether essential oils work, beyond them just 'smelling nice'. So I share these essential oils with the caveat that there is very little evidence, although no evidence of harm either, provided that you don't apply them directly to skin, or ingest them. I have a cautionary tale to share regarding the use of oregano oil. I read about the powerful antiviral properties of oregano for verrucas. Both of my children had stubborn verrucas on their toes, which did not respond to any conventional treatment and were frustrating as they both enjoyed swimming. I put one drop of oregano oil on a cotton bud and dabbed it carefully on my eldest daughter's verruca every day. It was painless and within two weeks, the verruca had gone. I then tried it on my younger daughter's verruca. Well… this was the child with the higher pain threshold (she had at that point been subjected to two years of chemotherapy and hundreds of painful procedures). She howled the place down for two hours. Was it her different immune system? More sensitive skin? Who knows – but from one parent to another – be careful. Natural products aren't necessarily 'safer'!

So, with all that in mind, I suggest you proceed with caution, using the oils in a diffuser if in doubt – as you can always turn it off – and don't apply them directly to your child's skin. The following oils have been known *anecdotally* to support rest, relaxation and sleep. I'll leave it to you to make your own mind up.

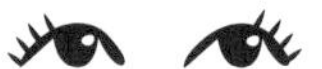

Essential oil	Reported properties
Lavender	Relaxing, may increase deep sleep
Bergamot	May lower blood pressure and induce calm
Rose	Anti-stress and anxiety, lifts mood
Geranium	Calming and relaxing, also reported to reduce pain
Clary sage	Antidepressant, and may reduce the stress hormone cortisol
Valerian	Anti-anxiety, may promote deep sleep
Jasmine	Can be helpful for insomnia
Neroli	Lifts mood, reduces anxiety
Orange	Reduces pain and stress
Ylang ylang	Reduces stress
Chamomile	Reduces anxiety and may help with insomnia
Sandalwood	Relieves stress and anxiety
Marjoram	Calming, and may help with insomnia
Vetiver	Anti-anxiety
Frankincense	Reduces stress, lifts mood

One user tip – if you dislike flowery scents, but want to try them out for their reported sleep benefits, try mixing with a woody oil. For example, if you mix geranium with sandalwood, it takes the edge off the floral note. I love mixing clary sage, ylang ylang and frankincense. For sleep, I like bergamot and vetiver. Have a play around and see what you like. From a practical point of view, if your child likes the smell, you may be onto a winner. It's virtually pointless trying to diffuse a smell they don't actually like. After all, the whole point is relaxation – it could be clinically proven to induce immediate sleep, but if your child hates it and starts fussing, they're not going to sleep any time soon.

Sleep red flags

While most of the time children have no significant underlying pathology to explain their sleep patterns, some children do indeed have a reason for sleeping the way they do, which can be identified, treated and resolved. See your child's doctor if you notice any of the following.

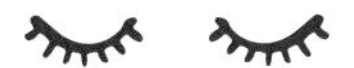

- **Mouth breathing, snoring or pauses in breathing.** This can be suggestive of sleep-disordered breathing. Some people suggest a tongue tie may cause a degree of sleep-disordered breathing, although evidence is still sparse to prove this. Other times it is enlarged tonsils, or another pathology. Either way, it needs to be investigated. This is normal during a respiratory illness, as children will breathe through their mouths if their nose is blocked. But if the mouth breathing persists even while your child is well, this warrants more investigation.
- **Your child is sleepier in the day than you would expect.** This can indicate that your child is not achieving restful sleep at night, which may be caused by an underlying sleep pathology.
- **Strange movements in the night.** I know this sounds highly subjective, but as the world expert on your child, you will know if something is unusual for your child. One-sided jerking, a new movement, or a movement that seems uncomfortable for your child are all examples. Get a video of it if you can, and show your doctor.
- **Poor weight gain/weight loss.** If your child is struggling with maintaining their weight, or gaining weight, your doctor should have a look at them. It could be nothing significant of course, but it's always better to get it checked out.
- **Feeding/eating challenges.** If your child excludes entire food groups, seems scared to eat, or eats a very limited range of foods (less than 20–30 individual foods) then it's time to call a specialist speech and language therapist and dietician. Nutrient deficiency can mess with sleep, and there may be underlying sensory issues.
- **Night sweats.** Some children are just sweaty, let's face it! However, if this is a new symptom for your child, it is worth getting them checked over. It could be that their sleep is being disturbed at night, but low blood sugar and some other conditions can also do this. Better safe than sorry.
- **Illness.** If your child has been under the weather for some time, with endless illnesses, it's worth getting them looked at by a doctor. It's normal for kids to get sick – their immune systems aren't fully developed – but if you feel worried, get them reviewed. Sometimes an acute infection will also mess with sleep – ear infections and urine infections don't always have obvious symptoms for instance.
- **Anything you're worried about.** This is wide open, but you are the best person to know if there's something 'not quite right' either physically,

emotionally, or mentally. There is a lot to be said for your gut instinct. If there's something you can't quite put your finger on, get them checked. It's not your job to diagnose – it's just your job to alert the people who can.

It's always worth ruling out the red flags before you get too far into your sleep investigations. If it's nothing, it's nothing, but it is simply not sensible to try to treat a health problem with a sleep solution.

Is my child tired?

Stick with me, I know this sounds like a daft question. But I'd like to encourage you to develop an attitude of curiosity about your child's tiredness levels. We sometimes interpret cranky, dysregulated behaviour as fatigue, when in fact it may be something else. I'm not saying it's *never* going to be fatigue: in fact, it often is. But just like adults, children can sometimes experience fatigue as a symptom of something else – such as stress, disconnect, overwhelm, or boredom. Just like adults, children can sometimes act up when there is something going on under the surface. Our stress can sometimes be *bigger* than our fatigue – which will prevent sleep.

I often speak to parents of infants about the different thinking filters we can put on – for example if we read about reflux, we may see all fussy behaviour through a reflux filter and interpret it accordingly. If we read about tongue-tie, we may see pulling off the breast or bottle, dribbling and clicking with a tongue-tie filter. But it's just as relevant for older children. If we put on the 'naughty' filter, we might see naughtiness instead of an unmet need. If we put on the 'grumpy' filter, we see grumpiness instead of hunger. If we put on the 'tired' filter, we see fatigue instead of boredom, stress or disappointment.

Your child may very well be tired, but I urge you to keep an open mind. Yawning can mean boredom and stress, as well as being involved in temperature control and other mechanisms.[8] Grey bags under the eyes may indicate a food intolerance.[9] Falling apart may mean too many new things happened today and it's all a bit too much. Just when that seems to make sense, of course, the reality is that humans are complex – we are sometimes tired *and* anxious, or tired *and* overstimulated.

You may have heard about the cola bottle analogy. Imagine a fizzy drink in a sealed bottle. As your child goes through their usual day at nursery, school, or home, little events will come along and shake them up. The lid is on the bottle, so nothing happens, but the pressure slowly builds. By the time they are home, in their safe space (with you), the lid comes off and the built-up pressure causes them to explode, like that bottle of fizzy drink that's been shaken up all day.

Why is this important? Well, because when children have unmet needs, those needs can sometimes override the need for sleep. Which means that while your child may be exhausted, if they are also dysregulated due to something else in their world, they may have a hard time falling asleep. Children use their parent as a secure base to manage the feeling of being out of control and stressed, which is why when they have a hard day, they may need you more. Being close to you means their own stress response system gets a break.

Overtiredness?

One of the things people can get confused about is the concept of overtiredness. Some people say that overtiredness is *never* an issue, while other people blame overtiredness for *most* sleep problems. But where is the truth? Can you ever be so tired and wired that you can't sleep? Well – yes and no.

Yes, because if you stay awake long enough, your circadian-alerting hormones will come into play and you will feel alert even though your sleep pressure is high. Also yes because when you are seriously sleep deprived, this causes your body physical stress. You know this already. If you have a serious sleep debt, you may feel run down, irritable and your immune system seems to take a hit. When your body's stress response is activated, then you release more stress hormone, which is relieved to some extent by sleep. Have you ever just been really worked up, but after a good night's sleep you felt better? Also, if you are really stressed, even though you might feel tired, sometimes it is hard to get to sleep, and when you do sleep, the sleep isn't always great quality, so you may wake up still feeling tired. This happens when we have chronic stress, anxiety, trauma or depression. If you are in this state, then yes, you can be exhausted, but not able to sleep. If this is true for either you, your child or someone you know and care about, then please reach out for some specialised help.

And no, because the brain is really good at making sleep happen when we are very tired. When sleep pressure builds and builds, it's a little like water boiling in a pan – think of tiredness being like a rolling boil, and

extreme tiredness being like the pan boiling over. When the pan boils over, you may see your toddler getting cranky and difficult, but sleep will usually still happen. In the stress state, you may need to calm your little one first, but they will still sleep. While some children probably could benefit from up to an hour or two of extra sleep, it is less likely that your child is *significantly* sleep deprived by several hours unless your child has a significant sleep pathology that is affecting their nighttime sleep quality. I think where the confusion comes is that when really tired, toddlers often get quite dysregulated (cranky/fussy/stressed) and then sleep can feel like a fight even though you *know* they're tired. Toddlers can also become dysregulated due to excitement. Have you ever been so excited you can't sleep?

I vividly remember my youngest, then aged six, on a long-haul flight. We had a layover halfway for a couple of hours and my littlest hadn't slept at that point for 20 hours. I kid you not: she was jumping up and down on an airport chair continuously for 30 minutes. Wired. But is this overtiredness? Or is it just excitement and nervous energy? Well, we can safely say she was sleep deprived, but had she not been excited and nervous, jetlagged and in a brightly lit room she would have slept. So, the issue for many children is not necessarily the fact that they are very tired, but what *else* is going on to stop them from sleeping.

So, the crux of it is this: if your child is a little late for their nap or bedtime, while they may be fussy, it is unlikely to be a total disaster. If they are actually missing out on a lot of sleep (see the chart in chapter 1 to check your child's total sleep) and getting dysregulated, then it is possible that sleep might be a little harder. But you definitely don't need to get bent out of shape about it. Look at your child's sleep over 24 hours, not from hour to hour.

Some of the common reasons your child may be wired at bedtime:

- Excitement
- Something new in their world
- Something they ate at their evening meal
- Nervous about something
- Big developmental changes
- Unresolved drama or argument at bedtime
- And many more...

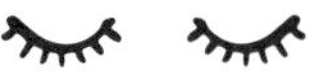

I have noticed that many people want to know exactly what is going on and *why* their child is behaving the way they are. I totally understand that. It's natural to want an explanation. But I have a truth bomb for you: you may never know. The reason may elude you. That doesn't mean you shouldn't bother trying to figure it out, but don't let it ruin your day, or evening. I've found that often, when the answer is not obvious, it's exhausting and frustrating to try to rack your brain wondering. Let it go. Sometimes you'll have a rough bedtime or a disrupted night for no obvious reason, and if you just accept this, you'll feel less stressed.

Sleep timings

You will also need to think about the timing of bedtime. 'Late' bedtimes are a subjective concept. What time do you think of when I say 'late'? Remember that you can only get a certain maximum amount of sleep in 24 hours. For many children, 10–11 hours overnight is about as good as it gets. Therefore, recommending early bedtimes in some cases may just set a family up for a very early start. A 7–7 schedule may simply be unrealistic or unachievable for many children.

Orla, aged three, has always gone to bed at 6.30 since she was a baby. But in the last couple of months, she has been waking up at 5am. One morning she even woke up at 4.45, ready for the day.

In Orla's case, getting older means a reduction in sleep needs. She may only need 10 hours of sleep, and if she is generally perky in the day, then this is not a true early rising problem, but a timing issue. Putting Orla to bed a little later every day should slowly sort this out. Doing this gradually is the trick. If her parents had kept her awake for an hour and a half later immediately, then Orla would have been very fatigued, and may still have woken early. But delaying her bedtime by 15–20 minutes every 2–3 days should gradually shift her body clock and help her to have a later start to the day.

When you are thinking about whether an earlier or later bedtime may be a sensible suggestion for your family, consider the age and individual sleep need of your child, and think about sleep in the context of how your child's behaviour and energy level is affected.

Remember that wake maintenance zone too – if you put your child

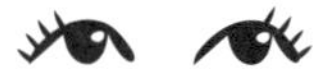

to bed *too early*, you risk them being hyper and alert. Weirdly enough, sometimes waiting for this to pass means an easier and quicker bedtime.

Bedtime routines

Don't worry, I'm not about to patronise you! I'm coming at this section on the assumption that you've had a bedtime routine for many months or years. You've already rolled your eyes at facile suggestions to try a blackout blind or give your child a stuffed animal at bedtime. That's not what I want to focus on. Sure, it's a good idea to have a predictable sequence of soothing activities, and keep the routine short and succinct, and age-appropriate. Those are all givens.

But I want to talk about the *purpose* of bedtime, and how and why it can get derailed. I want to talk about how we can prepare children for bedtime in a respectful way. Finally, I want to talk about how bedtime routines change as children get older.

The purpose of bedtime might seem obvious, but I think this can sometimes get distilled down to 'tricks to speed up getting your child to go to sleep'. Of course, that's the eventual aim, but if we dig into this a little, it's about far more than that. If we step away from the idea that bedtime is about getting the kids to go to bed, and embrace the fact that bedtime is time to calm, contain and connect, then it makes it less about the future, and more about what's happening now. This is important, because being present reduces stress. The future is less within our control than the present. When you stay here, now, you disarm the power of anxiety about what the future holds. The purpose of bedtime in the moment is to calm your child, and get them into the blue zone. Calming your child will ultimately achieve the other aim of a succinct bedtime. Containing your child in the moment allows you to hold space for your child's emotions and feelings. Sometimes worries, niggles and anxieties bubble up at bedtime, and as parents, we need to allow our children to express that (with words or otherwise) without digging into it and breathing life into the anxiety. Of course there is a time to discuss fears and concerns, but at bedtime, we need to allow our children to pour that into us, so that we can take that from them. Connecting with your child in the moment allows your child to feel safe, secure and unconditionally loved. When we calm, contain and connect in the present, we are less likely to be focused on why our child is *not* asleep – which let's face it, can be stressful and frustrating.

A Dad's perspective on bedtime

Thomas Piccirilli, Founder: The Dad Vibes

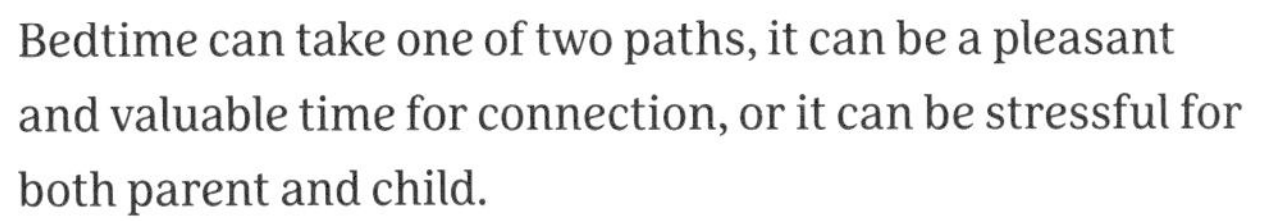

Bedtime can take one of two paths, it can be a pleasant and valuable time for connection, or it can be stressful for both parent and child.

If you've had a long or stressful day, it's easy to enter the bedtime routine in the wrong mindset. This may cause you to rush the bedtime routine, which in itself can turn an otherwise calm and pleasant experience into a stressful one.

My wife took 13 months' maternity leave, and during this time we decided that I would take the lead at bedtime. It was a fantastic opportunity for me to connect with our baby after a day at work. Yes, I was tired, but this wasn't comparable to my wife who had been looking after our little one for 12 hours straight. It also gave my wife an opportunity to have some time to herself and simply relax after a long day. From here it became the norm for me to do most bedtimes. As our baby grew into a toddler, the bedtime routine has certainly evolved. It's gone from a fairly simple routine (bath, a very short story, then sleepy time) to one that's a little more flexible involving lots of play.

Although our bedtime routine may kick off at the same time every night, there are so many factors that can impact how quickly our little one will drift off to sleep. Therefore it's really important that we parents communicate beforehand. Has our little one napped? For how long? When was his last nap? Has he had an active or a relaxing day? All of these factors can have an impact on bedtime.

Being aware of these things can allow us to mentally prepare for what's ahead. Some days, for whatever reason, we end up missing a number of important cues, for example: sometimes our toddler may want another book, sometimes he wants more playtime, or sometimes he just needs extra cuddles before falling asleep. If we miss these cues by racing to lights out, then bedtime can go awry very quickly. Even when he was much younger, a few times after a long day I started 'sleepy time' way too early, which led to him fighting sleep, getting stressed and eventually I'd have to tag in my wife to take over, as she was able to bring a fresh level of calm to the situation.

EXPERT VIEW

With this in mind, one of the best recommendations I can make is to treat bedtime as a time to *connect* with your little one. Reframing bedtime from a box-ticking exercise to valuable time for connection makes for a calm and relaxed experience. Ultimately we want our little ones to fall asleep from a place of calm, not stress. This is why having both parents (if possible) invested in bedtime is so important.

That doesn't mean that both parents need to be involved in the bedtime routine, but if both parents are available then by communicating, you're able to decide who's best placed to do bedtime that night. Who's feeling less stressed? Who's in need of that extra connection with their little one? On the flip side, maybe one of you really isn't feeling like doing bedtime: maybe you'd rather have a glass of wine, walk the dog, or just relax and take some time for you?

By communicating with each other and being honest, you're ensuring your baby or toddler will have the parent who's mentally ready for a relaxed bedtime. Try to remember that bedtime is a special time for our little ones and these moments won't last forever, so try to savour them as much as you can.

Social: @the.dad.vibes

When I talk about preparing children for bedtime, I don't mean putting their pyjamas on and cleaning their teeth – those are just tasks. I mean preparing them mentally. I mean calming their minds and bodies down, and I mean understanding that for children, bedtime is a 'goodbye'. Sleep is separation from wakefulness, our presence, and the fun of the day. Young children live in the moment, and at the moment of bedtime they are away from the other activities going on. They are astute enough to know that not *everyone* is going to bed, and therefore they are missing something (however boring and mundane that might be in reality).

They also do not have the life experience to realise that unless they go to bed and get some rest, tomorrow will be a disaster due to fatigue. Expecting a child to understand the ramifications of their bedtime delays in terms of the effect on their parents and the following day is unrealistic. I know it is as frustrating as anything to deal with bedtime drama, but your child is not doing this to annoy you. It simply does not occur to a young child that their delay of bedtime is inconvenient, draining or disrespectful.

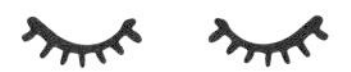

It is so hard not to take this personally, to not think 'I've poured myself out for you today. Now all I want is half an hour to myself.' I have absolutely felt this, and if you have too, then I'd be willing to bet you're in the majority. We simply cannot be all-patient and endlessly energetic all the time. You are human. But so is your child, and their behaviour at bedtime is almost always indicative of something. Instead of expecting things that are unrealistic, let me offer a few practical suggestions for how to prepare children for bedtime:

- Make sure the timing is right – a bedtime too late may mean a child who is falling apart and doesn't enjoy the routine. A bedtime too early means the sleep pressure is too low, or the circadian signals are wrong, and bedtime will be long and frustrating.
- Set the expectations in advance – communicate what is included in the package deal of bedtime. Let there be no surprises – children love to know what to expect.
- Communicate the components of bedtime in a way that is meaningful – many people assume that if a child is verbal, their cognition matches up to what they can say out loud. But this is not always the case. Some children are highly articulate, but their brains can get stuck computing the first few words while you've moved on to point four. For example, if we say; 'Go upstairs, sit on the toilet and then brush your teeth and I'll be up in a minute', they may still be processing the instruction to go upstairs when you finish speaking. They might then get upstairs and start to play, because they've forgotten, or not really heard anything else you said. As a parent, if this has happened to you, it's easy to see how this might look like your child has ignored your instruction and is messing about, or perhaps they need their hearing tested. It isn't necessarily that they can't understand, hear or are being defiant. They just may not have the processing speed and maturity to hold several instructions in their head simultaneously. That's one reason for keeping the routine the same. But that alone isn't enough. I assure you, at this moment in time, it's still sometimes a surprise to my children (aged seven and 11) that cleaning teeth and brushing hair happens every single morning before school. It takes time for these to be really well-established habits. Break the routine down into steps, ideally

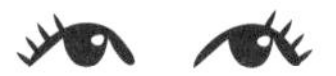

using pictures, and only give one instruction at a time – see what a difference that makes.

- Be firm, but kind with your boundaries – children learn where the limits are by pushing against them. To see if a limit is bendy, flexible, inconsistent, conditional on who gives it, or a brick wall, they push the boundaries. We will come back to this in chapter 4, *Little kids, big feelings*, but for now, it's enough to say that testing boundaries is part of the job description of being a kid. How else do they really establish the working rules? When you reframe limit-testing as a normal way of checking what your expectations are, it will feel less like defiance that tests your patience, and more like age-appropriate and predictable behaviour. It is absolutely possible – in fact, essential – to be both kind and firm with your boundaries. The firmer and more consistent the boundary, the faster your child will stop pushing on it to see if it's a bendy boundary. So if you have said you will read one chapter of a book, that's what will happen. When your child tests this by pleading and asking, you expect this, you are ready with your kind but firm answer of 'No sweetheart, just one chapter. But we can look forward to the next one tomorrow'. Firm does not mean draconian!
- Anticipate likely areas of negotiation in advance – expect your children to push the limits at bedtime. There will often be a curveball that your children throw you when you don't expect it. You have to get ahead of the curveball my friends! It's coming your way. At some point, they will announce that there is an important project they have forgotten about that is due in tomorrow. Or they simply must say goodnight to the dog one more time or they cannot possibly sleep. Or they have an itchy foot. Or an invisible scratch on their arm that is unbearably painful... or whatever. You can't prepare for all the randomness, but you can anticipate the most likely ones. Drinks, toilet trips, a favourite soft toy or their pillow a certain way are all fairly predictable, and you can have a stock answer ready for more random requests.
- Allow enough time for the process – children can sense when we are trying to speed through bedtime. Don't forget, sleep does not come easily if your child's foot is on their gas pedal. If you try to rush it, bedtime may backfire.

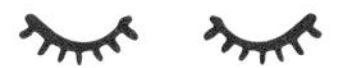

Finally, I know this is another obvious point, but as children grow older, the shape and style of their bedtime routine changes. It may be later, but there may also be more or fewer components to it. It may be less about the tasks of bedtime, and more about the calming of their mind. They may actually need you more. The niggles and worries of a three-year-old are very different to the niggles and worries of an eight-year-old, which are in turn very different to those of an 11-year-old. You may need to calm, contain and connect in a different way with your child as they get older. It may be less about a story and more about a foot massage as they share their frustration about school and friends and other 11-year-old sized problems.

Silly time

Silly time before bed? Does this sound like a bad idea? Well, hear me out. I have three main reasons for recommending silly time before bed, and by the way, this isn't just for four-year-olds – all children need a chance to let off steam.

Firstly, we can spend so much time thinking about calming children for sleep, that we can forget that kids have a lot of energy. In our busy modern lifestyles, it's hard to get enough exercise and activity. More physical exercise is usually a good idea for sleep, as this releases endorphins like serotonin, which in turn makes melatonin.[10] Serotonin production is also upregulated by daylight, so it's even better if exercise is taken outside in the light.[11]

But even with lots of activity, it's normal to build up stresses, strains, tensions and frustrations through our day – remember the cola bottle analogy (page 60)? Little people's problems might seem trivial to us, but they are a big deal to them. One way of getting the tension out is to move our bodies.

"Silly time before bed? Does this sound like a bad idea?... We can spend so much time thinking about calming children for sleep, that we can forget that kids have a lot of energy."

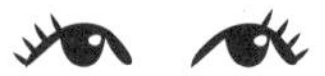

Thirdly, sometimes we do such a good job of keeping a calm household that there isn't enough excitement. It's hard to feel the transition to a calm state if you're already calm. I often talk about adding energy and dynamics to your child's day, to allow them to move between their zones. It's okay to be in the yellow zone and super-excited.

The reason I suggest silly time is therefore so that children can use up some energy, feel more physically tired, vent their frustration and then be able to move from a state of arousal to calm, to make bedtime feel like a distinctly different shift in energy level.

But what do I mean by being silly? Well, here are some ideas:

- Jumping around
- Chasing
- Tickle fights
- Pillow fights
- Races
- Obstacle courses
- Swinging on a swing set
- Playing football, shooting hoops, riding a bike
- Bouncing on a trampoline/space hopper
- Anything that gets your children squealing, laughing or smiling with their whole face

I know this sounds a bit radical. After all, you might have heard for years to not let your co-parent come in from work and get the kids all excited just as you're getting them ready for bed. I can hear the rumbling concerns about children being too ramped up to go to sleep.

This is where I need to explain that you will need to plan silly time in to your evening so that there is enough time for a distinct calm down before the bedtime. Sure, silly time in the bath when bedtime is in ten minutes may not be the best move. But silly time straight after the evening meal, followed by calm-down play and then bedtime? Now you're talking. Just give it go. It's amazing how often this helps with sleep, and also with connection and your child's emotional wellbeing.

Of course, to transition to sleep, you'll probably need to have a distinct calm down, and allow enough time before the bedtime routine starts to enable your child to come back down from the yellow or green zone to the

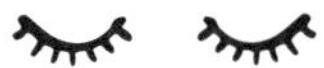

blue zone. You may well be wondering how to calm your child down after silly time. Here are a few ideas you could try:

- Yoga or pilates
- Colouring/drawing
- Finger knitting, sewing, or threading beads
- Lego
- Hiding toys (like plastic animals) in plasticine and asking your child to work the toy out
- Reading books
- Sitting down for a drink and a snack
- Sensory play
- Having a shower or bath
- Singing
- Taking it in turns to share the highlights of everyone's day
- Playing a simple card or board game

One factor to bear in mind is that silly time can become the favourite part of your child's day – which is obviously a good thing, but you may find it helpful to set some parameters around it. If your child struggles when fun activities come to an end, you could try having a timer, and manage their expectations by giving warnings about when silly time will end. This may be hard at first, but once your child realises that this time will be repeated every day, they will accept the end more easily. Just allow enough time for silly time, and calm down time before bed, and you never know – it might become your favourite part of the day too.

Sensory play

We are all sensory beings, and experience life through our senses. Some sensations can increase alertness, while others calm our stress response and make us feel more regulated. We all have different responses to sensory inputs, and sometimes a sensation that we find calming one day is irritating or alerting another day. The trick is to know and be aware of many sensory play ideas and gauge your child's response to them in a given situation.

You may find that your child likes many of these strategies, but not all on the same day. I know it would be nice if we could find the magic

Why read with your child?

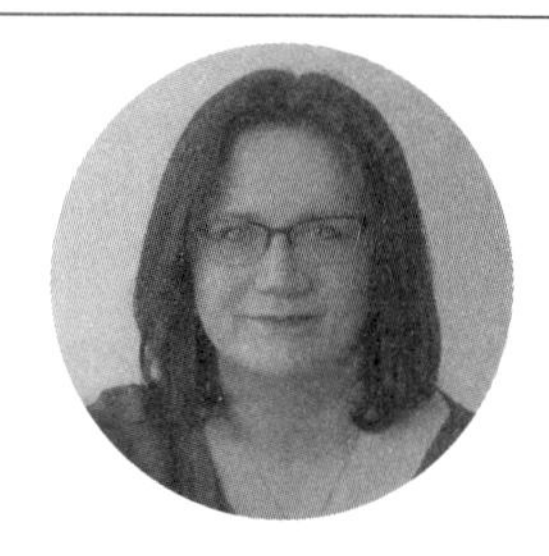

Caroline Zwierzchowska-Dod, parenting specialist, former headteacher and doctoral researcher

Most parents know that reading to children is 'a good thing', but why is this the case? There are, of course many reasons to do with learning the skills of reading – how to hold a book the right way up, how to figure out that the squiggles on the page have meaning, and which sound each one represents, as well as expanding the child's vocabulary.[12]

> *'Did you know that sharing books is the single most important predictor of later academic attainment from all the things parents do at home with their children?'*[13]

Sharing books in the preschool years has been closely linked with higher attainment scores through to late primary age. However, the benefits of reading with your child are much wider than learning literacy skills.

> *'Did you know that children's books contain more complex language than TV shows aimed at the same age group?'*[14]

Reading with your child often involves being physically close to them – it's an opportunity for snuggles and cuddles, holding them close, both looking at the book together and exploring it. The opportunity to spend time with your child is something else that parents really enjoy and both of these contribute to building the bond between you, which we call infant attachment.

Many parents find that reading can act as a calming activity which helps their child to self-regulate their emotions. Addressing concerns such as hitting out, worries about starting school or even big life changes such as bereavement through books can be a really effective way of helping the child to understand and process their own feelings, emotions and behaviours. Reading also forms a key part of many families' daily routines, particularly at bedtime. Here it serves a very different purpose from 'learning to read' – it helps signal that bedtime is coming and provides a crucial 'wind down' when parent and child are calm, often sitting or lying down together, without other distractions.

Should I read with my older child?

The majority of parents report reading daily with their child from about a year old until they are about seven years old, but by age 11, fewer than one-fifth of parents read with their children. However, research[15] shows that the role parents play in later childhood in supporting enjoyment and motivation with reading is linked to achievement, so reading with your tween as well as modelling reading yourself are important things you can do to help continue your child's reading journey.

How should I read with my child?

There are three key aspects to reading with your child that work really well from toddlers through to teens.

- **Read aloud** – reading books to your child that are a little above their own reading ability shows them that stories are to be enjoyed, and keeps them interested with topics and themes that they can't quite read for themselves yet.
- **Read together** – having regular family reading time enables siblings to read to each other, and different family members to share what they are enjoying. Show your child what you are reading and let them choose what to read to you. It helps reading to be seen as a relaxing activity, not just 'homework' to be endured.
- **Read and chat** – for all ages, talking 'around' the book rather than only reading the words on the page helps children to make connections with their lives and the world around them. It starts simply from birth – 'see the teddy in the book, you have a teddy too' and continues through the amazingly in-depth conversations you can have with your older children – I remember being amazed at how my 11-year-old linked *Alice in Wonderland* to leaving primary school and starting at secondary school, with all her feelings of being too big and too little all at the same time.

As children learn the skills of reading, it is natural to expect them to do more of the task of reading themselves, demonstrating their growing independence as readers, but keeping a mix of sharing books together, your child reading to you and you reading to your child is key in keeping the enjoyment which we know is key to creating life-long readers.

> *'Did you know that how much a child enjoys reading is a clearer predictor of future academic achievement than the family's socio-economic status?'*[15]

Showing how much you enjoy reading with them is an important way to help your child develop a love of reading.

How can I help my child to choose books?

There are benefits to children rereading old favourites and also in discovering new books. Rereading known books is a key skill in building up reading confidence and learning how stories are structured.

When choosing books, aim for some where they can read almost all of the text for themselves, to build confidence and reading stamina. Alongside this, children can choose more complex books that appeal to them – these can be read by the parent or older sibling to the child. Don't discourage children from picking books that are aimed at younger children, even though you might think they are 'babyish'. Reading easy texts builds confidence and you can make lots of discussion out of the pictures.

What happens if my child is a reluctant reader?

If your child isn't keen on reading to you, then focus on reading to them instead. Have lots of books around that are easy and that they are familiar with, including books with no words at all. Encourage them to tell stories and listen to stories including audio books. Try modelling reading yourself: 'I'll do dinner in a moment, I just want to finish the chapter'. The most important thing to remember is that focusing on enjoying reading is the most important thing, so let them choose books for you to read to them as much as possible.

Resources to support you and your child's reading journey

- **Book Trust** (and **BookBug** in Scotland, **Reach out and Read** in the US and others worldwide) gift books to children throughout their preschool years. They have some great lists of recommendations for different ages. www.booktrust.org.uk/books-and-reading/our-recommendations
- **Small Talk** is a lovely resource for the under 5s, focused on three themes: Chat, Play, Read small-talk.org.uk
- **Storyline Online** has hundreds of stories, all read by the authors or by celebrities. Think Jackanory for the 2020s. www.storylineonline.net
- From the master poet himself, **Michael Rosen**'s YouTube channel is stuffed full of poetry, songs and stories just for children www.youtube.com/MichaelRosenOfficial
- **The National Literacy Trust** hosts a wonderful resource for 0–12 year olds, with themed book ideas and activities wordsforlife.org.uk

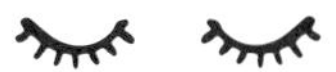

'sensory switch' that worked reliably and consistently, but you and I both know that life isn't like that. Experiment with some of these, and consider this your sensory play toolbox.

- Blowing bubbles
- Drinking a drink with a straw
- Bouncing gently on a yoga ball – either on their own, or if your child is too small, seat them on your lap.
- Wrapping tightly – try wrapping your child up in a blanket tightly and offering them a big bear hug.
- Rolling on the floor – encourage your child to lie on their back on the floor and raise their arms above their head and make themselves as long as they can. Then have them roll onto their front, and then over again onto their front, so they end up rolling from one end of a rug to another in a long thin pencil shape. This requires concentration and also provides some all-over pressure which can be calming.
- Flopping over a yoga ball – instead of bouncing, some children like to throw themselves forward over a yoga ball and just lie there. Keeping the ball from moving too much will require some core muscle stability and concentration, and many children find that being upside-down for a while is calming.
- Leaning against a wall and stretching – simply encourage your child to place their hands against a door or wall and then take a step or two backwards so they are bending forwards and leaning in. Get them to push as hard as they can against the wall.
- Having someone drum on their back – I call this the kiddy drumkit. Encourage your child to flop over a chair or lean against a wall and then use your hands to 'drum' or percuss their back all over. Some children like to make a noise while you do this – it will sound like a vibration due to the percussing, and many children enjoy that.
- Head, neck, facial massage – many older children like having a head massage. I often recommend a technique borrowed from Indian head massage that I call head 'raining' – you lightly use your fingertips to 'rain' on your child's head, and then follow up with circular massage over their temples, or wherever else they find soothing. Foot massages and hand massages are other options for children who don't like having their faces touched.

- Hair-brushing – while some children find knotty and tangled hair stressful, other children find hair-brushing really calming and regulating.

A practical suggestion is to try these activities at times of the day when it doesn't matter whether they work to calm or excite your child. Make a mental note of which activities are calming, and reserve these for calm-down time, or the bedtime routine. Activities that excite can be used for play time or silly time.

The idea behind all of these aspects of sleep is that they do not focus specifically on sleep. You're essentially trying to get all your ducks in a row before reassessing sleep. I normally suggest trying these passive strategies for a couple of weeks and then objectively reviewing your sleep situation. Sometimes, addressing these seemingly tenuously related elements of your child's day makes a big difference to sleep, without the stress of doing something different in the middle of the night. These strategies may not solve *all* your problems, but they may shrink them slightly. At the very least, even if you see no sleep improvement, hopefully you'll deepen the connection with your child, and know that you have optimised everything you can.

Cultural variation in sleep practice

There are many variations in sleep patterns and problems around the world. It is simply not accurate to report one single 'normal' way to sleep. The reality is that our ethnicity, culture, family and societal factors will all affect the way we sleep, when and how we sleep, our sleep habits, and even the length of time we sleep for. A very large sample of adolescents from 24 countries in Europe and North America found considerable variation in their total sleep time, with the longest sleep durations seen in Canada and the shortest in parts of Eastern Europe.[16] So, even a sample of 'Western' countries and cultures found significant discrepancies in sleeping habits and patterns.

It seems that sleep is not always clear-cut – there may be other wider socioeconomic factors that influence our habits. Another study looked at a sample of adolescents from a diverse college in the US where more than half the sample was non-white. Although all the teens were from the same geographical area, the non-white adolescents studied more, and also had more hours in paid work, and slept less than the white students.[17] This may suggest that other factors such as economic privilege, different work ethic and cultural expectations come into play, and affect sleep. If all the students had the same access to funds, would we see the differences in sleep change? I'm not sure, but it seems unwise to suggest that there may not be other factors involved.

A recent article[18] presents the assumption that white children have more problems with insomnia, and black children have more problems with obstructive sleep apnoea (OSA). I find this fascinating, but perhaps not for all the same reasons the researchers do. The black children were much more likely to bedshare, and the white children were much more likely to have problems falling asleep and staying asleep. What does this tell us? That white children have more behavioural sleep problems? Or that *all* children sleep better when in close proximity to their caregivers?

If we look at the study from the perspective that bedsharing is normal, and fulfils a need that children have to be close to their caregiver, then is it fairer to say that white children have sleep problems that are more about the social constructs of what is considered to be normal sleep (independent of parents), which may be out of step with their developmental and emotional needs? Is it also fairer to say that black children have more *actual* sleep problems – such as OSA? Does pathologising a way of sleeping and parenting mean that *not* doing it causes a different set of problems? So – if bedsharing is considered undesirable, is the choice between either a bedsharing 'problem' or a settling problem? If we reframe bedsharing as common and normal, then in fact, *not* doing it seems to cause problems because it is indeed normal for little ones to need reassurance, connection and parental proximity at bedtime. I'm not suggesting that you *have to* bedshare with your toddler, preschooler or older child – merely pointing out that those who did, didn't have the same problems with settling.

Sleep patterns can be specific not only to geographical location, but also to culture and ethnicity. For example, one study compared sleep patterns of children in Israel, but half the sample identified as Jewish, and the other half identified as Arab. The Arab children had shorter nighttime sleep duration, more sleep disturbances and later bedtimes.[19] It is therefore probably not reasonable to assume that all children in a geographical location – such as 'Asia' have the same sleep experiences.

Another study compared Japanese and Chinese children. This study found that Japanese children have more problems falling asleep, and Chinese children have more problems staying asleep.[20]

I feel privileged to teach and be in contact with so many people from around the world. Sleep and parenting practices in different cultures are so profoundly different that it is arrogant to assume there is just one way to sleep or arrange the sleep environment for a child. I asked people from several different countries and cultures to share their experiences of different sleeping practices.

'Where I come from, family and friends start socialising late in the evening and it is common to use a nap to rest up in preparation for a late night. Here in the UK, I don't often see naps used as a tool and I often feel I am viewed as a bit lazy when I do.

My family does take a nap every day and you wouldn't dare go knocking at a relative's door or making noise in the house between 1 and 3pm. Of course as older children and teens we didn't nap regularly so we had to whisper at these times. We were 12 cousins, so it was quite a challenge over summer holidays!' **Karina, Brazil**

'In my culture, it is normal to go home and have dinner late, so most references to sleep timings don't work here. I have tried to adapt all the recommendations to a later time but this makes it difficult when children are genuinely sleep deprived and overstimulated. I also know that many parents who stick with their late bedtime but do not find time for an afternoon nap are very sleep deprived.'
Nahia, Spain

'In the Netherlands it is quite common for the newborn to sleep in a crib in the parental bedroom for some weeks or months. Most babies move to their own room well before their first birthday. Bedsharing is still less common. Bedtime is relatively early (7pm–8pm) and we tend to have dinner early (around 6pm). The time between dinner and bedtime is long compared to other countries, which is thought to have a positive effect on sleep.' **Consuela, the Netherlands**

'In the UK there are so many expectations set for new parents today.

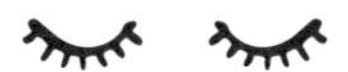

I don't know where it's come from, but I assume it's a part of the drive for the perfectionism of the developed world. While living in the UK I've felt the stark difference of a world full of competition, comparison and control in comparison to the developing country I grew up in.

Growing up in Jamaica – still a developing country – life is a lot simpler. Pressures come in their own way of course – but perfectionism is not one of them. Parenthood is much more led by your instincts rather than the need to be in control so you don't fail at something. Being a small island there is much more support – the metaphorical villages are very much alive and strong. There's support if you need it and the advice will still very much encourage you to feed your baby to sleep, contact nap and co-sleep with pride. Personally I slept in the same bed as my mom up until the age of 13. There was never any judgement to this and it's still seen as completely normal. I really think being aware of other cultural habits is so important. It reinforces that there really is no wrong or right – just what works for you and your family.' **Shanielle, Jamaica**

'Sleep in the Arab world varies from one family to the next. But in general terms most families are closely knit, and some people even live with extended families in the first few years of their marriage. This of course affects the way parents raise their children as everyone in the family tries to have their own expert opinion on the new baby. How to feed, burp and how a baby should sleep. Many mothers are taught about raising their child from their mother or mother-in-law who typically advise swaddling their baby tightly and formula-feeding the baby at night. Many people expect a baby to sleep through the night with minimum waking up time. Another factor to consider is that many people have a live-in nanny who helps a mother a lot with the children. Some let the mother sleep through the night and keep the baby with the nanny.

In the past couple of years many drastic changes have occurred as mothers have started to seek expert opinion on how to feed and get their child to sleep. Many new strategies have been suggested to families and a drastic positive shift has started to emerge. Mums are reading and researching breastfeeding and natural birth while they

are pregnant. They want to ensure the best for their babies, so many are taking classes. Many are asking about breastfeeding and sleep, and beginning to learn that whether breast or formula-fed, babies and children will still wake in the night.' **Ala, Kuwait**

'I was born and raised in the UK, but my parents are from India. They both grew up in very large traditional households, with many extended family members (grandparents, aunts, uncles, cousins) under one roof. Homes were spacious but open-plan – only one or two 'rooms'. Most members of the family slept out on the verandah, on 'takhts' or divans, which doubled as a seating area during the day but turned into giant family beds at night. My childhood home in London had enough bedrooms for us all to sleep separately, but my parents never insisted on it. To them, it was normal that I preferred to share the double bed with one of them until I was six or seven years old – and the other parent took the single bed in the room that was supposed to be mine! As I grew up, my expectations around family sleep were heavily influenced by Western cultural norms and when I had my first baby, I assumed she would sleep in a cot in her own room. It turned out both she and her younger brother had different ideas. Fast forward five years and here we are, all four of us, sharing a family floor bed just like my grandparents did with their little ones.' **Shazia, India**

'In my culture, bedsharing with your baby or toddler is a very foreign concept, even though it is normal for other African cultures, and it makes doing things differently quite challenging. People still expect babies to be in their own room from day one and to have consolidated nighttime sleep from very early on.' **Yolandi, RSA**

'Nobody really talks about sleep in my country. We have a lot of breastfeeding support because moms can get up to two years of paid leave and almost one year of unpaid leave, so a lot of moms try breastfeeding, and bedsharing is common. This is partly because a lot of people do not have enough rooms to put their children in another room. I often read that people bedshare because they live in a one-bedroom flat. I remember, when I was a child, we were sleeping

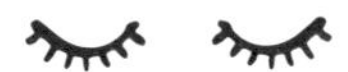

all in one room, just because we were only heating one room. But I also remember that we were going to bed after a song on the TV just before 8pm. Now it is a bit different, especially in the bigger cities. A lot of people finish work late, and by the time they get to the daycare to collect their children, it is after 7pm. A lot of the time they go outside to play, and especially in the summer, a lot of people put their kids to bed no earlier than 10pm, sometimes 11pm or midnight. Most people over here prefer to go to bed late and wake up late.'
Simona, Bulgaria

'In India, we see a lot of diversity with sleep. The urban population mostly go to sleep pretty late (after 11pm), and it's common to watch TV late. People also usually get up in the morning a little later (after 7am), and they do not nap. However, as you move away from the cities, people prefer to go to bed earlier (around 9pm), and wake up earlier, and they also commonly nap after lunch. Children usually follow the same patterns, so in the villages there is usually no differentiation between adults and children. However, there is a lot of difference between the rural and urban communities. Bedsharing is considered normal irrespective of whether the family is from a rural or urban area. Many babies also sleep in hammocks as well, and swaddling is very common.' **Prachi, India**

'I grew up in the UK but live part-time in South Africa. Over here, raising the child is the parents' job, but most people have nannies. Maternity leave is a maximum 12 weeks, usually has to start a month before the baby's due date, and is often unpaid. Usually the nanny will come and do jobs around the house (nanny/maid is very common) and the kids get to know her, and then the nanny takes over. The days are so long, so a child might be with the nanny from 8am until 6pm from a few weeks old. Most of our friends assume that babies will be in a cot in the parents' room, and will be bottle-fed at least at night, and they will stop night feeding after a few months. It seemed like the children were not meant to be mollycoddled, and there is quite a strict culture, of adults being the ones in charge and children do as they are told.

I thought this might be just certain friends who prefer a strict

routine, but I also have friends who are more child-led and they still have a nanny during the day, so they can work from home. It is expected that the nanny is an equal source of comfort.

I'm torn when I go, because I don't want anyone else raising our children, but also, does it take a village? Can you do both?'
Georgie, RSA

I don't know where you are from, but ask yourself – where do my sleep expectations come from? What is sleep like in my country and culture? Am I trying to squeeze my family's sleep into someone else's cultural norm? What would my grandparents say to me if I could ask them about sleep?

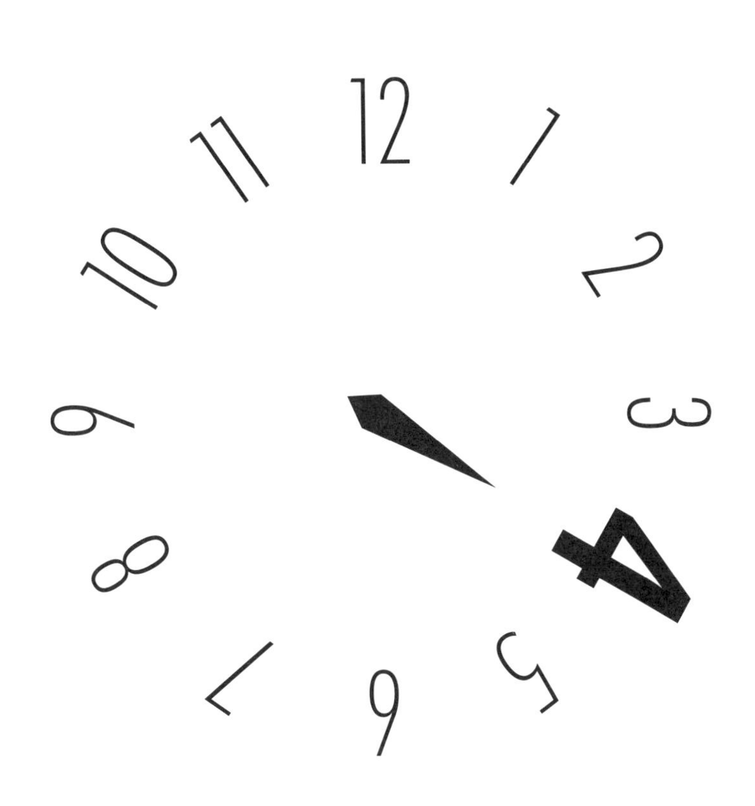

CHAPTER FOUR

LIFESTYLE FACTORS

Part of my 'back door' approach to sleep optimisation is to think of sleep as just one aspect of wellness. Of course, sleep is essential for our health, wellbeing and functioning, but it is also affected by those factors as well. Rather than addressing sleep head on, instead you could try to improve the family's lifestyle holistically and have confidence that, because sleep and holistic wellness are interlinked, sleep will passively improve in the process.

Exercise

Many parents find that their children sleep better after more active days. Over the last 50 years, we have generally become more sedentary. We use our cars more, and we travel further to take part in activities. I'm not judging by the way – this applies to pretty much everyone. Much of this can't be helped, but it means that we now need to be much more intentional with squeezing leisure and exercise in.

Many studies find that exercise decreases the amount of time taken to fall asleep, and increases the amount of deep sleep. It is difficult to say for sure what effect exercise has on sleep when the populations studied are mainly adult. Some studies have measured the effects of moderately obese people having 12–15-week programmes of exercise. The studies found that sleep was improved, but whether this was due to direct influences of exercise on sleep, or to weight loss and improvements in overall health and fitness, is hard to say. One study looked at the impact

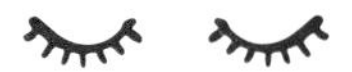

of regular exercise in adolescents, and found that it was beneficial for sleep,[1] but another study exploring the sleep and exercise relationship at ages three, five and seven years found that while this was true, as the exercise became more vigorous, sleep quality actually decreased.[2] The authors proposed that one explanation could be that if a child is exercising hard, they simply have less time for sleep. I suspect, as with so many associations, it could be multifactorial. I wonder, for example, if more active children sleep less simply because they are more energetic and need less sleep! In terms of recommending how much exercise is beneficial for health and sleep, it seems the jury is out. A recent meta-analysis that looked at a total combined sample size of over 70,000 children concluded that the recommended amount of exercise was inconclusive. So it seems we are going to have to exercise common sense and our parental judgement here!

Nutrition

If only it were as simple as me providing you with a list of foods to eat to instantly improve everyone's sleep and settling. While there are some foods that are notorious for containing some sleep-supportive vitamins or chemicals, I would be lying if I said that all you need to do to improve sleep is to eat these foods. However, nutrition in a broad sense really *is* important for sleep and wellbeing. Our bodies need fuel, and the fuel comes in the form of food and water. You may or may not know that most of your immune system is in your gut, and therefore, to maintain overall health, it's important to feed your gut with the right foods. Once in the gut, your body will start to digest food, making use of the nutrients and disposing of the waste. Bacteria in your gut help to break down and metabolise your food and also pass on important information to your immune system about your environment. Clever huh?

> "Rather than addressing sleep head on, instead you could try to improve the family's lifestyle holistically and have confidence that, because sleep and holistic wellness are interlinked, sleep will passively improve in the process."

Nutrition and child health

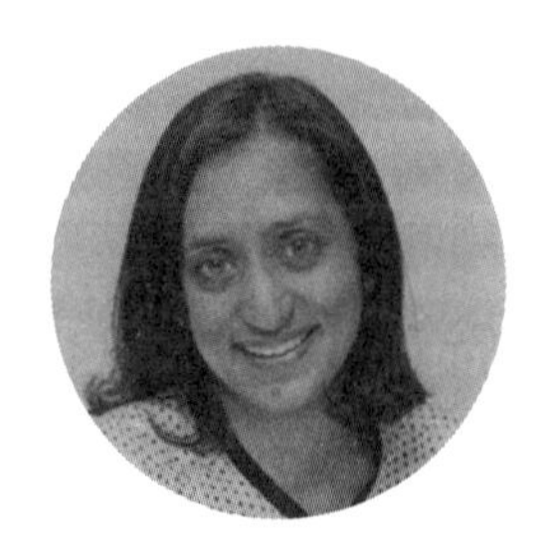

Dr Venita Patel, paediatrician, nutrition and lifestyle medicine specialist

The term 'food as medicine' has been used to describe the positive health effects of nutritious food, and the understanding that this helps prevent illness. It makes sense in children that good nourishment is fundamental for their optimal growth, development and immunity. This journey begins early, from pregnancy to infant feeding followed by weaning – setting the stage for future health, and also future appetite control and food preferences.[3]

What is the right diet for children?

Each stage of childhood has different nutritional needs, but there are certain aspects common to all.

The focus on vegetables is important right from the start of weaning, at around six months. A wide range of vegetables introduced before the age of 12–15 months allows babies to establish a taste for them. After this stage, some 'fussy eating' is common, so toddlers may need lots of tastes of foods before they accept them.[4]

Aiming for a variety of coloured vegetables and fruits, or 'eating the rainbow', helps ensure a good supply of micronutrients (vitamins, minerals and other plant nutrients or phytochemicals).

The rest of the plate needs a balance of:

- Wholefood carbohydrates (fibre-rich grains and root vegetables)
- Protein-rich foods (eggs, meat, fish, dairy, nuts, seeds, legumes and lentils)
- Healthy fats (avocado, olive oil, nuts/seeds, oily fish)

'Superfoods' vs 'normal' foods

While certain foods containing particular phytochemicals have been touted as having tremendous health benefits, it is generally more beneficial to include a variety of nutrient-dense foods. Seasonal and local vegetables and fruit will mostly have higher concentrations of nutrients. The more deeply coloured ones, such as dark green leafy vegetables, usually contain the highest micronutrient levels. There are also many foods beneficial for gut health, as we will find out below.[5]

What is gut health?

The concept of gut health is now very popular in the world of health, but what exactly is it? It usually refers to the huge numbers of different organisms, mostly found in the large bowel, called 'gut flora' or the bacterial microbiome. These bacteria have important functions, influencing digestion, immunity, appetite, weight, metabolism, allergies, hormones, brain function, development, and much more. A healthy adult has over 35,000 possible species of gut bacteria. Having plentiful and diverse gut bacteria usually means better overall health.[6,7]

What is the gut-brain connection?

The gut is linked to the nervous system and brain, through the long vagus nerve and some 'communicating' chemicals and hormones. It is thought that 90 percent of the 'happy hormone' serotonin is produced in the gut. Gut health is linked to behaviour, development, learning, mood and mental health. The gut microbiome has been studied in relation to neurodevelopmental disorders such as autism, and mood disorders such as depression. It is interesting to observe that children may complain of tummy discomfort when they feel emotional or upset.

Foods influencing gut health

Many factors influence the health and diversity of the gut microbiome. The number and variety of plant-based foods in the diet is a key factor. Recently a large study showed that eating over 30 different plants in a week results in the most diverse populations of gut bacteria, with significant changes seen in just 5–6 days.[8]

Conversely, refined or processed foods tend to discourage healthy bacterial growth. Having an imbalance of 'good and 'bad' gut bacteria (dysbiosis) may affect the gut lining permeability, resulting in 'leaky gut'. This is thought to play a part in issues such as food intolerances, allergies, eczema and autoimmune disease. Prebiotics are compounds, such as dietary fibre, which 'feed' healthy bacteria, thus increasing their numbers. Prebiotic-rich foods include onion, leek, garlic, Jerusalem artichokes, chicory root, apples, bananas, legumes, oats, bran, and other wholegrains. Probiotics are 'live' bacteria, taken as foods or supplements, with a positive effect on health. Fermented foods and drinks containing these bacteria include yoghurt, kefir, miso, natto, tempeh, sauerkraut, kimchi, apple cider vinegar, and kombucha. Numerous probiotic supplements are also on the market, with different combinations of bacterial strains.

Top tips for improving gut flora:

- Increase the *variety* of vegetables, wholegrains, legumes and fibre-rich foods eaten per week
- Eat prebiotic-rich foods daily
- Include some probiotic fermented foods or drinks daily
- Limit high sugar and processed foods
- Spend time in nature, as often as possible. Getting muddy is good!
- Exercise regularly – outdoors if possible
- Stroke your pets (or borrow a dog to look after!)
- Reduce stress levels
- Optimise sleep

Vitamins and minerals

Particular nutrients are important in children, and required in higher amounts during periods of rapid growth and development such as toddlerhood and adolescence. Nutrient deficiencies can impact all areas of a child's health and functioning, including bone growth, muscle function, brain and nervous system development, learning, behaviour and sleep. In the UK it is advised that babies receive vitamin D from birth, and all children from six months to five years have vitamins A, C and D as a supplement.

Vitamin D is essential for calcium absorption and bone growth, and all ages are recommended to take it as a daily supplement, particularly in the winter months and colder climates. Dietary sources: small amounts are found in eggs, oily fish, dairy and fortified milks and cereals.

Vitamin A is converted from beta-carotene in the diet, and is important for healthy eyes, skin and immunity. Dietary sources: orange/red/green vegetables, dairy, eggs.

Vitamin C has a range of functions including supporting immunity and healthy skin. Dietary sources: fresh fruit, especially citrus, and vegetables.

Other dietary nutrients

Iron is vital for healthy blood and oxygenation of the body. Iron deficiency has been linked to sleep disorders such as 'restless legs'. Dietary sources: meat, pulses, beans, tofu, green leafy vegetables, dried fruit.

Calcium is deposited in bone to give strength, and is also needed for muscle function. Dietary sources: dairy, beans, tofu, nuts and seeds, green leafy vegetables.

Some other important nutrients, often limited in the diet, are B vitamins and magnesium, which are needed for a healthy nervous system. Dietary sources include dark green leafy vegetables, nuts and seeds, beans, avocado and wholegrains.

Omega-3 fatty acids

Omega-3 fatty acids play a central role in child health and development. There are three main types: eicosapentaenoic acid (EPA), docosahexaenoic acid (DHA), and alpha-linolenic acid (ALA). These are required for healthy brain development and have an ant-inflammatory effect. EPA and DHA are primarily found in oily fish (salmon, mackerel, anchovy, sardine, herring, trout) and fish oil or algae oil supplement form. There is evidence of benefits of omega-3 supplementation in conditions such as asthma, ADHD, and sleep difficulties. There is also evidence of improvement in aspects of memory, learning and mental health. It is important to look for high-quality fish oils or algae oils, as these are less likely to become rancid.

Specific diets and allergies

Children being brought up on specific diets, such as vegetarian or vegan diets, or those with dairy allergies, benefit from a carefully planned diet to include the necessary micronutrients. Diets excluding dairy, eggs and animal protein may need extra supplementation with:

- B12
- Omega-3 fats
- Iron
- Vitamin D/Calcium
- Zinc
- Iodine

I would always recommend doing your own research or speaking to a registered nutrition professional, either a BANT-registered nutritional therapist, or a children's dietician or nutritionist.

Useful resources and books

- BANT (British Association for Nutrition and Lifestyle Medicine): bant.org.uk
- BNF (British Nutrition Foundation): www.nutrition.org.uk/healthyliving/lifestages/children.html
- Food & Brain Behaviour: www.fabresearch.org
- *Baby Food Matters* by Dr Clare Llewellyn
- *The Good Stuff* by Lucinda Miller

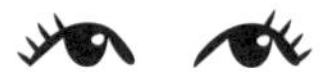

So, eating well is clearly good for everyone's health and wellbeing, as well as sleep. Rather than think about specific foods that are worth trying to incorporate into your diet, try to think about some general principles instead:

- A rainbow diet.
- As much fruit and veg as you can manage.
- When your child is *really* hungry, try to give them healthy, nutritious foods. That way, they associate satiety and the relief from hunger with foods that you would like them to eat more of. I know it's easy to grab the quick calories when kids are 'starving', but this may mean they more readily reach for the fast carbs when they feel hungry.
- Try to avoid highly processed food on a regular basis.
- Avoid foods that are bizarre and unnatural colours or are artificially flavoured.
- Try healthy swaps – brown or white/brown bread or pasta instead of white, grains like quinoa instead of rice, and natural yoghurt with frozen berries instead of flavoured yoghurt.
- Make sure you give your child a vitamin D supplement if they are under five, are darker skinned, cover their skin for cultural or religious reasons, or don't have much time outdoors.

But it doesn't always end there does it? Just because you provide a healthy balanced diet to your child, doesn't always mean mealtimes are a stress-free zone. While neophobia (fussy eating or rejection of new foods) is very common in young toddlers, if it persists beyond the toddler stage, it can be seriously annoying and worrying.

"When your child is *really* hungry, try to give them healthy, nutritious foods. That way, they associate satiety and the relief from hunger with foods that you would like them to eat more of."

Fussy eating and mealtime challenges

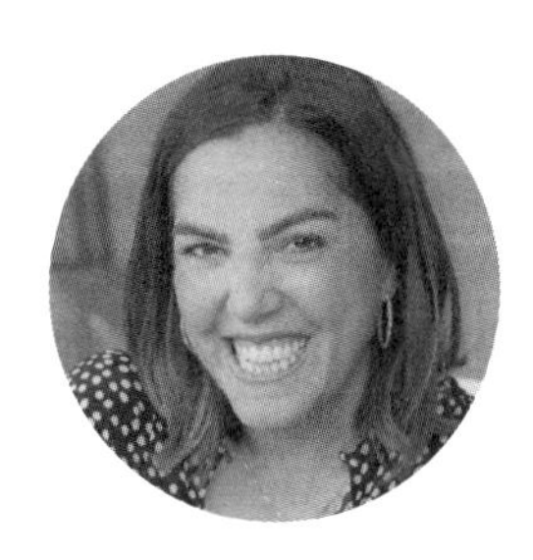

Stacey Zimmels, paediatric feeding and swallowing specialist, speech and language therapist, International Board Certified Lactation Consultant

Fussy eating is a relatively common phenomenon in children with studies estimating that 10–30% of preschool and primary school children are picky with their food.[9] It is thought to peak at the age of three[10] and for the vast majority of children it resolves over time. Fussy eaters will typically reject foods leading to a sub-optimal variety of foods in their diet.

Fussy eating is influenced both by your child's genetic make-up and also by environmental factors (something you can guide and shape). On a positive note, in the vast majority of cases there is no significant impact on a child's growth or nutrition despite them not having a varied diet, but when it comes to mealtimes it can often be extremely stressful for both parents and child. Common mealtime challenges include: food refusal, rejection of previously accepted foods, perception that the child hasn't eaten enough, which can in turn lead to pressure to eat, negotiation, bribery, punishment, distractions at the table and general frustration on both sides.

There are a range of strategies that can be introduced to reduce stress at mealtimes for both parent and child, and to support acceptance of new foods in the longer term.

1. Manage your expectations; particularly around portion sizes (they're often smaller than you may think). Also be aware of the impact of snacking/grazing between main meals and consider how best to manage your mealtime/snack schedules.
2. Trust your child and let them determine how much they want to eat. 'You provide, they decide' is a component of the 'Division of responsibility' feeding model by Ellyn Satter.[11] Following this approach removes virtually all mealtime battles and moves you away from habits that have crept in which can be unhelpful for long-term food acceptance. They include: pressure to eat, use of distractions, bribery or food rewards and offering alternatives.
3. Role modelling and eating family meals have been shown to have influence over intake of certain foods and also food preferences. This,

alongside positive and neutral (e.g. descriptive rather than emotional) language around food can lead to greater acceptance.

4. Expose, expose, expose! Parents often stop offering foods after they have been rejected by the child just a few times, but studies tell us that children require multiple repeated positive exposures to food before they may even taste it. Exposure can include looking at pictures of foods, picking out food in the supermarket, prepping and cooking it at home as well as seeing it on the family table or on their plate.
5. When introducing new foods select foods that your family eats regularly as these will already be familiar or choose foods which are similar in size, shape, consistency, texture, colour and/or taste to already accepted foods.
6. Avoid pressure and negativity around foods and eating. Pressure can include, coercion 'just have a bite', emotional blackmail 'if you were a good girl you would eat it because it took me a long time to make it', direct pressure 'you need to eat those carrots', bribery 'if you eat it you can watch TV' and negative consequences 'if you don't eat it then you won't have any TV time'.

There are instances when your child may not respond to the strategies outlined as they may have a feeding disorder which requires further assessment and more specialist advice and support. If your child has a developmental, sensory or autistic spectrum condition; if their intake is failing to meet their nutritional or growth requirements; if they have a medical condition limiting their diet, e.g. coeliac disease or food allergy, chronic illness, or if they have swallowing difficulties, then a specialist feeding referral is indicated.

There are a number of helpful resources for parents which may provide additional advice and tips to put the strategies outlined above into action:

- www.firststepsnutrition.org/eating-well-early-years for guidance on portion sizes and snacks.
- www.ellynsatterinstitute.org for a more detailed explanation and guide to the division of responsibility in feeding model.
- www.feedeatspeak.co.uk Stacey's feeding blog and online courses
- www.childfeedingguide.co.uk/parents for fussy eating tips and advice
- mymunchbug.com Parent books, courses and lots of free resources on her YouTube channel and Facebook page.

You can connect with Stacey on Instagram: @feedeatspeak

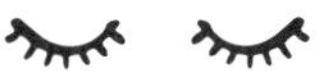

You might be wondering how fussy eating and food drama relates to sleep. Well, it does on a number of levels:

- Fussy eating is stressful and can erode relationships.
- Fussy eating may lead to power struggles.
- Fussy eating may be related to abdominal pain, or a parasitic infection (such as threadworms). Sometimes there is a medical reason that not only affects eating, but also health, which is why running this past your doctor is a good idea if you're concerned.
- Disordered eating may mean that children have micro or macronutrient deficiencies.
- Fussy eating can affect parent–child interaction.
- Food and eating are part of the bigger picture of child health and wellness.
- Significant fussy or disordered eating can make social interaction very difficult as restrictive diets can be difficult to accommodate and socially embarrassing.
- Fussy eating may be part of a broader sensory problem or neurodevelopmental condition (though of course the two conditions can occur independently).

Making food fun again, taking the pressure off and lightening the mood can all play a significant part in improving relationships, reducing anxiety and increasing the range of accepted foods.[12]

Activity, play and mental stimulation

All children need a balance of activity, calm-down time and mental stimulation. I'm not talking about sitting down and drilling your children on their times tables, or asking them to complete activities they don't enjoy. But all children need a variety of different stimuli to thrive and be mentally fatigued. I used to swear by the rule of 'five a day' for a good night's sleep:

- Right food
- Full love tank
- Physical exercise
- Mental stimulation
- Fun times

- **Right food.** As we've already found out, the interplay between nutrition and sleep is not straightforward. On one level, children simply need enough calories for maintenance and growth. If they are hungry they will not sleep well, struggle to get to sleep, or wake early. But even when they are well fed, micronutrient deficiency can cause havoc with sleep. Iron deficiency anaemia causes huge problems with falling asleep, the quality of sleep, and insomnia. Vitamin D deficiency is also known to cause sleep difficulty. On top of that, food allergies and intolerances cause abdominal bloating, digestive problems, reflux, abdominal pain and cramping, diarrhoea, constipation and, you guessed it, all this impacts their comfort and sleep. If you are concerned about your child's nutritional status, please talk to a suitably qualified medical practitioner, or consult a dietician.
- **Full love tank.** This is probably the biggest one. Children who have unmet needs in the day often wake in the night to 'fill their tank'. If you've argued with your child – try to make it up right before the wind-down period. If you know you've been busy and preoccupied, then invest in 10–15 minutes of high-quality one-to-one intensive time with them.
- **Physical exercise.** It's well-known that worn-out children sleep well. We bought a trampoline when our eldest daughter was 18 months – that night she slept through the night for the First Time Ever. It was a huge 'Eureka!' moment for us and we have never forgotten it. Is your child getting plenty of time outside, exposed to natural daylight, and running off steam? Do you find that they are literally bouncing off the walls, or are they tired by the end of the day? Children have varying levels of energy, with some being like little Labrador puppies, and others being more content to sit still. If your child fidgets, buzzes around, fiddles with things, hops about, or does laps of the living room – it's a fair bet they need more exercise.
- **Mental stimulation.** Children are naturally curious about the world around them. They have a thirst for knowledge and understanding. They like to fiddle and tinker with things to build concepts of how they work. Children need an opportunity to use their immense brains to apply reason and work things out. Give your child plenty of open-ended conversation – ask them not just 'what?' but also 'why?' and 'how?'. Ask them their opinion, give them yours! Talk

about the differences. Find out what interests your child and run with those ideas. Many parents have learnt through bitter experience that a frustrating, under-stimulating day at school or home causes dysregulation, boredom, frustration and poor sleep.

- **Fun times.** Play is the work of childhood and how children learn and develop. If they do not have the opportunity to let off steam, unwind, explore, get dirty, be themselves, be silly, and act their age – then they won't thrive. Make sure your child has plenty of opportunity to have fun, giggle, play, and interact with other children and you, in a way that meets their needs.

Here are a few ideas to help your children tick several of these boxes at the same time. Not all of them are suitable for all ages, but I haven't split them into suggested ages, as I have found over the years that putting particular play activities into age categories can feel restrictive, or lead parents to feel anxious that their child is somehow playing in the 'wrong' way.

Helping your child play, laugh and dance towards better sleep:

- Tickle fights
- Chasing and racing
- Football, netball and basketball
- Scavenger hunts – can your child find
  - five red objects
  - 10 items smaller than their hand
  - four differently shaped leaves
  - six things that begin with the first letter of their name
  - 10 items that are circular
- Jigsaw puzzles, shape sorters
- Taking apart simple gadgets and putting them back together again
- Learning to play a musical instrument
- Teddy bears' picnics
- Jumping on a trampoline
- Learning to draw or paint, colour by numbers
- Reading poetry, acting out a play
- Wood whittling, carving, construction
- Riding a bike

- Lego challenges
- Burying toys in putty, playdough or sand
- Water play
- Give your child cups, funnels, bowls and kitchen utensils and some dried pasta or rice

I'm not suggesting that this alone will be enough to help your child sleep well, but when you really wrap your head around the fact that we cannot look at one single factor (like sleep) in isolation, it makes sense to invest in something like activity and play.

Social interaction

The ease and way in which we interact with others can affect our confidence and wellbeing. We are social beings, and from infancy babies enjoy social interaction and being around people. As children get older, they increasingly enjoy time with people other than their parents, and benefit from making meaningful relationships with other adults and carers, meeting strangers from the safety of their parent's arms, and making friends.

It is widely believed that there are six stages of play:

Type of play	Approximate age range	What this looks like
Unoccupied play	0–1 months	Babies tend to try to make sense of their world by making movements, and are fascinated by everything they see, touch and hear.
Solitary play	0–2 months	Children play alone, generally because their language is limited and they are learning about themselves, others and objects through play.
Onlooker play	18 month to 2.5 years	Children are watching others playing in this stage. They learn a great deal by observing the play, activities and interactions with other people.

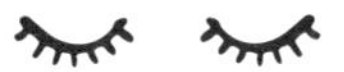

Parallel play	2.5 to 3 years	At this stage, children play side by side with another child. They may play with similar toys but there is no interaction between the children. They are learning about peers, but not yet ready to play interactively.
Associative play	3 to 4 years	Children at this stage will play with the same equipment, sharing and borrowing the toys, perhaps taking turns, but still playing independently. For example, there may be a group of children around a sand tray. All the children are using the toys in the sand together, but they are still playing independently.
Collaborative play	4 to 5 years and up	Children play in groups, usually coordinated by a 'leader'. They are able to communicate their goals for play – for instance, assigning everyone a 'part' to play.

A study of over 1,000 children aged 33 months found that there were two main predictors of whether children played with others – the sophistication of language, and their social competence.[13] It seems that children who are slower to acquire language, or who struggle with verbal expression, may tend to use exploratory play, rather than pretend play, for longer, and also tend to initiate less play with other children. This has implications for early intervention with speech and language. If you're worried about your child's speech, communication or play, please see your doctor or speech and language therapist, but here follow a few tips for encouraging speech.

Building a child's vocabulary through reading

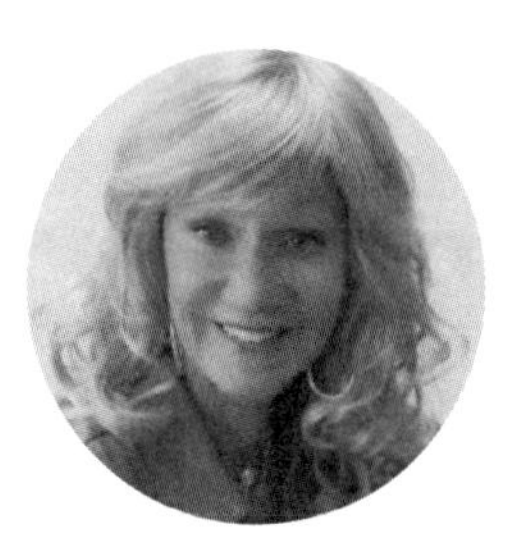

Professor Celeste Roseberry-McKibbin,
author of Love, Talk, Read to Help Your Child Succeed

One of the most helpful interventions for helping children with their speech is reading books with them. This can begin as early as you like, but it is never too late to start making this a daily habit. Foster a love of reading by having plenty of books around, visiting the library, modelling enjoyment of reading and reading to your child.

Make reading exciting and fun by using silly, dramatic voices. Be expressive! This is especially important for young children with limited attention spans. Read books your child is especially interested in. In kindergarten, my son Mark started hating reading and would have none of it because dyslexia made reading very hard. He would let me read aloud to him, though, and all he wanted to hear was Captain Underpants stories and Bible stories with bad guys (there are plenty of those!). Sound effects and funny voices kept him attentive and engaged.

Make reading a priority. Bedtime stories are especially good because they help children wind down and relax. Make it a special time of snuggling before they go to sleep. Sometimes children will want the same book over and over – that's fine!

Help your child figure out new vocabulary. Encourage your child to look at illustrations and pictures to figure out new words, but do supply the meaning if she starts getting frustrated.

As stated, be willing to read the same books over and over, but attempt to introduce new ones once in a while.

Take your child to the local library. Our local library had a sign-up sheet where you could register to read with Delilah the Dog. Mark just loved this, and it was very helpful in the early years when he was struggling with dyslexia.

An easy way to remember how to read with your child is to CARE: Comment, Ask questions, Respond, Extend (add words). You can read the actual book and CARE, or you can just look at the pictures and CARE. Either way, it's effective. For example:

Adult: Look at Thomas the Tank Engine going down the track. (*Comment*)
Adult: Where is he going? (*Ask a question*)
Child: He's going to see James.
Adult: Yes! He likes to see his friend James who is the orange train! (*Respond and Extend*)
Adult: Oh boy, I think James is glad to see him. (*Comment*)
Child: James happy.
Adult: James is happy because Thomas is his friend and they like having fun together. (*Respond and Extend*)

Here are some more specific ideas for building your child's early reading skills:

Before you start reading a book, look at the pictures and talk about them. Build pre-literacy skills by asking your child:

- How do you hold a book?
- Where is the cover?
- Who is the author?
- What do you think the book is going to be about?
- Point to the first page.
- Point to the first word.
- Will you turn the pages with me while we read?

Build on the child's previous knowledge. For example, if the story is about Dogzilla, you can say 'Do you have a dog? Do you know anyone who has a dog?' In another example, 'Look at that red fire engine. It has four wheels, just like a car. What does your Daddy's car look like?'

During reading, ask questions such as:

- Where should I read next?
- Where is the page number?
- Why did the character do that?
- What do you think is going to happen next?
- How does this character make you feel?

After reading, review the story by asking questions such as:

- What was the story about?
- What happened in the story?
- How did the story end?
- What was your favourite part of the story?
- Which picture did you like best? Why?

Start building your child's phonological awareness skills – awareness of how words sound. The very best way to do this is through rhyming, and I highly recommend Dr Seuss books! It's never too early to build print awareness skills – awareness of how words look. An easy way to do this is to start by having your child track print, or put his finger under each word as it is read. You yourself can put your finger under each word as you read.

Celeste's video 'Reading Picture Books with Toddlers' is here: www.youtube.com/watch?v=fAYBmNDlEBo&t=58s and 'How to Read to Your Child with Care' here: www.youtube.com/watch?v=kjiPMWM3i00&t=53s

Certain aspects of play, such as sharing, turn-taking and playing by the rules are usually only apparent in children aged four and upwards. This doesn't mean that you cannot teach a toddler about sharing, and having a turn, but it is a concept that may continue to cause stress and upset until they are cognitively and developmentally mature enough to negotiate play. If you think about it, this is quite a sophisticated skill. In Norway, all children up to the age of six may attend a *barnehage*, which is separate from mainstream schooling, and there is a huge emphasis on play and a child's right to choose the activities that interest them. One paper found that the more children played, the greater their sense of wellbeing. When given free choice of what and how to play, as well as whether to play indoors or outdoors, most children chose construction play, and spent about 70 percent of the time outdoors in the summer, and 30 percent of the time outdoors in the winter.[14]

Of course, children's play continues to mature and differentiate as they grow. As children get older, they may have less available free

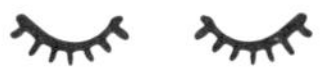

time to spend in play and activity due to being at school (unless they are homeschooled). But if possible, try to make time for organised activity with your older child too. A recent study of over 10,000 children up to age 15 found that organised leisure activities, whether they were individual sports, team sports, or arts were associated with a greater sense of wellbeing, fewer health complaints and better life satisfaction.[15]

One study explored the features of parks by the age of the children using them.[16] They found that in a sample of children aged three to 11, as children got older, they were more likely to access parks with more sports facilities such as skate parks, athletics tracks, tennis courts and swimming pools or lidos, rather than parks with swings, slides and seesaws. Another study exploring the use of Minecraft pointed out that video games can be used socially and intentionally, and there is an argument for separating out the types of screen use in children, rather than considering all screen time as equal.[17]

Hopefully you didn't need much convincing that play is vital, but the take-home message is that children need to play, as much as possible, and in a way that matches their interests. Play develops collaboration, empathy, tolerance and self-awareness. Which, of course, is what we all want for our little (and not so little) ones.

One of the aspects of raising socially competent children is helping them learn that not everyone is like them. There are a variety of books, podcasts and videos all geared towards developing cultural competence, fostering an attitude of anti-racism and tolerance towards people of other genders, sexualities, disabilities, cultures, ethnicities and faiths.

"Children need to play as much as possible, and in a way that matches their interests. Play develops collaboration, empathy, tolerance and self-awareness. Which, of course, is what we all want for our little (and not so little) ones."

Raising tolerant and inclusive kids

Kimberley Roberts (Nanny Kimbo) (They/Them)
co-founder of The Queer Parenting Partnership

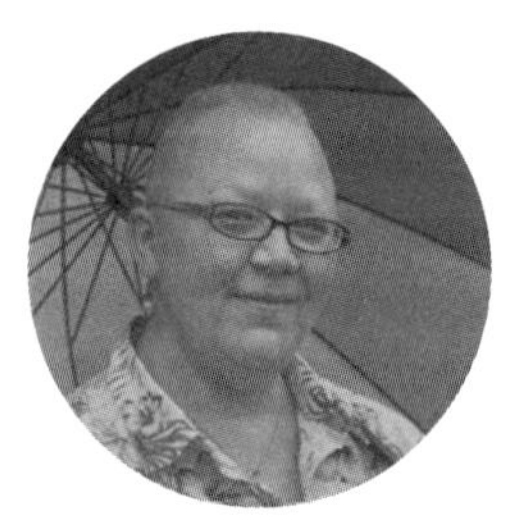

I am often asked 'at what age should I teach my child about *insert difference*?' My answer is always the same – from birth.

If your child has stories featuring black superheroes, LGBTQ+ parents, children in wheelchairs and so on, then you have already made incredible headway. Take your child to culturally diverse places. Watch diverse TV shows with them. Buy them dolls in a range of ethnicities. Parents and primary caregivers are the first teachers, so you need to model inclusive behaviours. If you are not behaving in an inclusive manner, your child won't either. If you are using LGBTQ+ stereotypes or slurs in your everyday language, so will your child. You may not think they're paying attention but believe me, they are!

Children are naturally curious and will ask questions. Sometimes those questions can come at rather inopportune moments and might make you feel uncomfortable. How you respond to the question is as important as the answer you give. If your child asks loudly; 'Mummy, why are those men kissing?' you may feel compelled to pull your child away quickly and hush them to save yourself and the men any embarrassment. This is teaching your child that two men kissing is shameful. Instead, address the question there and then with a simple response. 'Those two men are kissing because they love each other' is perfectly adequate. Your child may have a follow-up question, or they may be satisfied with that answer. If your child does have follow-up questions, be honest with them. Talk about LGBTQ+ couples in the same way as you would talk about heterosexual couples. Children don't need (nor do they want) graphic descriptions about what lesbians do in bed together, in much the same way as you wouldn't discuss the ins and outs of heterosexual sex with a very young child. Be sure to highlight and celebrate differences – don't fall into the trap of pretending that we are all the same because we're not. However, we do all deserve the same respect.

This early teaching is all the more important when you consider that your own children may grow up to be lesbian, gay, transgender or something else! Being careful with your language and attitudes now may make a world of difference if your child later wants to confide in you about their own experience. Rest assured that nothing in the world can 'make' your child LGBTQ+, and the best thing you can do for them is to support them and reassure them that you love them no matter what. If you feel out of your depth, there are therapists and organisations that can help you and your child to talk things through.

One of my favourite resources is Sex Positive Families. They provide parents and caring adults with education, resources, and support to raise sexually healthy children using a shame-free, comprehensive, and pleasure-positive approach. You will find all sorts of helpful information and workshops and even reading lists at sexpositivefamilies.com.

PFLAG is also a wonderful service for parents, friends and family of lesbian and gay people in the UK and they provide free information and support: www.pflag.co.uk.

www.parentingqueer.co.uk
www.thequeerdoula.co.uk

Family, motherhood and relationships

Children only really make sense in the context of the family and environment in which they are being raised. Supporting families is therefore a vital part of helping a child with their sleep. Identifying and managing stress and difficulty in the household can go a really long way towards reducing the tension in the home, which in turn leads to better sleep.

Many families are dealing with lack of support and overload. Some people have excessive interference from family members, while others have radio silence from their relatives. Some parents are raising children alone, and others are living far from family. Parenting is hard – we were never meant to do it alone, and yet that is the reality for many.

The cultural pressure of perfect parenthood
Dr Sophie Brock, sociologist, mother, and president of Maternal Scholars Australia

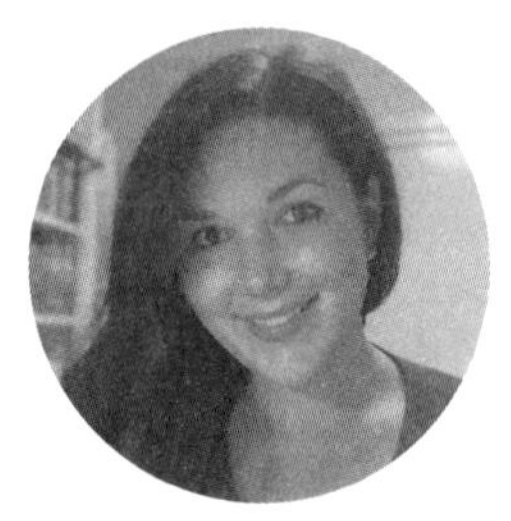

When we become parents, we experience enormous changes both physically and emotionally, relearning who *we* are in the process. But what is perhaps less recognised, is that not only do parents go through changes on an individual level, but they also experience shifts in how they live within our society. They *enter* the social and cultural realm of parenthood.

This is usually experienced differently for mothers compared to fathers. My work focuses specifically on mothers. I examine the pressures and 'shoulds' that come with motherhood, but of course you could also reflect on the ways that fathers are positioned. As an example of this, consider language and what it means when someone refers to 'fathering' a child, compared with 'mothering' a child. Often, the phrase 'fathering' connotes a biological relationship between a father and a child. On the other hand, 'mothering' is used as a verb, pointing to the connection and relationship between a mother and a child. This reveals a key distinction identified by foundational maternal scholars Adrienne Rich[18] and Sara Ruddick[19] and is a distinction that has been confirmed through decades of subsequent research. This distinction is between 'mothering' as a practice, and 'motherhood' as a social and cultural institution. Becoming a mother means you enter the realm of motherhood, and you carry out your mothering within that realm.

I find the analogy of a fish tank useful here. Think of the tank as the society that you live within, reflecting all of the 'shoulds' and expectations of motherhood. As an exercise you can engage in, draw a circle representing the fish tank. Now write on the outside of that circle all of the things you think it means to be a 'good mother'. Then draw a fish inside the tank. Think of this fish as the mother herself. She is mothering inside this tank of expectations, which is often coupled with a lack of support, resources, and community.

When you become that 'mother fish' within the 'motherhood tank' your experience of almost every aspect of life is impacted. This includes experiences of the workforce, family, friendships, health and legal systems, and various other places where we feel pressure to 'get it right' for our babies and children.

Some examples of what it means culturally to be a 'good mother' may be that she is endlessly patient, always puts her children's needs above her own, her children are 'well behaved' and 'good', she finds fulfilment in mothering, and she never gets angry or frustrated. There are many other assumptions that come with the idealised cultural image of what it means to be the 'good mother'.

The power of our social conditioning means that many of us equate 'good mothering' with fitting ourselves into a specific perfectionist mould. Yet there is always some collision between these ideals and our individual realities. This is because the perfect mother does not actually exist. She is an illusion, and yet she is sustained and upheld as a possibility by both our culture and ourselves. 'Failure' is inevitable when we are striving for this. What is also inevitable is guilt. We so heavily internalise the pressures of perfect parenting that we judge ourselves incredibly harshly. Trying to strive to meet this version of motherhood impacts our confidence, our sense of wellbeing, and even our life satisfaction.

If it *were* possible to be 'perfect parents' (which it isn't!) that reality would not be best for either our children, or ourselves. What our children need is connection with us, not perfection from us. This is where paediatrician and psychoanalyst Donald Winnicott's[20] concept of 'the good enough mother' becomes really useful. Winnicott and other researchers outline the ways our babies and child/ren's development, resilience, and sense of identity are supported by us *not* getting it 'right' in responding and attuning perfectly all of the time. Interestingly, there is evidence to say that embracing this style of parenting also benefits mothers' sense of identity, wellbeing, and fulfilment. Such effects inevitably then benefit her children.

When we accept our own imperfections and exercise self-compassion and care, we not only model this for our child/ren, but we send a powerful message that we can – and do – love and accept our child/ren for all of who *they* are. We release our children from the pressures of perfectionism.

If we can recognise and then challenge the 'social shoulds' of motherhood, we can start to reclaim our experience of motherhood, and imagine what we would like it to look like. We can seek liberation from the ideals that do not serve us and our families, to embrace the freedom that can come with good-enough mothering. This is ultimately a gift not only to our children, but to ourselves, our families, and our community more broadly.

Dr Sophie Brock is a sociologist who specialises in Motherhood Studies, and a single mother to her three-year-old daughter. Her work advocates for the liberation of mothers from the myths of perfect motherhood, bringing academic research on motherhood to the public forum. She offers online education through membership, courses, and individual mentoring, and hosts The Good Enough Mother podcast, to support mothers in reclaiming an empowered practice of mothering for themselves.

You can connect with her further on social media @drsophiebrock *and her website* www.drsophiebrock.com

How you feel about your own adaptation to parenthood can affect your other relationships as well. Reconciling the narratives we construct around our parenting, and how we perceive those who are co-parenting with us, can change our mindset and confidence. Relationships can be a source of strength, comfort, teamwork and cohesion. They can also be a source of stress, friction, antagonism and disagreement. Whether we are talking about the relationship you have with a partner or co-parent, your own parents, wider family members or friends, because we are built for community and relationship, we cannot help but need these people in our lives. Whether the relationships surrounding you are supportive or toxic, or somewhere in the middle, will greatly determine how you cope with the challenges of raising small humans.

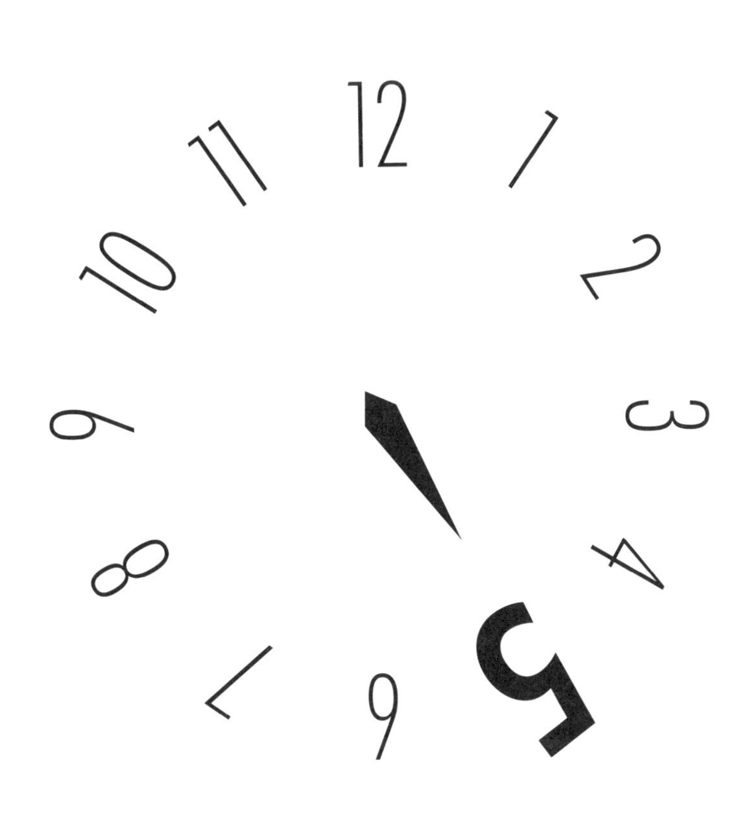

CHAPTER FIVE

LITTLE KIDS, BIG FEELINGS

Often, when I'm talking to parents of an older child, they will say something like 'my child has never been a good sleeper'. It's a simple enough statement, and I totally understand what they're saying in essence when they say it. But what does that mean? Do we mean that the child has not slept in the way that books, friends, and society at large expects them to sleep? Do we mean that it was difficult to manage and unsustainable? Or do we mean that it really was pathologically abnormal sleep?

When children are babies, they have a developmental, biological and nutritional need to wake in the night. They have emotional needs and very limited abilities to self-regulate. They may have a primitive autonomic ability to calm down, but if they become very dysregulated, they will wake and need support. All of this is sometimes packaged up as 'poor sleep'. We need to start by questioning our societal expectations and held beliefs about what is realistic for infants. Often, infant fragmented sleep is just normal. Hard, yes. But normal. When it persists into toddlerhood and beyond, is this an extension of the same 'poor sleep' markers then? Or is it something else?

The one thing that is constant is that children are always changing. As children get older, their sleep needs and the reason they wake up changes too. Perhaps the nutritional needs fade away. Perhaps the early problems of biological and developmental immaturity fade away. Perhaps they even have more self-regulatory abilities. But in many ways, they have even more needs than they did as babies. In this sense, sleep is a constantly 'new' problem. Perhaps children are not 'poor sleepers', but just little people with constantly changing and variable underlying needs that we need to manage at night. Sleep fragmentation is often a symptom of an underlying reason or cause, rather than a stand-alone sleep problem. By describing it as a 'symptom' I don't mean to imply that waking up is pathological. I simply mean that a child who has a need is likely to wake in the night and require your help.

It's often true that infants sleep the way they do because they are immature and biologically and developmentally unready to sleep for long consolidated bursts. As children get older, they increasingly develop this ability. So from a developmental perspective, they may be ready to sleep for longer stretches. But there may now be *other* reasons why they wake in the night. So in this sense, helping toddlers and older children with sleep is even more about digging into the other factors that affect sleep. The new issues that may arise might be to do with boundaries, big feelings, and emotional connection.

So could it be, in fact, that your child is not a 'bad sleeper', but simply a normal sleeper, who happens to have had a string of related, or maybe even unrelated, needs that cause them to wake in the night and need you. If this is true then I hope this lifts the burden of responsibility from you. Your child is not sleeping this way because you have caused it, or allowed it, or let it go on too long. The current reasons may not be related to the reasons your child woke as a baby. In this chapter, we'll dive into some of the emotional reasons your child may be waking more at night.

The emergence of a big personality

Children are not born a blank slate. They have an innate personality that is evident from birth, and to some extent, even before birth. Your child doesn't suddenly develop their personality. But as they get older, it certainly becomes more obvious, and some of the aspects of your child's personality may be considered more challenging. Don't forget though, that the same children that we might describe as high need during infancy, might be described as 'fun', 'playful', 'confident' or 'adventurous' toddlers. Those same children might be described as 'self-assured', 'independent', or 'ambitious' teenagers. The same characteristics that we find to be challenging in infancy can be the very character traits that we

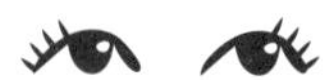

want for our children as they grow up. Back in the 1950s and 1960s there was some research around personality.[1,2] It seems that there are several personality traits that are present from before birth and manifest early on in your child's life. I developed a personality questionnaire based on these a while back, to help parents identify which aspects of their child's personality might be different from their own. Feel free to use this, and repeat for yourself. It may be that the aspects of personality you struggle to understand are those that are the polar opposite of your own tendencies. Read the statements and then place an 'x' on the dashed line to represent how strongly your child's personality matches the statement. For example, a cross on the extreme left for question 1 means that your child is very placid and low energy, while a cross in the middle means that they have equal periods of being placid and highly active.

1. Level and extent of motor activity

\- -

Placid, low energy — Highly active and energetic

2. Degree of regularity, of functions such as eating, toileting and sleep

\- -

Regular, 'clockwork' — All over the place, resists routine

3. Response to a new object or person

\- -

Curious, keen to interact, accepting — Wary of strangers, apprehensive, withdraws

4. Adaptability of behaviour to changes in the environment

\- -

Highly portable — Likes familiar environment, unsettled by change

5. Sensitivity to stimuli

\- -

Oblivious — Highly sensitive

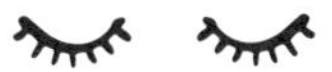

6. Intensity, or energy level, of responses

- -

Easy going | Dramatiser

7. General mood

- -

Cheerful, friendly | Cries easily, grumpy, hard to get a smile from

8. Distractibility

- -

Focuses on the task at hand without being distracted | Highly distractible

9. Attention span and persistence in an activity

- -

Able to concentrate on something longer than peers | Loses interest quickly

In general, the further to the right you have placed the 'x's on the dashed line, the more 'high need' that element of their personality is. The more 'x's you have on the right the more sensitive is your child's temperament.

NB: 'High need' children are not 'bad', or 'undesirable', and they will not necessarily struggle with relationships or tasks, but they *do* require more sensitive parenting, generally are more tiring to look after, and it may take longer to coax them into a new pattern of sleep.

Why is my child having a meltdown?

When your child has a meltdown, their big feelings exploding seemingly from every pore, not only is your child having the mother of all reactions, but we may have a number of reactions too. It's important to understand where your child is coming from, but to get to that, we first need to be calm and collected ourselves. If we are internally screaming, it's pretty much impossible to calmly help your child with their big feelings. So while we will get to your child, let's first focus on two common responses.

During a meltdown, you may go into intellectual mode: 'why are they doing this?'. It's worth running through a few likely triggers. Some children get really 'hangry' when they need a snack, or a meal. Some children get super cranky when they're tired or uncomfortable. But the truth is, you may never figure it out. The trouble with intellectual/detective mode is that we can do one of two things. Firstly, we can drive ourselves bananas trying to figure it out. If you've cycled through the usual suspects and you can't find an obvious trigger, then let it go. Otherwise you will be consumed with the why. Secondly, we can end up asking our child why they are doing what they're doing, or why they feel the way they feel, or why they did what they did. It's a natural response. But asking a child why they did something in the heat of the moment is not likely to yield a sensible answer. The chances are that a young child *doesn't even know*. Older children – I'm talking school age children upwards – *may* sometimes know and be able to articulate this. But even then, if they are raging out, they may just react viscerally. A meltdown is almost never premeditated. It's a response to overwhelm.

The second common response is that we may feel triggered and angry. This is especially likely if your own big feelings weren't managed with kindness and compassion when you were a child. If you were responded to with anger, ignored, sent to your room, spanked or made to feel ashamed of your outbursts, you may reflect some of those feelings in your response to your child without really even thinking about it. This deep subconscious response is hard to change, but the first step is to recognise this pattern. Once you are aware of it, you can interrupt the pattern by changing your behaviour. Many parents find that in the heat of the moment, they are too triggered and wound up to think clearly, so one practical solution is simply to leave the room to collect yourself. While putting children in time out doesn't teach them anything constructive about how to process their feelings or behaviour, it's actually pretty sensible to leave the room yourself if you're struggling. You're modelling self-respect, coping strategies and self-awareness when you identify that something is tipping you over the edge and you need to do something about it.

Managing our feelings as parents

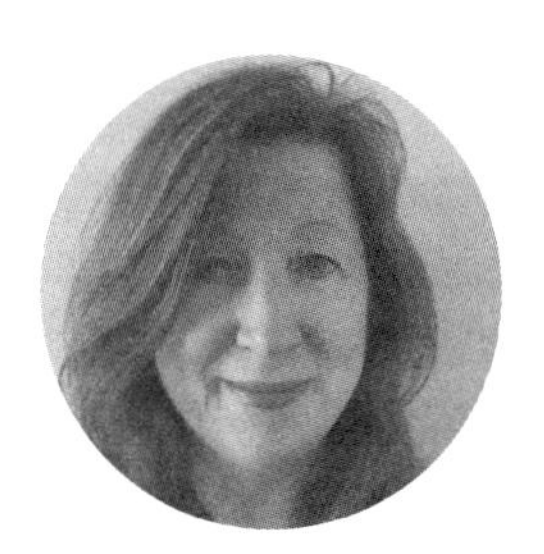

Julianne Boutaleb, consultant perinatal psychologist, director of Parenthood in Mind Consultancy

It's 5 am. You've not slept well and just as you've settled your baby, your toddler awakes. You take him into bed with you, hoping he'll settle too, but instead he starts tugging your hair and screaming. Heart pumping, the familiar rush of adrenalin. The red mist descends and before you know it, you're shouting. He's screaming even more loudly now. And you hear that critical inner voice saying 'Thought you'd never shout at your kids?'

Recognise this scenario? Well if you do, you're certainly not alone. Many parents hate to admit that they lose their temper with their children. And struggle to understand how quickly things can feel out of control despite their best efforts. It's definitely the aspect of parenting that most of us find most difficult. The expectation that we should be able to stay calm and regulate our children's emotions consistently, and the actual day-to-day difficulty of this in practice.

And yet research in infant brain development[3] clearly shows that children *do* need a safe, emotionally responsive adult to regulate their intense mood states. Certain parts of a child's pre-frontal cortex (the area of the brain involved in emotional regulation) are simply not mature enough for them to manage the 'big' emotions like fear or anger alone. In providing consistent containment of their children's big emotions, parents are 'active sculptors of their children's immature brains'.[4] But we also know that a parent's capacity to emotionally respond to their children can fluctuate and may be dependent on a number of factors such as:

- Our own experiences of being parented.
- Current factors such as how well supported we feel by our partner (if partnered), access to other parents or how much practical support we have.
- Other life stresses such as debt, unemployment or health issues.
- Issues specific to becoming parents such as sleep deprivation, mental health, hormone changes, birth trauma and feeding challenges.

The truth is that many of us are ill prepared for the intensity of our children's emotions and how viscerally they impact us. And rightfully so. Can you imagine how unlikely it would be for us to survive as a species if our infant's cries didn't jolt us out of what we were doing to feed them?

But being emotionally attuned to our children impacts our Autonomic Nervous System – for instance our breath, our heartbeat, muscle tension. Taking in and making sense of their distress means we are often emotionally dysregulated too. Our bodies may experience this as stress and in response elevate our adrenalin levels, speed up our breathing, and cause us to react more quickly or abruptly. And this means we need to regularly check in with our own emotions and stress levels as parents:

- Taking time to pause in a busy day with children is vital.
- Stopping to take a deep breath.
- Checking in with another adult.
- Having respite from childcare.
- Leaving the house.

All of these simple activities bring us back into a state of emotional equilibrium.

However, some parents may have internalised strong messages about emotions and emotional availability from their own childhood, and may experience their children's emotional outbursts as triggering. Commonly, parents may struggle with particular aspects of parenting related to their own childhood experiences. For example, a father who was told 'Big boys don't cry' as a child may struggle to soothe his crying child and may react angrily. Getting in touch with such emotions may mean that we are put in touch with 'unresolved residues'[5] from our own childhood. Instead of reflecting on and empathically responding to your child's distress, you may then feel like the mother in the first paragraph – overwhelmed, physically activated and emotionally reactive. Often just stepping back, counting to ten or taking a deep breath may be enough to regulate yourself, and allow you to repair the situation with your child.

But for some parents that might not be enough. If you feel you are regularly struggling with aspects of your relationship with your child, it is vital that you take time out to reflect on what is happening and how you can improve things. Alistair Cooper and Sheila Redfern, in their book

Reflective Parenting,[6] advocate the concept of the Parent Map. The Parent Map consists of three main parts:

1. Your current state of mind
2. Past experiences and relationships
3. Current influences

Perhaps you could think about your own Parent Map?

- Take time to think about your own influences growing up. What messages you internalised about certain emotions. How emotionally available your parents were in certain scenarios.
- Now think about your own child. Be honest about what aspect of your relationship is particularly triggering for you, such as when they throw a tantrum and you get angry. Or perhaps it's a particular scenario that you find hard, like getting them to school or dropping them at nursery.
- Reflective functioning – the ability to reflect on our own emotional experience and that of our child is one of the key aspects of reflective parenting. It's not about creating a perfect relationship with our children, but about being able to reflect on our feelings and theirs, and the times when our relationships with them feel tricky.

Our reaction may depend on our own emotional state, whether we are overloaded, and how much emotional capacity we have at the time. Understanding these triggering times when our children have meltdowns or tantrums, or are just struggling with the overwhelming big feelings they have, can be really transformative. If we can learn to be aware of how these situations make us feel, we might be able to put in place strategies to help us stay calm and in control. Finally, remember that we all mess this up on a regular basis. If you care enough to worry about this, I can pretty much guarantee that you're doing a good enough job.

Big scary feelings

Big feelings are part of the development of a child. The part of the brain that deals with functions like being rational, thoughtful, altruistic, logical, and solving problems is not fully developed until your twenties.

'Time-in' for tantrums

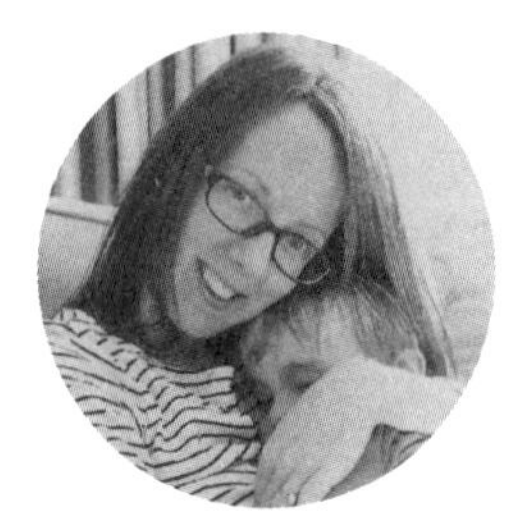

Dr Kimberley Bennett, PsyD Child, Adolescent and Educational Psychology

It can be helpful to reframe a tantrum or a meltdown as a stress response that erupts when children are overwhelmed by their emotions. Meltdowns are a normal part of childhood development that usually reduce in frequency when a child is around school age.

So why do they happen?

Your child's brain is still under construction. In the early years, young children operate from a largely limbic brain, and tend to be right-brain dominant (especially when emotional). This means big emotional reactions are to be expected at times when your child is overwhelmed or unable to cope with the demands of a situation. Sometimes the 'triggers' are obvious, like if your child is disappointed about having to leave the park, but sometimes the triggers are unclear; this can happen when a series of small incidents build-up and lead to a big reaction later on.

The area of the brain that is responsible for logical thought, decision-making, and emotion regulation is called the prefrontal cortex (PFC). This area is still developing throughout childhood, and, during a meltdown, the PFC temporarily goes offline. So even if your child has developed some skills in relation to emotion regulation, impulse control, or decision-making, they won't necessarily be able to access those skills when they are upset or distressed. A great book to learn more about this is *The Whole Brain Child*.[7]

As parents, what can we do?

We have all heard about time-out for tantrums... but what I believe is more effective is time-in. Time-in can still involve removing your child from the tricky situation, *but* time-in differs in that the parent remains physically and emotionally available to the child to help calm and soothe their anger, upset or frustration, and to encourage reflective learning when the child is calm.

One challenge can be that, when the sympathetic nervous system is activated during a meltdown, children often display a fight/flight/freeze response.

- A fight response might look like hitting, kicking, or throwing.
- A flight response might look like fleeing, hiding, or shouting 'Go away!'
- Freeze responses are more unusual in young children, and trickier to spot, but may involve a child withdrawing.

None of these responses sends the clear message to parents that your little one needs you close in those moments... but they really do. When children are distressed, their attachment system becomes activated, meaning that when our children are at their worst, that is when they need connection most. So during a meltdown we want to try to connect with our children in order to soothe their nervous system. Calming their nervous system by calming and regulating ourselves helps guide our child from a state of chaotic reactivity to a state of calm.

Empathy is one of our best tools to calm a dysregulated nervous system. Our children need us to try to understand them, to think about what they might be feeling, and to support them to make sense of their experience. '*You are so sad that we have to go home now. That makes so much sense. You were having so much fun!*' This emotional 'containment'[8] develops our child's ability to better manage their emotional experiences independently in the future.

How will my child ever learn?

It is only when your child is calm, when they are no longer reactive, that they will be able to learn. It is when we have soothed their nervous system that we can plant the seeds that support life-long learning. We do this by getting alongside our children and encouraging them to reflect on alternative ways of communicating their needs or dealing with a difficult situation.

It is helpful to remind ourselves that children are not always capable of independent reflection and problem-solving. Supporting our child during and after a meltdown is a neurologically-rich learning opportunity that develops their ability to self-regulate, reflect and problem-solve.[9]

Research suggests that punishment teaches our child all the wrong lessons, and actually increases undesirable behaviour.[10] On the other hand, loving guidance through time-in provides children with the support they need to understand and regulate their emotions. Over time, this equips them with the skills necessary to make different behavioural choices in the future.

For more information you can find Kimberley on Instagram or Facebook @the_psychologists_child or on her website at www.thepsychologistschild.com.

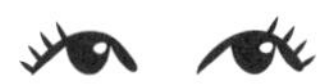

So whether your child is two or 10, they are not the finished article yet. Often, when a child is developmentally advanced, we expect more of their behaviour – but even for a bright child, their brain is still a work in progress. When they get scared, upset, angry or frustrated, they do not necessarily have the skills they need to calm down. There is no point in thinking that the level of the emotional outburst is relative to the problem they are reacting to, because your child is immature. So, if your child 'loses it' over their banana breaking, we might not think it's a big deal, but to them, it may well be. They simply don't know yet what things are trivial and what things really need to be worried about. That comes with life experience.

Hitting, biting, throwing...

Some children have a big body reaction to their emotions, and this can be really tough to deal with. I have noticed over the years that biting seems to be the most socially unacceptable behaviour, and the thing that parents worry most about. Of course it's never okay to hurt people, and children need to know that. But lashing out bodily is just an extension of screaming, shouting or crying on one level, and still needs to be managed with compassion.

Some children seem to feel emotions most acutely in certain parts of their bodies, and this may be why they use that part of their body to express whatever emotion they are feeling. For instance, they may feel it in their face – which might be why they bite. They may feel it in their hands, which could be why they throw toys or hit. Or they may feel their emotions in their feet, which could be why they stomp or kick. They might feel their emotions in their tummy or all over their body, which may be why they throw themselves on the floor, arch their backs, plank, or heave.

If they do use parts of their body, you can help them use that part of their body in your calm-down solution. For instance:

- For children who bite, spit or shout – try blowing bubbles, singing, breathing, crunching on an apple, chewing gum (if safe and age appropriate), 'chewellery' (chewable jewellery) and sucking on a straw.
- For children who stamp, kick and jump around – try consciously stamping out the angry feelings, marching around the room, star jumps, football, leg stretches and foot massages.

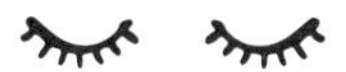

- For children who throw, hit or punch – try clapping hands, finger dancing, punching a pillow or cushion, or stretching out the hands to make a starfish shape.
- For children who flail, heave, plank, arch or roll on the floor – try percussing their back, firm wrapping in a blanket, and encouraging them to take deep breaths into their tummy.

Emotion coaching and emotional intelligence

Emotion coaching, coined by John Gottman in the 1990s, is a communication strategy used by parents of children of any age to help them understand their emotions, manage their stress response and regulate themselves under stress. There are many aspects to successful emotion coaching, including helping children to find the language to express what it is they are feeling, validating the feelings that children have, and being empathic to children with big feelings. Emotion coaching has been shown to improve children's social behaviour, as well as helping them to regulate their stress response.[11]

Emotion coaching is something that any parent can learn to do, and you may be surprised by how much it transforms not only your child's emotional responses, and self-regulation, but also your relationship with your child. I recommend reading John Gottman's book[12] for more detail, but as a starting place, these are the five steps to become your child's emotion coach:

1. Awareness
2. Connection
3. Listening
4. Naming emotions
5. Finding workable solutions

The first step is to be aware that a range of emotions is normal. There are no 'good' or 'bad' feelings. It's normal to feel happy, sad, angry, confused, bored, excited, scared, jealous, or thoughtful. All emotions are valid and important, and becoming aware of how both you and your child are feeling is important. Your child may express emotion with language, facial expression, behaviour, or body language. Learn to observe both the evidence of a particular emotion, and also the shift in emotions.

Next, when you notice that your child is experiencing an emotion that

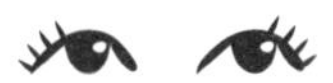

they may need help with, try not to dismiss it, but use this as an opportunity to help your child learn more about their emotional state. Allow your child to talk about their emotions, and help them to find a way to manage them before it all descends into ugly crying, snot, and meltdown.

Thirdly, make time to listen to your child, and validate the emotion that they're feeling. Remember they don't have the same perspective as us. My daughter told me about a crisis at school recently. It seemed to be a big deal, so I braced myself and asked her to tell me more. 'Our games teacher always picks the same children to be on the team. I'm actually a really good defender, but I never get a chance.' In the life of a child, this is a big deal. While our adult perspective tells us that in the grand scheme of things there could be a whole load of reasons why this might not be a problem, it's important to a child. I could easily have said, 'Okay, kiddo, well, just let it go', but instead, I said: 'Hmm, I'm guessing you didn't feel great about that?'. She then told me that she felt disappointed and angry, and a little sidelined. She hates injustice, and this felt unfair, yet she felt powerless to challenge the teacher. These emotions are valid and meaningful, and moreover, provide an opportunity to learn that this stuff is part of life and growing up, and that there may be ways to handle this situation that provide life skills.

Next, name emotions. Providing a name for the 'thing' that your child feels helps them to know what they're experiencing. Have you ever had a pain or a medical problem, but felt a little better once it was diagnosed and given a name? Even if it's a stupid name, like *Adenovirus* (yes, that really is the name of a virus!), many people feel a little better. Partly this is because when there is a name for something, we know it's a 'thing'. Someone else has had it before. We know a little bit about it, and we might even know the right treatment. It's a little similar with emotions. That ugly burning fiery feeling in your belly – that's anger. The bubbling seething feeling that makes us want to huff and flare our nostrils – that's resentment. And so on. Having a name for an emotion gives children a hook to hang those feelings on. It's like a placeholder for a time when they may feel something similar.

Finally, help your child find a solution for their emotions. This is not to say that there is always a solution. In some cases, children (just like us) want to offload, without being given a solution. That's okay. For example, I suggested that my daughter could go up to her teacher and ask if one time maybe she could have a shot at being on the team. That suggestion didn't fly. Sometimes kids don't want a fix, they want to dump their feeling

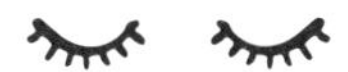

on someone. That's part of the parental job description. But other times, especially with younger children, they may need a better solution than just sitting with the feeling. Depending on your child's age, developmental stage, cognitive ability, language and problem-solving skills, you could ask them if they can think of a solution. For example, you could say: 'It looks like you're bored. What could you do about that?' Or, 'I can see you're angry. Shall we stamp around the room together?' Or, 'I know you're frustrated that you can't play with your sister and her friends. Can you think of something else we could do instead?'

If your child does something that crosses a line – such as hurting someone, then you can still follow this process. You need to first connect with and calm your child. There's no point reacting immediately and going straight for the consequence (or the lecture that we all love to impart sometimes). You need to connect, calm and contain first, then name the emotion, validate that, and help your child find an alternative. For example: 'I'm here, I love you. I know you're angry. Shall we sit together for a while till you feel better?'. Once your child is calm, *then* you can reinforce the boundary. 'I can see you were very angry, but we don't kick or hurt people. Let's find something you *can* kick if you feel angry like that again.'

This process is not something you will get 'right' every time. You're human, and sometimes you will react in the heat of the moment. That's totally understandable. You can help your child, even in those moments, by owning your own imperfections, forgiving yourself and helping your child to see that not only do you not have it all figured out, but you have solutions for when you mess up too.

Limits and boundaries and how this relates to sleep

What do limits and boundaries have to do with sleep, you might wonder? Well, it will be pretty hard to enforce a limit – any limit – overnight if your child doesn't experience limits in the daytime. We cannot compartmentalise nighttime and daytime behaviour. Limit-testing is a normal part of childhood. As children get older and more developmentally mature, they are able to consider ever-increasing aspects of morality and ethics. Peter Singer calls this the 'expanding circle',[13] which refers to the idea that children initially make decisions based on a very small circle of influence: their home, bodies, toys, and parents. As they get older, this circle of consideration expands to friends,

teachers, and their wider family. It is many years until children develop altruistic skills, such as the ability to refuse a plastic straw because it may end up in the sea and harm turtles, or choose not to eat foods that contain palm oil because of deforestation. The nuance of the degree of concern may vary according to a child's upbringing, peer influence, and exposure. For example, whether a child cares as much for someone they have never met, as they do their grandparent, or whether they care as much about a fly being swatted and killed as they do about their pet being unwell.[14] These moral decisions seem obvious to us as adults, but a child's world is relatively smaller, and the maturity required to make these decisions is a work in progress.

Limit-testing in younger children

Until these moral decisions are intuitive and innate, children are not always aware of the impact of their actions or behaviour on others. They also don't know what the rules and social conventions are until they encounter a boundary. I often explain to families on a practical level that the way a child finds out whether the boundary is flexible, or rigid, is by pushing it. They may go right up to the boundary, push it, shove it, lean in to it. They may try to make the boundary move in different ways. They may see if the boundary is different depending on the context, or the person they ask. Essentially, they are trying to work out how bendy the boundaries are. The bendier your boundaries, the more you will experience limit-testing behaviour.

One scenario I encounter a lot with parents who have chosen to raise their children responsively, gently and respectfully, is a struggle with boundaries. It's really hard to say no to a child. They sometimes get upset or even appear devastated. When our babies are tiny, their needs and wants are the same thing. When needs and wants become separate is a little murky. But certainly by toddlerhood your child will have clearly demonstrated that they have wants. Some of the wants are easy to say no to – such as sharp knives, running in the road, climbing in the bath alone. But the grey areas are a lot harder to figure out.

I've also noticed that for very understandable reasons, sometimes parents avoid certain places or situations that are likely to involve a conflict. For instance, I have known families to avoid going out because of a battle over the car seat, or their child insisting on sweets in the supermarket every time they go down the confectionary aisle. I totally appreciate that these daily struggles are stressful and demoralising. Sometimes avoiding a situation is the right thing to do to preserve everyone's sanity and dignity. But if you are avoiding lots of places, consider whether you might perhaps be missing an opportunity to help your child learn about limits. I know it's super embarrassing to have a screaming toddler in a public place when you say no to what they want, but believe me, you will not be either the first or the last person to manage this particular parenting delight. So don't always avoid the troublespots – consider them an opportunity to practise the boundaries.

Lastly, while it is important to have firm and clear boundaries which you uphold consistently, if you are continuously fighting with your child you are picking too many battles. Reflect on whether the most common arguments are over trivial things that you could address in another way, or whether they are the deal-breakers. If they are the deal-breakers, then think about how you could get your child more involved in the decisions about the house rules.

Some tips:

- Mean what you say and say what you mean!
- Decide what your absolute limits are calmly, with your co-parent. These should be the absolute deal-breakers – i.e. hitting, shouting, swearing and so on.
- If at all possible, get your child involved with the rules – even if they just colour in the rule sheet.
- Try to anticipate likely areas of negotiation in advance.
- Make sure you have plenty of quality time, so your little one doesn't have to act up in order to get your undivided attention.
- Avoid sarcasm and double negatives.
- Maintain eye contact when possible.
- Use a normal tone of voice.
- Keep track of when you and your child fall out – is it always the same time of day? Are they hungry? Tired? Bored? Are you rushing? Are you giving enough warnings about activities coming to an end, or changing? Note the triggers and times, and see if there is an obvious pattern.
- Try not to shout – this just gets everybody's hackles up. Try stage whispering, or singing what you feel like yelling instead. A great

resource is the Orange Rhino website: theorangerhino.com

- If you've told your child what the boundary is, remain firm *and* kind. Remember to connect and empathise with your child's frustration/ sadness/anger, but don't budge.
- There is a time and a place to either respectfully ask, or present the non-negotiables. For instance, if your child is refusing to clear their plate, or get in the car seat, or stay still while you change their nappy, try turning your request around by using language of assumption. So, you might say; 'I see you're not ready for playtime yet. *After* you've cleaned your plate away, then we can play.' Or, 'I know how much you want to go swimming. *When* you've got into the car seat, we can go to the pool.' Or, 'I know your nappy is making you feel uncomfortable. *When* you lie down, we can make you clean and dry.' We are not using language that suggests options or choice, but the words are still kind and respectful.

Limit-testing in older children

Most of us accept limit-testing behaviour in little ones. But if your six, eight, or eleven-year-old is testing the limits, this can feel like a whole new ball game. Limit-testing in older children may indicate a need for control, whether that is control of a situation, material possession or property, or to control your emotions or response. Sometimes, our response is exciting, or entertaining, or they enjoy the power of arguing with an adult.

Some tips:

- I know it's hard, but try to stay calm. Rising to the bait will probably inflame the situation.
- Allow your child to tell their side of the story.
- Practise reflective listening: 'Okay, so what you're telling me is that you feel like it's unfair that you have to tidy your room by yourself, because your little brother gets help to clean his room. Is that right?'
- Validate how your child is feeling, without condoning their action: 'I can see that you're upset, and I'm sorry about that.'
- Make sure your older child has plenty of quality time and feels unconditionally loved.
- Help your child understand that people have different realities, and two people's perceptions of a single event can both be right at the same time.
- Beware of language loopholes.

- Try to avoid it being about winning and losing – this makes children feel either too powerful, or powerless. Strategies such as forcing children to apologise, or admit they were wrong, are unlikely to be constructive.
- Build self-esteem, encourage independent thinking, and give opportunities for responsibility (more in chapter 5).
- Be authentic and flexible with boundaries. Sometimes, they need to be changed as children get older: 'It wasn't okay that you shouted at me when I turned off the computer game. But I've been thinking, and I guess the screen time allowance needs to go up a little now that you're eight. What do you think about a one-hour limit instead?' This way, everyone's dignity is maintained, and you model the reality of having to reconsider, be adaptable and also to be humble enough to say that something you did is no longer appropriate.

It might sound odd to consider behaviour, boundaries and consequences, but you'll find that respect, and developing that attitude of being both kind and firm, will filter through to bedtime boundaries as well.

Love tanks

Imagine that your child has a tank that can be filled with love, warmth and affection. As we go through the day, experiencing the ordinary stresses, frustrations, ruptures and limit-setting, as well as separation, the love tank gets a little emptier. Little acts of kindness, responsiveness and compassion fill it back up again.

When a child's love tank is dry they tend to instinctively seek out parental proximity and attention. Their need to procrastinate, control and negotiate is sometimes a sign that they are seeking connection and a refilling of their love tank.

I often explain that there are two ways to fill a love tank – trickle-charge it, or super-charge it.

Trickle-charging is through spending plenty of quantity time with a child. It doesn't all have to be high-energy, intense, focused time, but just hanging out all day, sharing life, will fill a love tank.

But of course, many parents work, and trickle-charging is not an option. This is no time for guilt, but time to get pragmatic and solution-focused. If you're not with your child all day, never fear – that's the point of super-charging. With super-charging, you spend a short amount of time that is highly focused and undistracted. Even just 10–15 minutes of quality time per day makes a huge difference.

One of my favourite tools are the love languages. Dr Gary Chapman and Dr Ross Campbell wrote the hugely popular book *The Five Love Languages of Children* in 1997, proposing that we all have a preferred love language:

- Quality time (hanging out together, one-to-one playtime, going for a hot chocolate together)
- Acts of service (fixing a broken toy, helping a preschooler to tidy up, helping a preschooler to get dressed)
- Touch (massage, cuddles, breastfeeding, wearing your preschooler)
- Affirming words (telling your preschooler how special they are, how much you love them)
- Thoughtful presents (this doesn't have to be a bought present – it could be a shell, pretty rock, or a little piece of origami)

Children feel most loved and connected with when we communicate with them using their primary love language. When we know a child's primary love language, we can love-bomb them to fill their love tank regularly to stop it running dry.

The transformative part of the love languages is the idea that we tend to express love with our own love language – which is not necessarily the way our loved ones most feel loved. We can also wound most deeply by using someone's love language – for example, withholding touch for a child whose love language is touch, would be more damaging than if their love language was words.

The other reason I love the love languages as a tool is that they're good for everyone. All relationships can be helped or healed with more sensitive use of the love languages. Consider how you could use this knowledge in a transformational way in your other adult relationships. All of us sometimes feel like our love tank is running on empty if people communicate their love to us in a love language that is not one we relate to. I've not seen any research on this, but my experience has been that sometimes our love languages can shift at times of transition. My love language prior to having children was quality time. Post kids, it is acts of service. Can anyone relate? My feeling on this, which, as I've noted is anecdotal only, is that as our deepest needs change, so too can the ways in

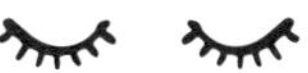

which people can most effectively show their love for us.

Try to work out what your child's love language is to most efficiently refill their love tank. Here are some ways to try to tell what their love language is:

- If they can understand this question, try: 'When do you feel most loved?'
- Since very young children are often naturally egotistical, you could try asking them how they make sure Mummy/Daddy feels loved. They are likely to suggest something that *they* relate to.
- You could also try: 'What was your favourite part of today?'
- If these questions are too tricky (especially for younger children) then think about how your child communicates love to you. Are they super cuddly? Do they like just spending time with you? Do they find you little presents, like rocks, snail shells etc? Since we tend to instinctively demonstrate love to others using our primary love language, it's a good bet that this is your child's love language.
- If it is really unclear, then experiment with all of them and see which one seems to connect the most.

Don't forget, love languages can fluctuate, and it's common to have a primary and a secondary love language.

Separation anxiety

Separation anxiety is not just for babies. Children can go through numerous phases of separation anxiety in their lives. When they start a new daycare, nursery, school, or a major change is upon them, this can trigger another wave of anxiety about saying goodbye or leaving you. Common times for disruption include moving to a new house, and having another baby. At any of these times, it's normal for your child to need extra reassurance. If your child seems extra sensitive to saying goodbye, my suggestion is to meet their need for connection. As with all other phases, it will pass. You cannot rush children out of these developmental stages. They have to run their course.

Shyness and anxiety

At times you may wonder whether your child's separation anxiety is normal, or whether it is morphing into social anxiety or shyness. Shyness can be particularly difficult for children if they struggle to make friends.

The difference between normal separation anxiety and social shyness in children

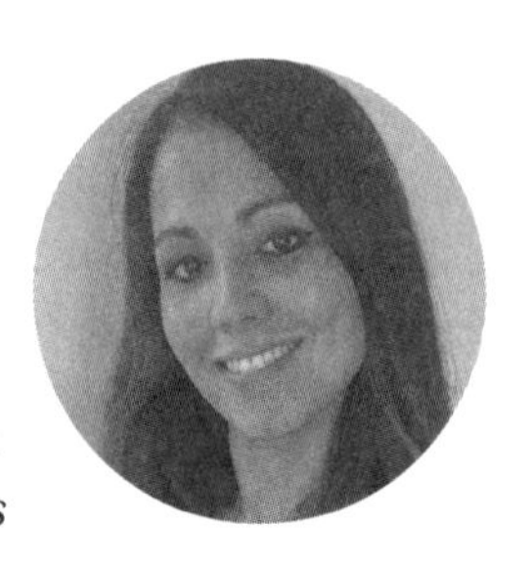

Dr Martha Deiros Collado, clinical psychologist with family therapy training and expertise in paediatrics

Separation anxiety and shyness often overlap during childhood but they are distinctly different. Separation anxiety is a normal part of development and all infants and toddlers experience this at some point throughout their life. Separation anxiety may look like:

- Difficulty being away from parents or other loved ones through signs of tearfulness and behavioural outbursts
- Worrying about harm to loved ones when apart
- Worrying about danger to themselves when separated from parents or loved ones
- Difficulty leaving the house to go to school
- Difficulty falling asleep or sleeping through the night
- Experiencing physical symptoms that look like signs of illness (e.g. tummy aches, headaches, and pains and aches)

How parents respond to separation anxiety can have an impact on children's secure attachment, which in turn can influence the intensity to which a child shows social shyness. Overprotective parents may teach their child to be inhibited and fearful of new and unexpected situations, whereas children who have not developed a secure attachment with their caregivers may feel greater anxiety when in new situations and be more likely to show shy behaviour.

Children who experience social shyness may appear inhibited in unfamiliar situations or when interacting with new people. They might seem socially withdrawn and have a strong preference to stay close to safe adults and prefer to stay 'on the sidelines' rather than join in with others.

Most children experience social shyness at some point or in certain contexts. Many children grow out of social shyness as they get older, although some may continue to show shy behaviour in certain contexts as adults.

How social shyness may inhibit children from making friends, and the impact on their self-esteem

Social shyness may reduce a child's opportunity to develop or practise social skills. While they stand watching the action from the sidelines they often miss out on participating in activities with their peers. This reduced engagement means they miss out on practising social skills that may help them boost their confidence and limits their experience of positive feedback after engaging in fun activities with others.

As a result of these limited opportunities and interactions, social shyness can reduce children's confidence in their social skills and impact on their self-esteem. It can invite Anxiety to show up when they meet with peers or are faced with new and novel situations tricking them into believing that they will be 'judged' or 'get it wrong'. For some children Anxiety may show up as blushing, physically shaking or having a stammer and this can feed into a vicious cycle where children may start to avoid social situations to stop the feelings of Anxiety and social discomfort. Over time, children's confidence and self-esteem may start to shrink and, as their social interactions become more and more limited, it further perpetuates the shy behaviour.

How to help children who are shy or unconfident

Words are powerful and children tend to live up to the labels they are given. Labelling a child as 'shy' to them and/or others can create a narrative of the child's identity that can be difficult for them to break away from. One of the first steps in supporting children who experience social shyness is to not call them 'shy' or offer the label as an unchanging aspect of their identity.

Instead, talk to your child about their experience in social situations without placing a label on it. Be empathic and stay curious about what holds them back from engaging with others in certain situations and be open to the labels they put on this. Try not to run to 'fix' the situation, instead allowing for their experience to be heard without judgement. Using words like 'I noticed...' and naming what you see without judgement, alongside using 'I wonder...' to offer ideas and give your child permission to say how they felt, can be useful.

For example: '*I noticed* you chose to stay with me at the party rather than go and join in the games. It is okay if you prefer being with me for a while because I am always happy to be with you. You are such a fun kid, *I wonder* whether something was getting in the way of joining in the fun. Did something make you feel a bit scared or worried?'

Or: '*I noticed* you watched the game from the bench the other day. I know how you much you love running around. *I wonder* whether you knew the rules of that game or maybe something was different about yesterday that made you hold back?'

Once a child has started to open up about their experience all you need to do in the moment as a parent or caring adult is to acknowledge and validate their experience. It may be that children need support with overcoming feelings of anxiety, or perhaps they need some skills building in areas of social communication and interaction. Problem-solving what needs to be done next can only happen when children feel heard, seen and understood.

Finally, children learn the most through watching behaviour rather than talking about it. If you have a child who experiences social shyness, modelling confident behaviour and demonstrating skills that help to overcome anxiety in social situations is crucial. You can bring this alive in everyday situations by being more explicit about what you are doing and how it is making you feel. Some simple examples of this may be:

- Talking to a stranger – e.g. 'Oh I felt so nervous talking to that lady in the park. I didn't want to stop and talk to a total stranger. It would have been so easy to walk away but I am glad I stopped she was so nice wasn't she? And she told us about that festival that is coming up, we would have never known about that! Sometimes doing something a little scary feels good afterwards.'
- Getting out of your comfort zone – e.g. 'I have a presentation to do at work tomorrow. I am feeling so nervous, I always feel scared before a presentation and this one is online with so many people I don't know! Ugh. I hate this feeling... But I know I can still do this. I am going to take a break and go for a run first to make me feel a little more relaxed and then I am going to practise running it online with my friend just to make sure I know how to use all the buttons.'

Simple strategies for helping children make friends

Useful strategies will vary depending on each individual child and the unique circumstances and stories of their lives. Some simple ideas to try may include:

- **Do some social skills coaching.** Social skills do not come naturally with children, they need to be learnt. And if a child experiences social anxiety they have probably had a limited experience of what social interactions look like and may benefit from a little more coaching than others. You can use everyday conversations at home to think about this or even use 'social scripts' to rehearse situations. Aim for small, incremental steps that develop your child's social skills and confidence in applying them. This means teaching children the conversational skills of starting a conversation, exchanging information, and interacting. For example:

- Giving eye contact and smiling
- 'Hello'
- 'My name is...'
- 'What is your name?'
- 'I like playing with...'
- 'What do you like doing?'

- **Practice makes perfect!** To make the steps above 'real' to your child you can use role play with toys and take the position of the child who experiences social shyness. Use different scenarios and practise some of the conversational skills you have shared with your child. Children tend to find it easier to speak up through role play and you may witness or hear your child say words of encouragement or boost the confidence of the teddy that is holding back!
- **Prepare your child.** Before going to a party, park or social situation, talk to your child about what is going to happen. Let them know you understand the situation may bring up fear or make them feel uncomfortable and problem-solve together ways your child may be able to manage this. For example: 'So this afternoon it's your cousin's birthday and she is having a few friends come round. I know you find meeting new people a bit scary. What do you think will help you join in the fun? Is there anything you want to practise or try out before we go? I am always here for you.'
- **Build up their confidence.** Encouraging opportunities for your child to meet with peers in a safe situation can help to boost their confidence. Setting up a playdate at home with one or two children can help them practise social interactions in an environment that gives them control and helps them feel safe. Encouraging one or two extracurricular activities that have structure and allow for self-expression can be really helpful in boosting confidence, skills and abilities. For example, try individual or team sports, Scouts/Brownies, music, drama or creative groups. Make sure they are activities your child enjoys and is good at as this will help them engage with the activity and, over time, with others who have the same interest in common.

- **Be realistic.** Not all children are social butterflies, and that is okay as long as it does not impact on their quality of life or interfere with activities they would otherwise enjoy. Some children only have a few close friends and that can be very normal. Be guided by your child. Encouraging friendships is important, as is learning to sustain them. Also remember that social shyness often resolves and/or may not show up in all contexts so don't be surprised if your child finds an activity that makes them shine, or hits an age that helps them become surprisingly outgoing and comfortable in social situations.

You can find Martha on Instagram @drmdc_paediatric_psychologist or read more about her on her website: DrMDC.co.uk

Building confidence and self-esteem

Building confidence in children. How do we do this? Well, it seems to come naturally to some kids. Others seem to have to work harder. This may be down to temperament and personality. But there are certainly things you can do to foster confidence and boost self-esteem in your child.

1. **Help them to develop a growth mindset.** This is a concept coined by Carol Dweck,[15] and refers to the importance of praising effort, not achievement. A fixed mindset says 'I can't do that'. A growth mindset says 'I'm finding this hard, but with a little practice, I can learn'. I have a fixed mindset about technology. I panic when someone suggests a new platform, piece of software, or app that I have to learn how to use. I *assume* from the outset that I will not be able to do it. Having a fixed mindset can rob you of the chance to try something that might be good. Dweck points out that just praising effort is not enough either. Just telling a child 'well done for trying' won't help if they continually struggle. Fostering a growth mindset also means helping children to come up with strategies or a different approach so that they can learn from mistakes. For instance, 'You worked really hard for that spelling test, good for you. Next time, shall we try a different way to learn to try to do even better?' A growth mindset enables a child to learn that knowledge and mastery of something is not something that is set

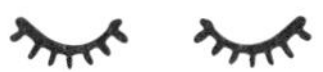

in stone, but can be developed and improved. This is important for confidence, independence and self-esteem.

2. **Help them accept failure.** Having opportunities to lose and have emotional support with this is really important for a child's confidence. Try turn-taking games, memory games or races (don't always let them win!). If children are scared to fail, they are sometimes reluctant to try. When children know they can lose in a safe space, and retain their dignity, they are less scared of trying. But always failing is pretty demoralising too! Build your child up by helping them to learn a skill. Whether this is catching a ball, learning a simple song, or managing to complete an obstacle course, winning (with humility) is also good for kids. Some activities, such as martial arts, teach self-control, empathy and respect, as well as strength and conditioning. This can be a good activity for a child as it teaches perseverance and growth.
3. **Give them responsibilities.** When children feel useful, valued and important, this can really boost their self-esteem. Learning to work as part of a team has long been known to encourage children's confidence and facilitates friendships, though not all children realise at the time that this is a major benefit of the exercise.[16] Ask your children to help regularly in the home, and help them to understand the importance of their contribution.

You may wonder what this has got to do with sleep – well, when children learn that they can learn to do things, it increases their confidence and decreases anxiety. This may in turn reduce problems with sleep caused by low self-esteem and anxiety.

Supporting speech and language

Finally, some frustrations can arise due to delayed speech or problems with hearing. I know *all* of us wonder at times whether our children have selective hearing loss, but sometimes they really are struggling. Other times, they struggle with comprehension, or hearing instructions or requests in a busy or distracting environment. Children who are struggling with speech or communication sometimes find it hard to regulate their emotions, or have to rely more on body language and behaviour to get their point across. You can find some tips to encourage speech on the next pages.

Encouraging speech, language and understanding in toddlers and preschoolers

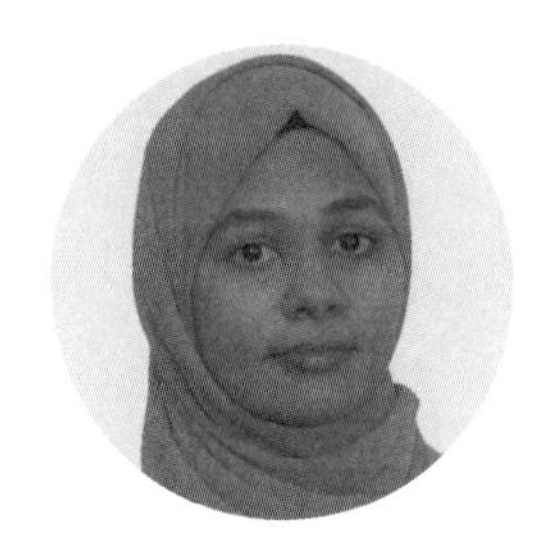

Aishath Zimna Hussain, audiologist and speech and language pathologist

Most people are aware that speech and language development is a crucial part of every child's development. Delays in speech and language can lead to frustration, social impairment, emotional problems and behavioural challenges.

Speech/language delay is when a child does not develop speech and language skills as we might expect for their age and stage. It is important to identify and address these problems early to minimise the consequences. If you are working on improving your child's speech and language skills, or if your child has a speech and language delay, here are my top six tips to support them:

1. Limit screen time and spend more time playing and talking with your child. Playing is the 'work' of a child. A child who is not playing and interacting with others is unlikely to be learning as well as they could be.
2. Read, read, and read books. Try touch-and-feel books, pop-up books and books with colourful real pictures. Let your child flip the pages. Read together and use an animated voice to get your child's attention.
3. Do not focus too much on academic concepts like numbers, letters and shapes if your child is not yet talking or they are using only a few words. Instead teach functional words that your child can use in everyday life.
4. If possible, let your child spend time and play with other children. This will improve social skills and language skills.
5. Use the same words or phrases in the same way, in the same activity repeatedly, for example; during bath time, meal times, bedtime and so on.
6. Get your child's speech and language skills evaluated by a licensed speech and language pathologist/therapist (SLP). You could also check their hearing, as sometimes speech delay may be worsened by hearing difficulties. An SLP will give treatment recommendations and if speech therapy is necessary, it is important to start early as early intervention leads to better outcomes.

If you feel your child has a speech/language problem, always trust your instincts and get professional help or additional information until you are satisfied.

Not all children with speech/ language delays will require speech therapy. Whether a child needs speech therapy or not can only be decided after a comprehensive evaluation. In the UK, your GP or health visitor can refer you and your child, or you may also choose to seek private support. There are many websites and Instagram accounts you can follow for additional support. Just make sure you get information from trusted resources – such as qualified speech and language therapists/pathologists.

You can find Aishath on Instagram at @speech_therapist_audiologist

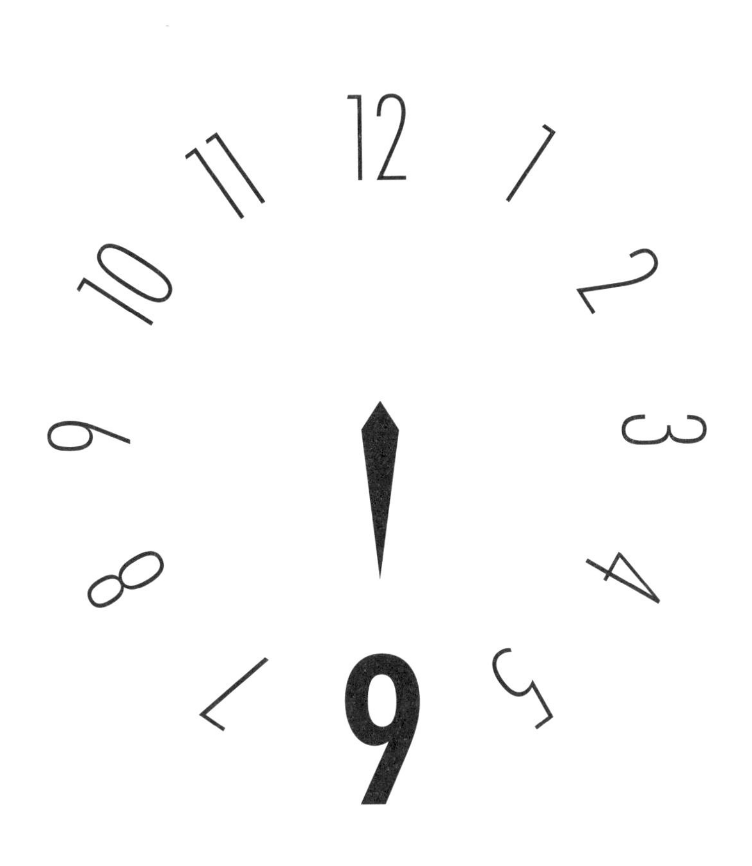

CHAPTER SIX

THINGS THAT BUMP, WALK LEAK AND YELL IN THE NIGHT

The medical term for conditions that cause us to walk, talk, or generally do interesting things during sleep is parasomnia. Parasomnias are events that occur either as we fall asleep, during sleep, or as we wake up. Although parasomnia sounds like a scary word, these conditions are all pretty common in children, and are usually benign. Some parasomnias occur mainly during deep sleep, while others are more prevalent during dreaming (REM) sleep. Many parasomnias are genetic, self-limiting and will resolve themselves, though one or two of the conditions in this section warrant further investigation and referral by your child's doctor.

Nightmares, terrors and confusional arousals

Nightmares are vivid and frightening dreams that usually occur during REM sleep. Since most dreaming sleep occurs in the second half of the night, your child is most likely to have a nightmare in the small hours of the morning. Almost all children have nightmares at some point, although they are more common at times of disruption or stress. Some children suffer from recurrent nightmares. They will often wake a child up, and the child usually has good recall of the nature of their nightmare.

Most children grow out of nightmares spontaneously. Until they do, reassurance and comfort are the best tools to manage them. It's absolutely appropriate for you to go and sit with your child, rub their back or give them a hug if they are scared or distressed. I once met a family where the dad had a ritual of looking inside cupboards, under the bed, and in the toy chest for the zombies that his daughter was worried about. Looking for monsters is not a great idea, as this can reinforce the possibility that they might exist. A better strategy is to validate the fear, but bring your child back to reality. For example; 'Wow, yes that does sound scary. I can imagine that you would be frightened if there was a zombie in your room. But you know, the great thing is that zombies don't exist. So they aren't something we need to worry about.'

Consider whether there are any potential triggers for bad dreams – such as TV shows that your child may be exposed to. It doesn't have to be something they are intentionally watching – they could just be passing the TV when something they shouldn't be seeing comes on. Check which books they are looking at, or are reading. Try asking if there's something that your child wants to be removed from the room. I remember needing to take a certain big brown bear on a one-way trip to the charity shop after my eldest told me that he was 'nice in the day, but scary at night'.

Sometimes, the worst thing to be frightened of is the fear itself. Some children become scared of being woken by a nightmare, which can make them reluctant to go to sleep in the first place. Logically, if you don't go to sleep, you can't experience something frightening. It makes perfect sense really.

Worry toys

In many cultures around the world, there are various traditions for easing anxiety about bedtime. All of them essentially help a child to deal with something that is worrying them in a more tangible way. This might be something at school, home, or fear of going to sleep, or of nightmares.

- **Worry dolls** are a Guatemalan tradition. They are tiny dolls inside a small drawstring bag. Traditionally, a child tells each doll a worry, and then places the dolls inside the bag under their pillow. In the morning the worry will be gone.
- **Worry eater** – this is a plush toy. It comes in many different colours and designs, and even different sizes. It has a friendly face, and a zip-up mouth. You or your child write down something that is worrying them, and place it inside the worry eater's mouth. As the parent, you just have

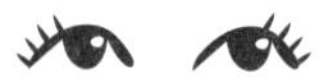

to remember to take the worry out before they wake up! I once forgot to do this and had to think on my feet. In case this happens to you, I told my daughter that since that was a pretty big worry, it might just take the worry eater a little bit longer to chew it up. You'll be glad to know I got away with it! You can buy these toys from various companies. Sorgenfresser make a lovely variety of different worry eaters.

- **Dreamcatchers** are a Native American tradition, from the Ojibwe tribe, and they are used as a talisman to protect sleeping people from bad dreams and nightmares. Native Americans believe that the night air is filled with both good and bad dreams. The dreamcatcher traps the bad dreams and allows the good ones through the spider-web design. They are hung on or near a child's bed, and are usually small, and made of materials like leather and feathers.
- **Bad dream spray** – you can make a special bad dream spray out of water, a couple of drops of essential oil, glitter and food colouring. Ideally get your child involved in making it, and act as though you've researched the right recipe. Spray it a few times around the room at bedtime. You could invent a bad dream banishing song for extra nightmare-busting power if you like.
- **Worry jar** – finally, you can adapt these ideas and use a worry jar. This is a nice idea for a child who feels better once they have spoken about or written down their worry. You simply write down the worry or thought on a piece of paper, fold it up, and put it inside the jar, rather than throwing it away. This may be more appropriate for a child whose thoughts and worries need validating, rather than binning.

Finally, one option for recurring nightmares is to create an alternative ending to the nightmare. One family I worked with had a child who was having recurrent nightmares about the family house burning down. What had an almost immediate positive impact was talking to her about how the dream was happening inside her head, and therefore she could change the ending. She liked unicorns and rainbows, and so her parents and I discussed how they would help her imagine (during wakefulness) that the smoke was in fact cotton candy/candyfloss, and the flames were actually rainbows that you could slide down and land on the back of a unicorn. It worked instantly.

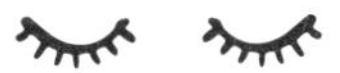

Night terrors

Night terrors are alarming, loud and disruptive nocturnal events that occur during deep sleep (you're more likely to see these in the first half of your child's sleep). They occur in about 5 percent of children, are often genetic, and they usually make their first noisy appearance around the preschool age.[1] Children may thrash around, sit up, shout, scream, and talk nonsense. They may also sweat, pant and have a rapid heartrate. It's common for them to yell certain phrases, such as 'stop it', 'don't do that', 'get off' and so on. This leads a lot of parents to worry that their child has been frightened by something during the day. The good news is that night terrors are not a sign of psychological disturbance. One of the defining characteristics of a night terror is that children usually have absolutely no recollection of the episode the next day. During the terror, they may have their eyes open, but they are often completely unaware of what's going on. I know they look horrendous, but you really don't need to worry. Just be there for your child, and make sure they don't hurt themselves by getting out of bed and wandering around. There is no need to try to wake them: in fact, this can make them very irritable when they *do* wake.

Night terrors are also more common at times of excessive fatigue. Since they occur during deep sleep, and we get more rebound deep sleep with excessive fatigue, they can be more likely if your child is a little low on sleep. They are also more common at times of stress, disruption or a big change. You may be more likely to see sleep terrors if your child is unwell, or has another type of sleep disorder such as sleep apnoea. Finally, they seem to be more common when a child is beginning to learn how to hold their bladder overnight. I run into many families whose child starts having terrors when they are just on the cusp of being able to stop wearing nappies. One option is to lift them to the toilet for a 'dream wee'. I must stress that this is generally not a recommended approach to potty learning, but if it stops a pattern of predictable and distressing night terrors then you at least know that the terror is due to the potty learning process. It may be worth reducing fluids before bedtime if this keeps happening.

Confusional arousal

This is another type of sleep behaviour that I call the timid little sibling of the night terror! They are more common, and seem to affect almost 20 percent of 3–13-year-olds.[2] However, because they are less alarming, it is likely that far more children experience them, but just never bring it to the attention of a medical professional. They also occur during deep sleep, so like the terrors, you are most likely to see them at the beginning of the night, but usually they are less loud and scary.

Children will commonly sit up, look slightly baffled, and say really strange and nonsensical things. My youngest daughter was very prone to both terrors and confusional arousals, and I've lost count of the bizarre and frankly humourous things she has said in her sleep. She once said 'I don't like the circles, they make the numbers go funny'. Another time she said: 'I hate the blue bunny'. We've never had a blue bunny, I hasten to add....

Lastly, some children are frightened of the dark (frankly, some adults are too!). This fear often appears for the first time in the toddler years, but it can come on at any age and is particularly common when children's imaginations start to run wild. Children can imagine frightening objects or scenes when there is no light to dispel those fears. Of course, the light has to be right though. Some lights can cast eerie shadows that are even worse than full darkness. Some nightlights can be stimulating or scary. I have seen lava lamps that look scary in the night! Most artificial light is on the 'blue' end of the light spectrum, and this will inhibit melatonin production, so you'll want to aim for a red-light nightlight to avoid this problem.

You could try experimenting with turning different lights on – perhaps there is a landing light, bathroom light, or a light in another room that could cast a small amount of light into your child's room to prevent it from being pitch black. You could always turn this light off once they have fallen asleep if it bothers other people, or you find that your child wakes early because of the light.

Head-banging

This is a type of rhythmic, repetitive movement that up to a quarter of children under one engage in. The prevalence of head banging or other body rocking movements tends to decrease as children get older and

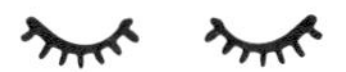

these behaviours are not usually anything to worry about. Head-banging and body rocking movements seem to be most common as children drift off to sleep, and are thought to be a primitive form of self-soothing.

If your child only ever bangs their head as they are going to sleep, it is almost certainly nothing to worry about, and will probably go away spontaneously. Head-banging is something that toddlers occasionally do when they are bored, angry or frustrated during the day, and the way in which we manage this is important, as sometimes the way we handle it can reinforce the behaviour. Head-banging can be worrying for parents, especially if your child bangs their head on the floor and gives themselves a bruise. Try if you can to use your emotion coaching strategies and offer your child an alternative place to bang their head, such as a cushion. Drawing attention to it may make it worse. It's a totally understandable reaction to react with immediacy, alarm or even panic when your child whacks their head on a wooden floor. Rest assured though; while alarming, they do not usually inflict anything more than a bruise on themselves. If you are concerned about head banging, please discuss this with your doctor, who will be able to advise on the best referral for more support if it is needed. If your child also has a neurodevelopmental condition or developmental delay, they are more likely to head-bang,[3] but head-banging in and of itself does not indicate that your child is developing atypically.[4]

Sleepwalking and talking

If you've ever thought your child was peacefully asleep, only to hear them crashing around, or even walking right up to you, it can be a pretty surprising experience! Sleepwalking is pretty common,[5] in fact, one study found that 15% of 5–12-year-old children have sleepwalked at least once and the chances of it happening increase if both parents sleepwalk.[6] There are two main concerns with sleepwalking – safety and inappropriate behaviours. Although uncommon, some children crash into furniture, fall, or injure themselves. I knew one girl who managed to break her arm during a sleepwalking episode. I knew a little boy who used to urinate in his mother's handbag. Rather frustratingly, this happened a number of times, and required a lot of new handbags...

Clearly, the main action if you have a sleepwalking child is to try to make the room safe. Consider the following:

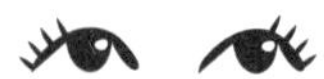

- Use a stairgate to stop them falling downstairs.
- Make sure doors and windows are shut, or have safety catches.
- Clear a space around your child's bed, so they have a clear passage to the door.
- Consider using a baby monitor if your child does this frequently, so you have a chance of hearing when they get up.
- Hang a little bell on their door so you can hear when they open it.
- Ensure furniture is secure and not likely to be tipped over if pulled or climbed on.
- Try stirring your child about 15–20 minutes before they usually sleepwalk. Clearly this is only a useful trick if the episodes generally occur at the same sort of time. If there is some variability, stir them just before the earliest time they usually sleepwalk. You don't need to fully awaken them, just rouse them enough so that you see their breathing change, or they make some movement or noise.
- Don't wake them, just guide them back to bed. Like the night terrors and other deep sleep parasomnias, your child will have no recollection of this the next day.
- Like night terrors and confusional arousals, sleepwalking is associated with sleep routine disruption, excessive fatigue, stress, and illness, so try to maintain a regular bedtime routine and good sleep hygiene.

In many ways, it is helpful that sleepwalking tends to occur at the beginning of the night, when there is a chance you are still awake unless you've had an early night. If you are concerned about your child's sleepwalking, unsure whether it is sleepwalking or another problem, or they have other sleep-related concerns, please make an appointment with your child's doctor.

Sleep-talking is very common, and pretty self-explanatory. The main difference between this and confusional arousals is that while a child may mumble incoherently during a confusional arousal, they may say relatively sensible things when sleep-talking. My father apparently used to play games of Monopoly in his sleep! Your child may be amused the next day if you tell them what they said, but they will have no recollection of talking in the night.

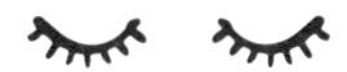

Bedwetting

Children achieve nighttime dryness at different rates. There are many approaches to potty learning – from elimination communication, to using reusable/cloth nappies, using disposable nappies and the choice of whether to use pull-ups or training pants. The purpose of this section is not to evaluate various approaches to potty learning but to help parents manage bedwetting.

Bedwetting, or nocturnal enuresis, usually decreases by age. A formal diagnosis is not usually made until after a child's seventh birthday, since it is so common in young children. It can, however, be very distressing as well as embarrassing and inconvenient for older children, who may feel unable to stay overnight at friends' houses or go on residential school trips. Enuresis can occur after a period of nighttime dryness, or it may be that a child has never been dry at night. Children with enuresis do not wake up with bladder fullness, and also do not control the flow of urine during sleep. They may wake up wet, cold and uncomfortable.

There are many reasons why some children wet the bed, including:

- Differing rates of developmental maturity. Usually, with age, children begin to control their bladder. As children get older, they begin to release a hormone called vasopressin which reduces urine production. This hormone is circadian linked – it's actually pretty clever if you think about it for there to be a mechanism by which we don't make as much urine overnight. However, some children seem to produce less vasopressin,[7] and occasionally are prescribed it by a doctor if the enuresis is persistent.
- Children with developmental delay or neurodevelopmental disorder can take longer to achieve nighttime dryness.
- If children are excessively tired, they may have more deep sleep, which is harder to be roused from. They are thus more likely to wet the bed. This is also more likely if they have a sleep disorder which reduces the quality of their sleep, such as sleep apnoea.
- Some children have very small bladders, or a malformation of the urinary tract.[8] They may also have a urine infection (whether acute or chronic).
- Enuresis is strongly associated with constipation. Impacted faeces press on the bladder, reducing the capacity and causing the bladder to

void more often.

- While wetting the bed is not a psychological or psychiatric condition, it is more common during times of stress, upheaval or distress, or if these events occurred early in a child's life.[9]
- There is a significant association between allergy[10] and other atopic diseases such as asthma and eczema.[11] The mechanism for this association has not been conclusively proven, but it is hypothesised that the bladder may be irritated by a foreign protein. It might be worth keeping a food and bedwetting journal to see if a pattern emerges.

Bedwetting can be especially tiresome as it can go on for years. It's frustrating for children, and also for parents. Here are some tips:

- Avoid caffeine: tea, coffee, cola, energy/sports recovery drinks, chocolate and cocoa-containing foods such as brownies, chocolate cake and so on.
- Maximise your child's fluid intake in the day, but then restrict fluids two hours before bedtime.
- Keep a bedwetting and food diary to see if there is an obvious trigger, such as types of food, or volume of liquid.
- I know it's frustrating and the extra laundry can be brutal, but try not to punish or shame children for wetting the bed. It's hard to be patient at 2am if your child comes through to tell you they have wet the bed, but making them feel bad is unlikely to help.
- I would also avoid the use of sticker charts for dryness, since this is something your child cannot help, so this strategy may make them feel worse.
- Try lifting your child to the toilet at your bedtime (sometimes called a 'dream wee'). This is not a great long-term strategy, as it won't actually help your child learn to hold their bladder. However, it may be useful if, for example, you know your child has had a lot to drink, has eaten something you know makes them pee in the night, or if they are unusually tired.
- Ensure your child does actually go to the toilet before bed (some children say they have when asked, but don't actually urinate, or get to the bathroom and then forget to go!).

- Ensure your child has a good diet, is not constipated, and takes plenty of exercise.
- Try getting your child to sit on the toilet and urinate, then stand up, pause for a moment, and then sit down and try again, in case they have not completely emptied their bladder.
- From a pragmatic point of view, waterproof sheets are essential! Try layering your sheets so that you only have to strip off the sheet and waterproof sheet, and the clean sheets are ready underneath.
- You may wish to use pull-ups when travelling or during a phase that presents additional stress.
- Take your child to their doctor to make sure they do not have a urine infection. Some children may be prescribed vasopressin, and others may have success with a pad which detects moisture and sounds an alarm. Over time, this can train a child to wake up to use the toilet, rather than sleeping through urinating.

If your child is older, bedwetting can be really crippling socially, but the good news is that although some of the treatments for enuresis can take a long time, they are usually effective, so please do ask for help for your child.

Tooth-grinding (bruxism)

Tooth-grinding and jaw-clenching in the night can be remarkably common, and the noise it makes is particularly unpleasant to anyone listening! It may not cause any problems, despite the sound, but it is worth asking your child's dentist to check their teeth to make sure that the teeth are not being ground down – which can eventually happen if bruxism continues for a long time. It is not clear how common tooth-grinding is, as there are no universally agreed diagnostic criteria, but some dentists suggest that if it has been occurring for 3–5 nights per week, for more than six months, and there is facial pain or wear on the teeth, then the child probably has a diagnosis of sleep bruxism.[12]

Bruxism is associated with allergy, anxiety, teeth-crowding and dental malocclusion (overlapping teeth). Certain conditions – such as attention deficit hyperactivity disorder (ADHD), autism spectrum disorder and Down's syndrome seem to be associated with high rates of tooth-grinding. Finally, bruxism is more common alongside conditions like

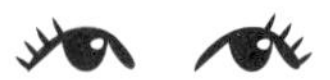

sleep apnoea, so have a listen for strange noises during breathing and mention this to your child's doctor.[13]

Bruxism may also cause headaches, jaw pain and sensitive teeth – which very young children may have trouble articulating. You may need to watch for other signs that they have facial or head pain, such as head-banging, rubbing their jaw, pulling their ears, or refusing to eat.

Sometimes changing your child's sleep position if you hear them grinding their teeth may be enough to stop the behaviour at the time, or if your child does end up wearing down the enamel on their teeth, their dentist may fit them for a mouth guard to prevent further damage.

The red flags

While you may want to run any of the parasomnias past your usual doctor, there are some conditions that do definitely need to be checked out. These include:

- Strange movements in the night – including jerking, twitching, and excessive limb movements.
- Snoring
- Mouth-breathing
- Pauses in breathing
- Noisy breathing
- Night sweats
- Anything you are worried about

Remember, as the parent of your child, you are their expert. If something doesn't feel, look, sound or smell right, then get it checked out. As a paediatric nurse, I had a very brief spell in the paediatric emergency department. Every child who came through the department had their reason for attendance recorded. One of the recording codes we used was 'parental concern'. It's absolutely appropriate to seek medical advice if you're worried, even if you can't articulate the reason for your concern.

Restless leg syndrome (RLS) and periodic limb movement disorder (PLMD)

RLS and PLMD may occur in 2–4 percent of children, though it is likely that this is an under-diagnosis, because not every child is seen by a

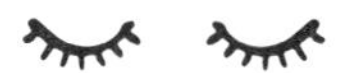

doctor and officially diagnosed. The rates of these movement disorders are higher in children with attention deficit hyperactivity disorder (ADHD), and it appears that the disorders may also be genetic. Both conditions involve an urge to move a limb or limbs and can really disrupt sleep. They are often worse after inactivity, and also associated with iron deficiency, particularly if your child's ferritin is low. Ferritin is a marker of long-term iron stores, and while not all anaemic children have RLS or PLMD, many children with these conditions are found to have low ferritin. In these cases, prescription iron supplementation can help.[14]

Both of my children were wriggly in their sleep, but the difference between the one with PLMD and the one who was just wriggly, was that my wriggler was wriggly all day. The child with PLMD wasn't especially wriggly, but every night would moan and flail in her bed, and in the morning it looked like she'd had a fight with her duvet. Iron supplementation stopped this completely within two months.

If you're not sure whether the movement you see your child making is just them being wriggly, or something else, then please ask your doctor. Your job is to be your child's parent, not to diagnose them. It's really helpful for your doctor if you can videotape the movement. I worked with one family who used an outdoor animal camera that they relocated indoors to capture footage of their child squirming in the night! Other families use a video monitor, or sit by their child's bed with their phone if it happens at a predictable time.

Snoring, noisy breathing, mouth-breathing and sleep apnoea

This section is one that comes with an almost blanket recommendation to seek medical support. The only exception is a child who mouth-breathes or snores only during a cold/flu. It's normal to mouth-breathe when your nose is blocked, but if your child commonly mouth-breathes, or snores, definitely get it checked.[15] Pauses in breathing should always be checked by a doctor – your child will probably be referred to an ear, nose and throat (ENT) doctor to check for causes, such as large tonsils and/or adenoids.[16] Sleep apnoea is a condition where someone (adult or child) experiences pauses in breathing or shallow breathing that last from 30 seconds to several minutes. These episodes may occur 5–30 times per hour. Sleep apnoea is more common in overweight children, black children, children with large tonsils or adenoids and children with

Down's syndrome. It is characterised by the following features:

- Mouth-breathing and snoring
- Daytime sleepiness and irritability
- Bedwetting
- Intermittent airway collapse
- Gasping
- Turning blue at night due to decreased blood oxygen saturation
- Poor school performance
- Hyperactivity (caused by poor-quality sleep)
- Nighttime waking
- Faltering growth

It's pretty obvious that this is one of those conditions where you can't try home remedies. You'll want to make an appointment, and it is really useful for your doctor if you have a video. Don't worry too much if the picture quality is poor in the dark – it's the sound your child makes when they are sleeping that is really helpful in guiding the right referral. The current guidelines[17] recommend referral to an ENT specialist, and possible sleep study to confirm sleep apnoea.

If your child is diagnosed with sleep apnoea, they may have it further classified as central sleep apnoea, obstructive sleep apnoea, or complex sleep apnoea. They may be referred for adenotonsillectomy, and if that doesn't work, some children may need to wear a continuous positive airway pressure (CPAP) mask. This is a non-invasive form of ventilation also used in intensive care for preterm neonates. It maintains a constant stream of air into the airway which forces the airway to remain open. You know how hard it is to initially blow up a balloon, but once there is some air in the balloon, it gets much easier? This is a little like the way CPAP works.

Not all children with sleep-disordered breathing are diagnosed with sleep apnoea. Like so many conditions, there is a spectrum of severity, with mild snoring at one end, and severe sleep apnoea on the other end. Your child will need to be diagnosed properly to get the right treatment.

Night sweats

Night sweats in the absence of environmental temperature change are

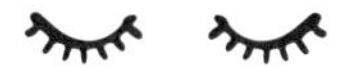

relatively common, more common in boys, and may not suggest anything other than a particularly vivid or scary dream. However, they are associated with other conditions which is why this symptom probably needs to be checked out. Night sweats are more common in children with asthma, eczema, allergy, sinusitis and other allergic diseases, as well as respiratory illnesses. They are also more common in children who have hyperactivity disorders.[18] Finally, they are associated with obstructive sleep apnoea, so have a listen for snoring, mouth-breathing or other strange noises. There are some more unusual causes of night sweats as well, but your child's doctor will be best placed to assess the whole picture and run any tests or make any referrals they need.

Illness and sleep

It's unfortunately a fact of life that children get sick. You've almost certainly by this point spent a few nights sitting up with a snotty or coughing child. Some people reading this will have a child who has been more seriously unwell, or who has a chronic condition or disability. There's no doubt that illness affects sleep. Respiratory illnesses, including coughs, colds, croup, and chest infections, are especially notorious for ruining a few nights' sleep. Having a blocked nose, dry mouth, cough, sore throat, headache or painful ears is very disruptive to sleep for obvious reasons. I wish I could give you a solution to manage these situations so that they do not disrupt sleep, but honestly, meeting your child's needs, accepting several days of sleep disruption, and then getting back to normal when you can is really all you can do.

Chronic conditions are more difficult to manage in many ways, not least because your child may not 'get over it' in the same way that they recover from tonsillitis. While children with a chronic condition are sometimes managed so well that they don't become acutely unstable, it will be something that is in the background of your child's life. Some of the most common chronic conditions include asthma, eczema, diabetes, cerebral palsy, sickle cell anaemia, cystic fibrosis, epilepsy and allergy.[19]

Supporting children with chronic illness is also complex because it involves all the family. Siblings as well as parents are affected, and all this can cause stress and difficulty. Some general suggestions of practices that are associated with better outcomes in chronic illness include:[20]

- A high warmth, low criticism environment. This is generic advice, but it is found that in homes where there is more warmth and less criticism in general, children's health outcomes are better.
- A collaborative approach to supporting the child's involvement with the illness management. This needs to be age appropriate – so a two-year-old with diabetes needs a lot more help to manage the diet, insulin and monitoring regime than a nine-year-old with multiple food allergies, but both children will need parental support.
- Help children understand that they are not alone and that keeping them well is a shared responsibility. Sometimes, as children get older, we give them more responsibility for managing their illness, but research has shown that this may lead to poorer outcomes, including lower levels of self-care by children.
- Establish an attitude of teamwork, which helps children feel like the burden of illness and care is not all on them.
- Provide a helpful family environment, including modelling good selfcare, healthy eating and exercise.

Of course, the other problem with illness is that it tends to invade other areas of life, such as self-esteem, social relationships, and family functioning and stress. Frequent hospital trips or admission to hospital can be worrying, boring, expensive, disruptive, triggering and frustrating – sometimes all at the same time. If you, your child, or your family is struggling with any of these aspects, then please ask your child's healthcare team for more support. It may be that you are eligible for more help, financial assistance, adaptations or psychological support that might make life easier.

Both chronic and acute illness, as well as some disabilities, can affect sleep. Rather than provide highly specific ideas for certain conditions, this is a collection of ideas from my experience as a children's nurse, sleep coach, and mother of a childhood cancer survivor:

- Accept the fact that your child may need you more during periods of illness or instability. Letting go of the expectation that their sleep should remain unaffected will free you from unnecessary additional frustration.
- Make sure with your doctor that your child is on all the right

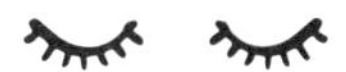

medication. If they are itchy, uncomfortable or in pain, they definitely won't sleep as well.

- Stick to your family routines as much as you can. Even if you are in hospital, negotiate with the nurses looking after you to avoid disrupting your child's usual patterns. Not all procedures can wait, but you'd be surprised how many things can work around you if you communicate your preferences.
- Remember your own self-care. If you are worrying about and caring for a child who is unwell or complex to care for, this can take a massive toll on you. Make sure you have people you can talk to, activities you find relaxing, and support from professionals as well as friends, family and your co-parent.
- Include any other children you have just as much as the child with an illness or condition. Siblings are often affected almost as much as parents, and can experience feelings of jealousy, anxiety, loneliness and frustration.
- Try to do as many 'normal' things as you can so that life is not all about managing illness. Obviously this depends a lot on exactly what you have going on, and your child's condition, but staying positive, and keeping normal activities going, is important for everyone's mental health.
- Organise respite care if you're exhausted. Exhaustion takes many forms – it can be physical fatigue, of course. But it can also include emotional fatigue, fatigue from being asked the same questions and constant medical procedures and interruptions to normality. Fatigue can also come from being in different environments and having to adapt our patterns of normal. So, even if your child is sleeping well, you may need a break to just do something normal. I remember someone – I actually can't even remember who – coming to relieve me in hospital when my daughter was awaiting the news of whether her cancer had relapsed (it hadn't by the way!). I felt like I should be with her constantly, but actually, the stress of the situation made me snappy and irritable and I was probably not helping her anyway. Driving home enabled me to cry in private (I didn't want to show my then five-year-old how worried I was) and have a bath in peace. Make sure you take care of yourself – you cannot pour from an empty cup.

In a general sense, trying to stay as healthy as you can, as far as that is in your control, is likely to help sleep to be optimised. This includes mental health as well as physical and emotional health. Not allowing illness to fully control your life is a discipline in many ways. You cannot always control whether illness or medical complexity happens, but you can choose how you react to it, and what structures and supports you build around your family when it happens. You can choose:

- Your diet
- Exercise options
- Your own sleep hygiene
- The way you think about your situation
- The support and offers of help you ask for and accept
- Your friends
- What hobbies are helpful
- Your self-care options

Finally, you can choose to be grounded in the present. Anxiety and worry are future-orientated, as opposed to fear, which is a response to an immediate threat.[21] Worrying about the what-ifs can reduce your energy levels and rob you of living in the moment. Many people use meditation, guided relaxations, yoga or pilates, journalling, mindfulness, or positive affirmations to get them through these stressful times.

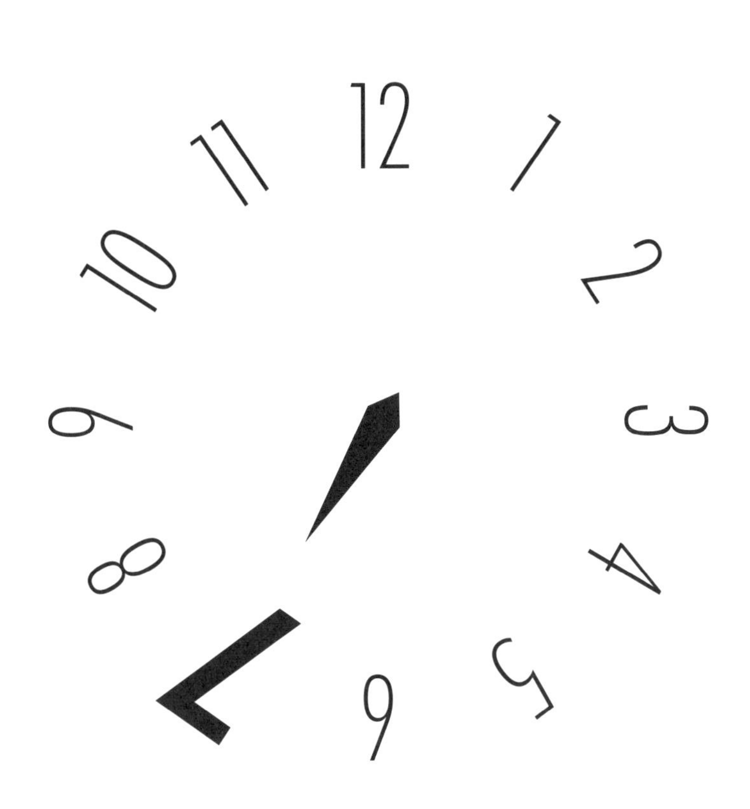

CHAPTER SEVEN

BIG CHANGES, BIG DEALS

Being sleep deprived is never much fun, but when there are situational stresses and big changes, it can feel like sleep is the straw that breaks the camel's back (in this case, yours). Sometimes stressful events such as relationship breakdown, house moves, and illness can worsen sleep. Other times, they are not necessarily the cause of the sleep drama, but merely in addition to sleep fragmentation and deprivation.

I can't possibly know what your exact situation is. Our lives are busy, complex and sometimes messy.

But I probably know what the overarching problem that all difficult situations have in common is, and that's why these tips will apply to you even if I don't mention the exact scenario you're facing. You see, what all situational challenges have in common is *stress*. Of course, the thing that would really help when you have a lot on your plate is a good night's sleep! Which may be the one thing that you can't make happen. But the truth is, a lot of people come at this problem from the wrong way around. Many people focus on trying to get their child to sleep, so that they can all calm down a bit. But what if I suggested that you flip this on its head? Instead of trying to get your child to sleep to reduce your stress, try focusing on maintaining calm, to facilitate sleep.

As you know from chapter 3, you can't sleep with your foot on the gas pedal. What I mean by that is that sleep does not occur in a stress state. You probably know that your stress response is always waiting in the background, ready to act if needed during a fight, flight or freeze situation. When the threat or stress passes, your body can stand down,

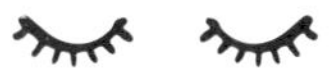

and move into the 'rest and digest' or parasympathetic state. Sleep occurs in the parasympathetic state, and not in the stress state. This makes a lot of sense if you think about it. If you had to run for a bus, escape a scary situation or react to someone being threatening, that is no time for a nap.

The problem is that when we are in a stressful longer-term situation, our stress response can become activated on a more long-term basis. Essentially, our gas pedal is down more than it should be, leaving us feeling wired, on edge, and anxious. It's much harder to calm down, never mind sleep, when we are in this state. This means we will probably not get as much sleep – because feeling stressed can mean that we lie awake worrying. We achieve less good quality sleep – because anxiety can change the state of sleep we achieve and leave us feeling unrefreshed in the morning even if we manage to sleep. But also, the stress response itself is tiring, so we may feel more rundown than usual.

If we add in a child waking up, the situation can reach breaking point, because our reserves at this point are depleted due to poor quality and insufficient sleep.

But how are children affected by these situations? Well, of course children can find stressful situations stressful. But they also pick up on the vibe and the tensions, and they take their cue from those they trust. This is where we can make a positive impact. If you focus on trying to get your child to sleep, you may not manage it, because there are many other factors at play, not least your own stress response, and theirs. Instead, if you shift your priority to trying to calm both you and your child down, you may find that sleep improves without you focusing directly on sleep. At the very least, you may find that your child's sleep stresses you out less.

I can't promise that all your stresses will be gone, but sometimes, knowing what to concentrate our efforts on can reduce unnecessary stress. Focus on the aspects of your child's care that are within your control, and you will be able to let go of factors that are difficult or impossible to change. This can bring some peace and calm in the chaos.

Starting nursery/school

Starting nursery, childcare or school is a major milestone for your child. Not only is this about their cognitive development, but also about relationships, peer interaction, separation from you, making friends, learning about structures and systems, new environments and new boundaries.

Choosing childcare

Rosie Joyce, early years specialist and parent coach

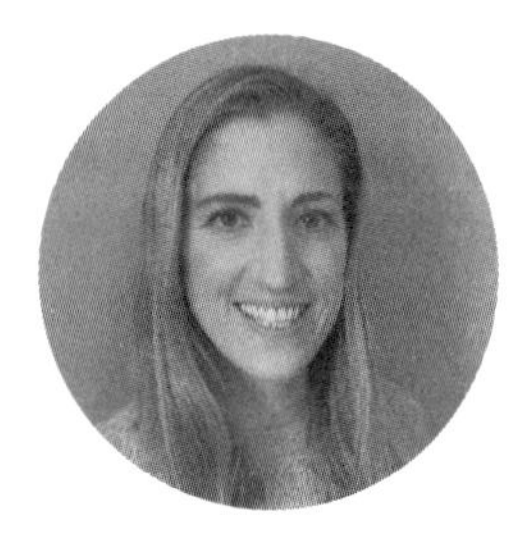

If you have ever chosen a house to buy or rent, you will know that often, what you first think you want is not actually what you need. You may go in to things with a location and price point in mind but rarely are these two things your deciding factors in the end. It is a *feeling*, a culmination of instinct, practicality and alignment. It takes visiting a few places, and realising what you *don't* want, before finding 'the one'.

Why am I talking about houses, when I am here to talk about childcare and school? Because the premise is the same. The decision is huge and once you have spent the time searching, you may find that what you initially thought you wanted is not what you find you need. You would never rely solely on a friend telling you which house to buy, and the same applies to making childcare choices. What *you* feel matters and whom *you* feel connected to will be unique.

Whether you are somebody who is keen to return to work or not, choosing your childcare can become a big event. It is very common for people to put it off until the very last minute, or to feel some level of urgency and sign up to waiting lists for the most 'popular' nursery they have heard of. I urge parents to think differently and go in to things slowly and with less expectation. It is totally acceptable to explain that you are visiting lots of different types of childcare provision. As childcare providers this is music to our ears because we want parents to feel fully confident about their choice from the start. This is always about what is best for your child and only you can decide that.

As I said, location and price are important, but there is a lot more to it. When you visit the different childcare providers, go with an open mind and ask lots of questions. As you collect the different answers you will begin to see clarity and feel a connection to a certain place. Great childcare will be different for everyone and your instinct is valuable so trust it implicitly.

Common concerns when looking for childcare will be around maintaining your child's routines as well as there being a level of continuity with life at home. Remember, your child's routine will change over time and the setting may need to do things differently to home, but it is transparency about this that is key and helps to build trust. A great provider will be fully responsive to your queries and concerns and should reassure you that they understand and will be able to help your family through the transition.

It is very normal to feel mixed emotions before, during and after your child transitions in to childcare. Having made an informed choice you will feel some level of calm and relief, but you may still be worried about the separation, how to maintain connection with your child and how it might change them. All childcare providers will have a system whereby they keep you up to date. This will differ between providers, and depend on how many children they have and the system they use. This is definitely something worth asking about on your first visit.

Separation

It may feel upsetting that your child will be building an attachment to somebody else while you are at work, but actually you can feel proud about facilitating a safe environment for them, enabling them to build this very important skill. Building just one or two strong, secure attachments in the early years will provide a blueprint for your child going forwards, and they will likely find the next transition (e.g. to school) easier. You and your child's key worker will be showing your child how safe they are making transitions, and that leaving one another for periods of time can be positive – and importantly, that you always come back.

In the run up to the transition there are some things you can do to alleviate stress and prepare yourselves.

- Journalling your own thoughts can be incredibly useful in order to get straight in your mind how you are feeling.
- You can create a little book for your child with pictures of their new setting, their key worker, the toys they will enjoy and being collected. Outline each page using simple sentences about what will occur, in a 'first, then, next and finally' type structure and read this together in the week prior to starting.
- Your provider may ask you to provide information for them, but if not, you can do this activity with your child: make a collage with them, sticking down pictures of things, people and places that are important to them. This will help your child feel part of the process and that the people there are interested and want to know all about them. They will feel proud

showing their key worker, and it will give them something to bond over.

The first day

Depending on the age of the child, you may wish to use some of these ideas to help your child feel connected throughout the day.

- If permitted, your child can take a comforter, or scented piece of cloth.
- The invisible string – tie an imaginary string to your child's clothes and one to your clothes in the morning and explain how you will be connected by the string all day long.
- Cuddle button – draw or stitch a 'cuddle button' somewhere. Tell your child when they press the button you will be thinking about giving them a big hug.

Be sure to tell the key worker if you have tried any of these methods in the run-up to the transition so that they can monitor and reinforce your sentiments.

Looking after yourself

During times of change, emotions can feel heightened. Much of this can be anticipation (worrying about what ifs) and therefore we can in some ways start to manifest possible issues. This is very hard to manage but hopefully, if you have done lots of the work mentioned already, you will feel as calm and prepared as you can be.

You will become a container for your child's emotions as they transition to childcare, and as you pass them over to their key worker, their key worker will take on that role. Therefore you must take time to consider yourself in all of this. Expect that this process will leave you feeling emotionally drained whether they settle well or not. If you do not have to rush off to work, make a plan for yourself. If you are taking care of yourself you will be better equipped to manage your child's emotions.

If there are tears at drop-off, it is easy to feel heartbroken. However, to rationalise things for parents, I like to explain my escalator analogy. Both the bottom and the top of the escalator are safe and really fun, but the anticipation as you ride up the escalator can build as you prepare to jump off at just the right time. That moment can be a little wobbly, but once you've made the leap and are safe at the top you can relax. This is exactly what it is like for children in those moments as they are 'passed' between you and their key worker. The first time they ride the escalator (or go to childcare), these feelings of anticipation will feel more intense, but more times they do it, the less wobbly the transition will be.

After the settling period

Once your child seems to be settled in to childcare it is easy to relax and feel relief, but there are a few things still to consider that may crop up and surprise you. As they build resilience in their new life, your child will also be trying to regulate themselves in the new environments in front of new people and manage the energy levels required. There will be new sensory input, new routines and boundaries and new faces to become accustomed to. In response, there will be some level of disturbance from all of this which can reveal itself in the weeks after starting childcare, such as through sleep disturbance, emotional meltdowns or physical outbursts. Again, navigating these periods of change teaches integral life lessons, and it is our responses that matter.

Now is a time to really hone in on your child's basic needs, ensuring your child is fed and watered more often and that they have more rest when possible. This may not always mean sleep, but providing more downtime will help your child feel reconnected and 'filled up'. You can do this through calming or sensory activities, reading, listening to relaxing music and providing lots of touch and affection to fill up what they might be lacking when they are busy in their childcare setting. Cutting back on extracurricular activities or too much interaction for a few weeks is usually helpful. Acknowledging your child's feelings and labelling them, e.g. 'I see that you are feeling very overwhelmed because you have been very busy today', can help your child feel understood and unashamed for their outbursts or deregulation. Holding space for them and showing empathy will really help them through.

Social: @rosie.orchids.and.dandelions
Website: www.orchidsanddandelions.co.uk

New siblings

Expecting a new sibling can be a momentous time for a child as well as you. You might feel worried about how your eldest will feel if another sibling comes along. You may well be anxious about whether you will be able to love your new baby as much as your first. Or have you thought about whether your eldest will even like their new sibling? These fears and thoughts are normal and common.

Many parents worry that the issue of sharing your time, attention and love will be hard for siblings. One thing is for certain: at some point, sibling or no sibling, your child will have to learn to share. They will be okay. As children get older, they are increasingly able to do different and more varied activities. They are also often more willing to play with or be cared for by more people. Of course there will be times that feel chaotic and relentless, with everyone needing you at the same time, and your own needs being shelved in that moment. You will get through it though, and so will your children. They will learn many important lessons that are invaluable for their coping ability, resilience and character.

Another major anxiety is that you cannot love your new baby as much as your older child or children. Not everyone falls in love with their new baby immediately (whether it's your first or your fourth). Bonding is a process that takes time and builds in intensity. You don't have to love your older child less in order to love your new child. Your heart doesn't make room for your new baby, it sort of expands. Although you will love your children the same, you will also love them differently. It's okay to find one of your children difficult in some moments, while the other is relatively easy. It's normal to not *like* your children at some points as well – you're not a bad parent if you feel like this.

And before you worry that your eldest won't like their sibling – here's a spoiler: they will definitely fall out. 100 percent guaranteed. They will fight and squabble and drive you nuts. They will argue over things you couldn't possibly imagine anyone could argue about. They will probably hurt each other at some point. And at the end of the day they will still defend their sibling to the last person standing. That's what siblings do.

Many people tell me they feel guilty about having another baby, that it's almost like they're 'cheating' on their first. But know this: giving your child a sibling is a great thing. It will teach them patience, empathy, and compassion. They will learn to wait, take turns, and

Helping children adjust to a new sibling

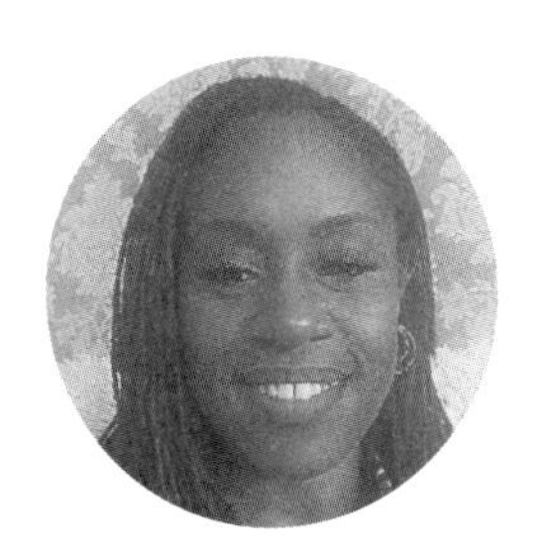

Charmaine Walters, infant sleep educator and night nanny

Helping your toddler get used to a sibling doesn't need to be stressful. While adjusting to a new normal can be tricky, I find toddlers can handle most things well when they are well prepared for them and supported emotionally during the changes.

Put yourself in your toddler's shoes for a moment: You've had your parents' undivided attention your entire life (even a couple of years is still their whole lifetime). You've not had to share your parents' time and attention with anyone. This tiny person comes along and steals the spotlight from you. You're no longer the centre of attention.

How would you feel? How do you behave when you feel sidelined? I feel angry. I can feel jealous. I feel unwanted. My feelings are hurt... but I'm an adult so I can think rationally, know that my feelings are temporary and know that I have not been permanently replaced. A toddler may feel all the above feelings and more. *But* a toddler doesn't have the thinking skills or the verbal skills to understand and communicate those feelings. Those feelings can manifest themselves in temper tantrums, outbursts and misbehaviour instead.

Having worked in early years for over 20 years I've learnt some simple ways you can prepare and support your toddler when the arrival of a sibling is imminent and also for when the baby arrives too.

Before the arrival of the baby

- Talk to your toddler about the new baby. Your toddler may not be able to communicate verbally, but their comprehension surpasses their ability to express themselves with words. Talking to them about the new baby coming will help prep them for when the baby arrives and give you opportunities to help them come to terms with the changes and get an idea of how they might feel about it.
- Take your toddler to your baby scan or appointments if possible – so they can see the baby or hear the heartbeat of the baby.
- Include your toddler in shopping trips to buy items for the baby and allow them to choose some of the items needed.

- Read story books about babies arriving and what happens to help them build a picture. Read these stories repeatedly before the baby comes and once the baby arrives too. Try:
  - *The Berenstain Bears' New Baby* by Stan & Jan Berenstain
  - *What about Adjoa* by Rachel Buabeng
  - *Babies Don't Eat Pizza* by Diana Danzig.
- Allow your toddler to talk to your baby bump and feel the kicks during your pregnancy.
- Point out babies on TV or when out and about. If friends or family members have babies allow your toddler to see and touch the baby. Use words to help your toddler understand that new babies need to be looked after and cared for.

Once your new baby arrives

- Allow your toddler to visit mum and baby in the hospital if having a hospital birth.
- Get a gift for the baby from the toddler and vice versa (get your toddler a toy from the baby) and exchange these gifts as a way to introduce baby and toddler to each other.
- Allow your toddler to help you care for the baby if they're interested in doing so. Simple tasks like fetching the nappy or getting the baby's dummy from another room can help your toddler feel included and important. They love that!
- Schedule some 1-2-1 time with your toddler away from the baby for just you and them and spend quality time together. Even just 15 minutes a day together can make all the difference to your toddler.

The goal is to help your toddler feel a part of the journey. Showing them the role they will play in the baby's life and supporting them emotionally can help smooth the transition to life as an older sibling. Validating their feelings through emotion coaching will help them understand any new feelings that pop up and help to prevent the new emotions from overwhelming them. They may feel jealousy or anger at the arrival of a new baby. These feelings are normal. Label those feelings for your toddler and acknowledge and recognise that change can be hard for them, but that you are there to support them.

Website: www.soundlysleeping.co.uk

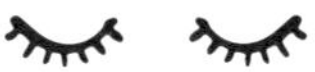

share. They will have a playmate, a comrade and a partner in crime.

Don't feel guilty. Expect number two with excitement. Great (and, also hard, irritating, frustrating and hilarious) things are coming...

Children's mental health

According to global data, 13–23 percent of children and young people have a mental health challenge that they live with.[1] Mental health problems and sleep problems can go hand in hand: mental health problems can cause sleep disturbances such as insomnia, fragmented sleep and poor quality sleep, but sleep problems can also exacerbate mental health problems. Additionally, some of the factors that seem to be associated with mental health problems are also associated with poorer sleep – such as chaotic or irregular family lifestyles.[2]

Children at risk

Unfortunately, some children seem to be at greater risk of suffering from mental health problems, including children who are refugees and children living in poverty, especially when this is associated with widespread problems such as economic recession and unemployment.[3] Other risk factors include high levels of conflict at home,[4] neurodevelopmental disorders,[5] the presence of parental mental health problems, and children with a more 'difficult' temperament.[6]

Trauma and sleep

There are many different classifications of trauma, including interpersonal trauma, domestic violence and community trauma, exposure to natural disasters, chronic trauma, early life trauma and complex trauma. Sleep disturbances are one of the diagnostic criteria of post-traumatic stress disorder (PTSD), although not all trauma-exposed children will develop PTSD.[7] Adverse childhood experiences (ACEs) are not necessarily the same as traumatic events or experiences, but it seems that the more ACEs a child has, the worse they sleep. Other research suggests that the younger the child is when exposed to certain trauma, such as a natural disaster, the worse their sleep problems.[8]

Childhood trauma and ACEs

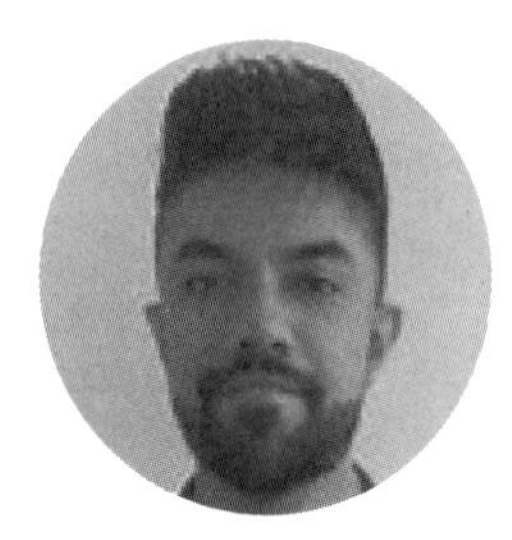

Dr Shafraz Kazia, paediatrician and mental health advocate

The early years lay the foundation for our physical and mental health.[9,10] The brain develops at an explosive rate, forming more than one million connections per second in the first three years of life.[11] Think of it as a complex gadget with wires firing impulses from one circuit to another. What we experience from conception to adulthood literally shapes the trajectory of our health and wellness. This includes our emotions, intellect, personality, learning and even our ability to cope with stressful situations. But what happens to these connections if there is a sudden jolt of electricity that may alter the network in our brain permanently? This is called trauma.

The Substance Abuse and Mental Health Services Administration (SAMHSA) defines trauma as resulting from 'an event, series of events, or set of circumstances that is experienced by an individual as physically or emotionally harmful or life-threatening and that has lasting adverse effects on the individual's functioning and mental, physical, social, emotional, or spiritual well-being.' Back in medical school, the image that came to mind when we heard the word trauma was of broken bones and blood. But what about trauma that seeps into the very matter of our minds, the hidden effects of which we experience in our bodies decades later?

Human babies are the only mammalian species that is entirely dependent on their primary caregiver in the first 1,000 days of life. Neuroscience tells us that 90 percent of brain development happens within the first three years outside the womb, so a child's caregivers help to build their brain's foundations. The optimal ingredient in building a healthy brain is unconditional love. Infants need attention, love, hugs and secure relationships – this promotes healthy brain development, bonding, attachment and positive mental health.

Babies learn how to interact with the rest of the world by observing and mirroring their caregiver's behaviour and facial cues. Powerful research from Romanian orphanages has shown us how the brain can physically shrink in size without love, relational consistency and responsive caregiving.[12] This in turn may have detrimental effects on cognition, learning, memory, sleeping patterns, physical development and infant mental health.

Although babies do not have the ability to lie down on a couch to discuss their feelings with a therapist, infant mental health can be described as 'the young child's capacity to experience, regulate and express emotions, form close and secure relationships and explore the environment and learn'.[13] It is generally difficult for our society to imagine a young child in the room capable of having their own thoughts and we often fail to address the child as a person in their own right.

Imagine not being able to verbalise your feelings, but still being able to read your caregiver's behaviour, especially when it's negative. How would this play out in your behaviour? When babies are clingy, or can't sleep well, we turn to sleep- training, or spend an absurd amount of money trying to fix the situation, when in fact the problems may stem from our own childhood trauma, lack of social support and perhaps marital discord.

What happens to our bodies when we go through trauma? How do we understand it and overcome its effects? In the past two decades, there has been growing evidence of the burden of Adverse Childhood Experiences (ACEs). These are instances of stress and trauma during childhood. The research suggests that exposure to childhood trauma before the age of 18 is associated with negative physical and behavioural health outcomes.[14]

ACEs happen as a result of physical, sexual or emotional abuse or neglect and exposure to chronic environmental stressors such as living in a household affected by domestic violence, caregiver incarceration, substance abuse or parental mental illness. However, there are also many protective factors that may act as a 'cushion'. The research suggests that the risk of health issues increases if you have encountered three or more ACEs in the formative years. Hence, the higher the dose of trauma, the higher the incidence of experiencing negative physical and mental health later in adulthood.

When our brain senses a threat in the environment, our fight, flight or freeze response is activated. The hormones adrenaline and cortisol flood our body, there is increased blood flow to our muscles, our heart rate increases and we may even sweat. We are ready to run away from the threat, although we can sometimes want to fight it or our bodies may freeze.[15]

Science suggests that some amount of stress may be healthy for development, but prolonged exposure to the stress hormone cortisol can lead to toxic stress, when our stress response systems go into overdrive and fail to go back to baseline levels. This can be felt across multiple systems in the body, from weakening the immune system, to causing heart disease, stroke, diabetes, cancer, depression and being highly prone to suicide.

Besides this, trauma can also change the way our DNA is read and translated. The emerging science of epigenetics is revealing how our health is shaped by chemicals that lie on our genes and can act as on and off switches. Thus trauma can trigger both physical and mental illness, especially if we are genetically predisposed to certain diseases. Furthermore, research shows that grandmothers can genetically pass down allergies that are caused by cigarette smoking to the next three generations.[16,17] Trauma can also potentially be passed on to the next generation.[18,19] In addition, pervasive long-term environmental factors such as poverty, systemic oppression, bullying, racial injustice, climate change, homophobia and sexism among others can potentially augment these effects in the body. Research suggests that minorities have suffered these consequences for generations.[20]

Is there a way we can mitigate these negative effects? What if you are now aware that your child has one or more ACEs? In graduate school, I was introduced to how to measure resilience – the ability to bounce back from a negative situation. Sometimes it only takes one adult to alter a situation involving trauma and toxic stress: if they provide a safe and secure environment and teach healthy coping skills, this cultivates resilience and improves the outcome after trauma.[21,22]

I believe that we need to take a public health approach to create awareness about childhood trauma and ACEs. Healing is a daunting journey and early recognition can go a long way. If we want to break the cycle of intergenerational trauma, seeking out practitioners with knowledge of best practice in infant mental health, who can carry out ACEs prevention and screening can be very helpful. Learning about the science behind attachment parenting and healing, and pursuing a healthy relationship with your child can be life-changing. As a society, we need to move away from the traditional model of mental health and accept that our experiences and social determinants of health play a huge part in shaping our overall health.

So is there hope for individuals who live with trauma? Absolutely yes! Children and adults may recover from ACEs by firstly recognising the problem, and then addressing the issue in a holistic manner with the right resources. We can promote better emotional and physical health to overcome ACEs by maintaining supportive relationships, good sleep hygiene, optimal nutrition and even engaging in therapy, spirituality and mindfulness.[23,24] These simple yet effective practices have been scientifically proven to reduce stress hormones and inflammation in the body to diminish the effects of toxic stress. Parents need support now more than ever.

It is never too late to change the way you parent and to be more attuned to your little ones. The journey can be a powerful one that changes our perspective, as we become stronger, wiser and more resilient. That gives us hope for a better future.

How to support mental health

There are several strategies that are proven to be supportive of optimal mental health. This is not to suggest that *not* providing these will lead to mental health problems, or that if you incorporate all of these strategies, you will definitely prevent problems, but they may be areas to consider.

- Good quality diet.[25]
- Positive and consistently supportive family relationships are known to be a great buffer.[26]
- While face-to-face support is considered preferable, not all children meet the criteria for referral into children's mental health services, and when they do, there may be a long waiting list. One alternative that seems to show promise is the use of self-help strategies for anxiety, depression and disruptive behaviour. These include written guides, online study and cognitive behaviour therapy.[27]
- Building parental self-esteem and confidence, and helping parents enjoy parenting.
- Social support structures – both for parents, and also helping children form meaningful friendships.[28]

House moving

Moving house can be exciting. It is also right up there in the top ten most stressful life experiences. It's really common to move house with small children. You might be looking to move to a larger place, so you can spread your wings. Or perhaps you're moving somewhere smaller, to reduce monthly outgoings, or maybe you're going rural to have some more space to run around. Whatever the reason, it is a major upheaval. Whatever benefits there are, there will be some emotional and psychological costs. I am a veteran house mover. I was born into a military family and lost count of the number of times we had moved house by the time I was 20. It was at least 18... As you can imagine, I've picked up some survival tips along the way.

Children's worlds are pretty small. They have limited life experience and their home and their familiar places and faces form part of their metaphorical security blanket. Moving house can really shake up your little one's world. Don't forget, they haven't looked at the pros and cons like you did. They haven't been planning the heck out of this house move for as long as you. They haven't got the same forward-thinking and future-oriented goal-setting ability as you. It's definitely going to be weird for them. But fret not, there are things you do to make this easier.

Whether your child's sleep has deteriorated as a consequence of a stressful life event, like moving house, or it is about the same as ever, and you are struggling more in the context of the situation, there are many small changes you can make.

1. **Try to find ways to create calm.** Try meditation, mindfulness, music, or journalling. Some parents find having a bath with their child calms everyone down. Work on making your environment soothing and relaxing. We are sensory beings, so tap into as many senses as you can. Many people prefer dim lighting, as well as pleasant smells, and reducing the volume of unnecessary background noise. Staying calm in the midst of moving house might take a practical turn, like going and staying with relatives while your partner deals with the worst of it. Or perhaps the children could go on a tactical holiday to Grandma's while you move. Remember to ask for help, accept offers of help, and call in favours. This is no joke – you need all the help you can get.
2. **Maintain connection.** Children who are stressed and not sleeping usually need more connection, not less. Provide plenty of reassurance, and one-to-one time. Keep the connection going through the chaos and your child will not feel as unsettled.
3. **Keep things familiar and safe.** When the environment is necessarily

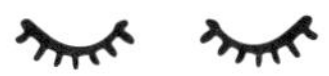

chaotic, such as during a house move, or moving between separated parents, keep familiar routines going, and keep comforting objects or loveys close by. It can also help to have some items of clothing that smell familiar. You can use the same essential oils in a diffuser in a new environment so that your new home smells familiar. You could avoid washing their bedding so that it doesn't smell clean and new. You could put them to bed in the same PJs they wore in the old house.

4. **Keep a bag of essential items nearby.** This might include toys, changing bag, snacks, and crockery and cutlery. Plan your first meal in your new home so that you don't have to cook, and make sure you all have a change of clothes. I can pretty much guarantee that the clothes you want will be hard to find for a few days otherwise!
5. **Reduce small situational stresses.** I'm not saying that you can stop stressful things from being stressful, but try to reduce the total stress load. For example, make sure you have the items you need close by. Keep similar items together. Pack things you know you will need every day in a suitcase so that they are easy to find. Hire packers if you can afford to – it massively reduces the stress of packing things up for several weeks, and reduces the chaos to just 48 hours.

Moving house is super exciting, and as long as you expect a certain level of disruption, your child's sleep will get back on track once you're settled and less stressed.

Fostering and adoption

We become parents by many different, wonderful routes. The reasons for parents choosing to adopt or foster are also many and varied, and I do not pretend to know your situation, and the details of your journey so far. I imagine you've had many months or even years preparing for family life through adoption or fostering. Children who have experienced different, sometimes chaotic, or multiple homes can have additional reasons for their sleep dramas, as well as all the usual ones.

The implications for children's sleep in fostering and adoption placements

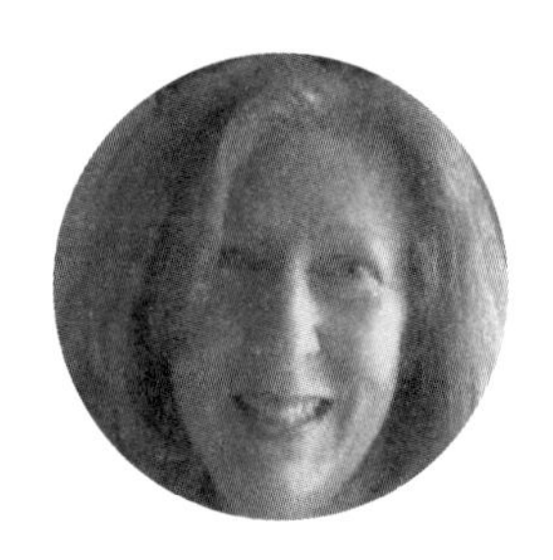

Sheila Franklin, independent social worker, holistic sleep coach

Trigger warning: this passage contains information about child abuse and neglect that some readers might find upsetting

Children who come into foster care and/or are placed for adoption will have had a range of experiences in respect of bedtime, sleep and waking up. They will bring those experiences with them into the foster or adoptive home. Looked-after children may have come from backgrounds that were chaotic, neglectful or abusive. As a result, bedtime and sleep may have become associated with negative experiences. The bedroom may have been used as a punishment, the sleep environment might have been cold and dirty, children might have been punished for wetting the bed or left crying alone for extended periods. For some children, devastatingly, bedtime and nighttime may have been a time when they were most at risk from sexual abuse.

Instead of a warm, safe haven, the bedroom and nighttime may have become a place and time of fear. If bedtime has become associated with feelings of fear and extreme anxiety its approach is likely to leave a child in an alert, hypervigilant state, not the calm drowsy state conducive to falling asleep.

While not all children coming into care will have had negative experiences around bedtime and sleep, bedtime and falling asleep may be a time when those children feel the separation and loss of their birth family most acutely.

Fostered and adopted children might display a range of behaviours in respect of sleep, as a result of trauma and disordered attachment. They might be unable to settle at bedtime, struggle with the separation of going to bed, wake up during the night or very early, experience nightmares and find transitions difficult, including the start of the day when they wake up.

A fundamental part of supporting foster/adopted children with bedtime and sleep issues is to address the underlying causes. 'The Secure Base Model', developed by Gillian Schofield and Mary Beek,[12] can provide foster parents and adoptive parents with a really helpful framework for addressing the anxiety and lack of trust caused by insecure attachments. The Secure Base Model is drawn from attachment theory[29-33] and includes five dimensions of care giving: *availability* which helps the child to trust; *sensitivity* which helps the child to manage their feelings; *acceptance* which builds the child's self-esteem; *cooperation* which helps the child to feel accepted, and *family membership* which helps the child to belong. If foster carers and adoptive parents would like more information on how to use The Secure Base Model, 'Promoting Attachment and Resilience – A guide for foster carers and adopters on using the Secure Base Model'[34] is a valuable resource.

There are many ways foster carers and adoptive parents can encourage and support attachment and the following suggestions are just some of them. Introducing and involving children in the family routines and rituals is an important step in helping them feel as if 'they belong'. It can be really helpful to explain to a child from the beginning how the household works, e.g. a drink and snack when coming in from preschool/school, putting out school clothes the night before, having a story and a drink at bedtime, and so on. It can also be beneficial to find out what the child likes and incorporate some of that, where possible, into the family routine. Having photographs of the child on display, alongside photographs of other children in the family, is another way of promoting that sense of belonging.[35]

Having a regular routine with mealtimes, bedtime and getting up in the morning is really important. Consistency, predictability and reliability enable children to know what to expect and when. Using a calendar, picture chart or social story can help children to predict and anticipate what is going to happen and can help reduce anxiety around transitions.

Some children who have missed out on early nurture can become 'stuck' at an earlier emotional stage, which means they behave as a much younger child would. For these children responding to their emotional age as opposed to their chronological age will help them move through those missed developmental stages. For an older child this might mean having a bedtime routine which might be thought appropriate for a younger child – a warm bath with bubbles, warm towel, cosy pyjamas and dressing gown, a nighttime drink, a cuddle and a story will be of benefit whatever the age of the child.

Bedtime can be a good time to read stories that remind children of being safe and loved as this can be really reassuring. Some older children might regress and want a bottle of milk and a dummy at bedtime, especially if that is part of the nighttime routine for younger children in the household.

While some foster carers and adoptive parents might be worried about the appropriateness of this with older children, it is usually short-lived and it can meet a missed developmental need.

Storytelling, in the context of Life Story Book work, is an important way of helping a child to integrate their past into the present, in order to help them to move into the future. However, more general storytelling can also be really powerful, helping build attachment, as well as helping children learn, talk about and manage emotions. Storytelling involves the process of speaking and listening and provides a natural way of learning about feelings and relationships. Because it is not a one-way process, but an interaction between the storyteller and the listener, storytelling can echo some of the things that take place with healthy attachments, such as eye contact, emotional attunement and turn-taking.[36]

Reading to children boosts educational attainment, but storytelling also provides parents and caregivers with an opportunity to teach children about the world and how to deal with it. Books such as *Owl Babies*, and *Can't You Sleep, Little Bear*, both by Martin Waddell can be invaluable in helping young children begin to explore and name emotions.

Not all children who are adopted or fostered experience abuse, neglect or trauma. Some children have a nurturing early foster care experience. It is certainly not true that all children will bear the weight of negative early life experiences, or that these will be equal for all children. As with so many aspects of development, the ways in which children cope with and respond to their early life experiences may be (to some extent) influenced by genetics, resilience, temperament and other buffering factors. For many children, simple strategies may be enough to help them adjust. However, I want to acknowledge the very real lived experiences of other children who may need more support. Some of these strategies may also be appropriate (with advice from your child's medical and mental health team) for children who have experienced other forms of trauma.

Therapeutic interventions for fostered or adopted children with developmental trauma

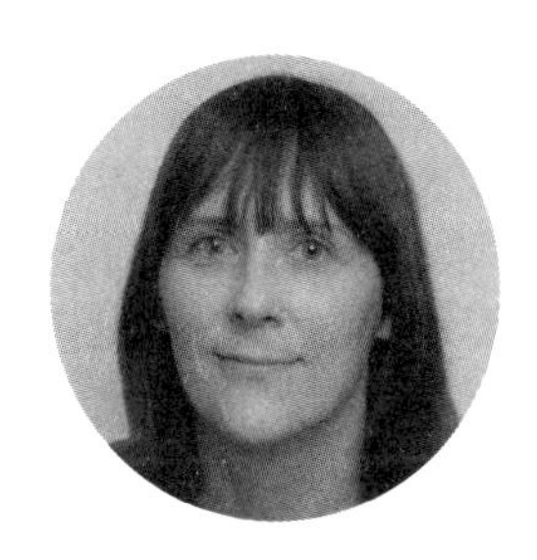

Tessa Scully, paediatric occupational therapist, somatic experiencing practitioner

Children who have experienced developmental trauma often have difficulty with participating in activities of daily living, and as a result sleep is affected. Common issues include insomnia, restless sleep and nightmares.[37]

Developmental trauma is a type of trauma which has occurred in the context of a relationship, over time (not a single event trauma), usually in the context of abuse and/or neglect. This results in 'a biological system which keeps pumping out stress hormones to deal with real or imagined threats leading to physical problems including sleep disturbances'.[38] Stress responses can occur in the womb, and also during the neonatal period, which explains why even children who were subject to a care order from birth can still have trauma and show difficulties with their arousal states and responses to stress. The child may not have a verbal narrative of their experience, but their nervous system and body is still affected.

> *'Trauma is not in the event itself; rather, trauma resides in the nervous system.'*[39]

Children with a trauma history often have a reduced capacity for dealing with stress – their 'window of tolerance' (coping zone) can be far narrower. This means that it takes less stress to trigger them into a survival response such as fight or flight (hyperarousal) or freeze, dissociation or shutdown (hypoarousal). Many children will fluctuate between these states while also remaining hypervigilant – scanning the environment for signs of danger. This is often true at night when they may have had to stay alert in order to stay safe. They also often have fluctuating responses to sensory stimuli and can 'go from being in a heightened state of arousal to collapsing/sleeping. This would indicate over-stimulation has occurred which has then led to shutdown.'[40]

Children who may have been exposed to the same danger may respond differently in terms of their survival responses and attachment strategies (often evident in sibling groups), so be mindful that the same approach will not always work with different individuals.

Holly Van Gulden[41] writes about permanency as a crucial stage of attachment, which is often missing for children who have had inconsistent early parenting experiences. Permanency is the sense of the parent or caregiver still existing when out of sight. As you can imagine, if this is lacking then separation anxiety will be elevated and sleep disturbed.

Many fostered and adopted children have complex needs, with many influences affecting their ability to emotionally regulate and therefore sleep well. In addition to their unique trauma history, other common factors include sensory processing difficulties (this may be associated with traumatic experiences, but is not always due to trauma), neurodevelopmental difficulties and the effects of prenatal alcohol/ substance exposure. Unfortunately, it is not always easy to access support to identify, confirm or rule out these additional factors. However, intervention is more likely to be effective if both the child's trauma and neurodevelopmental issues are understood.[42]

Common reasons for children to have difficulty with sleep at nighttime

- Attachment triggers: fear of separation or fear of further rejection.[43] Early experiences related to nurture and comfort (or lack of) can be triggering.
- Bodily (somatic) symptoms, painful memories which often are recalled at night.
- Anxiety about transitions and upcoming changes, fear of moving to a new home/placement.
- Previous exposure to domestic violence leading to persistent hypervigilance.
- Sensory processing difficulties including hypersensitivity and sensory-seeking patterns.

How children present with sleep-pattern disturbances as a result of early trauma and loss

- Heightened anxiety before contact sessions resulting in not being able to sleep or sleeping too much (shutdown response due to overwhelm).
- Pattern of not sleeping well correlating with school attendance, no

problem sleeping in school holidays or weekends.
- Anxious about novel sounds (hypervigilance and auditory hypersensitive).
- Only being able to sleep if a parent or caregiver is present with them (separation anxiety).

What helps?

The good news is that there are ways to help and support these children. It often involves going back to how you might approach gentle sleep for an infant in terms of being responsive and attuned to their needs, supporting them by reading their cues and helping them to feel safe. Indeed, children who have had limited or inconsistent experiences of early attunement in infancy will continue to have difficulties with recognising and interpreting their own internal body signals (interoception), so will do best when they have an attuned parent or caregiver to support them to make sense of their sensations and feelings.

While these children often thrive on predictability and professionals often encourage a routine, perhaps it is most helpful to consider making a predictable response rather than being wedded to a strict routine, as this may get in the way of responding in a gentle and warm way. This is important if you find yourself becoming stressed because your plan is not working!

Finding ways to regulate yourself as the adult is crucial. Your presence is often your greatest tool: by connecting with and providing a feeling of safety in your child, their survival responses will then reduce. Daniel Siegel writes about the importance of children feeling 'safe, seen, soothed and secure' in *The Power of Showing Up*[44] if you would like to explore these concepts further.

Supporting children to be regulated in their body before bedtime

- Engaging children in activities involving *muscle effort* can have a down-regulating effect. Provide opportunities for physical play involving muscle effort and heavy work such as crawling through a play tunnel (pop-up or Lycra) and hanging from a pull-up bar.[45]
- Regular *one-to-one time* with the adoptive parent or caregiver where your child chooses the game or activity – even 10 minutes of your undivided attention can work wonders.
- Play *games that involve separation* and being 'found', including hide and seek, peekaboo (when this stage has been missed, you will find that even

older children will enjoy this infant game), and pushing toy cars back and forth between you that 'go' and 'come back'.
- *Develop permanency by providing transitional objects* to evoke the sensory memory of you, in order for them to maintain sensory contact with you when apart.
- *Reduce screen time* at least two hours before bed.
- Story massage – this can be a way to *introduce safe and nurturing touch* (for fostered children, your social worker can advise whether this is appropriate for individuals). Always seek permission from the child when touch is involved and be guided by the child's response (some may say yes but appear uncomfortable, which is a sign to stop).
- Draw an outline of a gingerbread man on an A4 or larger piece of paper and ask the child to shade with different colours what they are sensing and feeling in their body. This can be a way to process some of their day before bedtime. They will usually give meaning to different colours, for example, drawing yellow squiggles in the tummy area might mean anxiety. There is no right or wrong way to do this exercise; it works best if you are not suggestive.
- Teach your child to *regulate their heartrate* by placing their hand over their heart, which can be calming (for some). You can do this with them by modelling on yourself and if appropriate, you may put your hand on their heart too.
- Tuck a child in with a top sheet underneath their duvet – this can help some to feel more contained and give the sensory feedback they need to settle for sleep (though this will be too much for some individuals). Some children even benefit from a sensory compression sheet (made of Lycra).

What do families say?

> *'We have a pull up bar in a doorway at home (so our daughter can hold on to the bar and hang by her hands). The nights that we forget to get her to hang from it before bed are the nights we struggle to settle her for sleep. She often seeks this out herself now throughout the day to regulate herself and will remind us too!'*

> *'I often do a squishing game with him, making him into a sandwich with cushions, this helps to calm him enough to be*

ready for bed. He also replicates this by the number of soft toys he likes to burrow under to sleep with.'

'Introducing reflexology via the story book helped her to start to accept comfort from me, now she will seek out a hug.'

'Doing a gingerbread picture before bedtime with me helped both of us to identify the feelings he was having and the nightly tummy aches went away once he got it out on paper.'

Tools and books to read with your child

- *The Scared Gang*[46] helps your child to understand survival behaviours via the different characters, learn about sensory-based activities and foods to support regulation.
- *The Invisible String*[47] introduces the concept of being 'held in mind' and not forgotten, promoting connection for your child when they are not with you.
- *Once Upon A Touch*[48] introduces massage via story. Children engage well and often generate their own ideas too.
- *The Mouse's House*[49] introduces reflexology for calming children at bedtime via story.

Holly Van Gulden also has a series of short clips on YouTube which explain concepts of permanency and related themes. Look for the CoramBAAF Adoption and Fostering Academy Channel.

There are some excellent resources for understanding the needs of children affected by prenatal alcohol exposure at www.nationalfasd.org.uk

Consult an occupational therapist for guidance about addressing tactile sensitivities and for safe guidelines on use of other tools you may have heard about such as weighted blankets. If your child has experienced trauma and you suspect there are sensory processing difficulties, seek support from an occupational therapist who has knowledge of working in a trauma-informed way and has ideally trained in Sensory Attachment Intervention. Your child's sensory, attachment and arousal patterns can then be profiled and bespoke guidance given on how to provide an enriched environment. For more information see www.sensoryattachmentintervention.com

Conflict between parents about breastfeeding (or another aspect of parenting)

I have a number of conversations every year with parents who are seeking sleep support, but the real issue is a breast/chest-feeding debate between parents, or close family members. Occasionally the issue is bedsharing, or a broader objection to gentle parenting in general. This is a tricky issue to navigate, and requires a fair bit of open-mindedness and honesty. It's not all that uncommon to find that two parents have different views on parenting, bedsharing and breastfeeding beyond infancy. I think it is worth trying to work out what the underlying issues are.

Difficulty adjusting to the reality of the changes in relationships after having children can be a major reason for conflict. Sometimes it is easier (or just different) for the breastfeeding mother or birthing parent to adjust to and accommodate the changes. Some fathers or partners who return to work soon after the birth of their child have less time to process these changes. For those who don't have a chance to adjust, some have told me they can feel sad and confused that a major, life-changing event just happened, but they have to get up and go to work, just like they do every day. There has been a seismic shift in the dynamics, and yet without time to process that, some partners can feel bewildered.

Your partner may have postnatal depression. This can lead to negative or anxious thoughts, as well as an inability to see the positives. Partners can experience birth trauma as well, or your partner may be struggling with their own self-esteem, as Mark Williams explains on the next page.

"It's not all that uncommon to find that two parents have different views on parenting, bedsharing and breastfeeding beyond infancy. I think it is worth trying to work out what the underlying issues are."

Fathers' mental health matters too

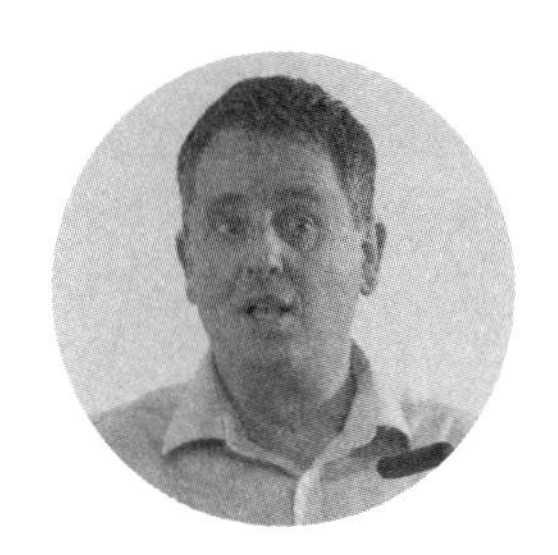

Mark Williams, author, TEDx speaker and mental health advocate

With the biggest killer in men in the UK being suicide, and new fathers being up to 47 times more at risk, it's important to include fathers in perinatal mental health services. The evidence shows that one in ten fathers suffer postnatal depression, with professionals feeling that this is an under-reported figure due to men not seeking help thanks to continued stigma. We also know that up to 50 percent of people looking after a partner with postnatal depression also suffer depression.

Due to a lack of screening, fathers may hit crisis point some time after the postnatal period. Therefore, they are often diagnosed with generalised anxiety and depression, but the root cause is not always identified.

It has been reported that 39 percent of new fathers are in need of support (Mental Health Foundation, 2018). One in five are socially isolated and lose close friends in the first year of fatherhood (Movember, 2019) and 73 percent are more concerned about their partner's mental health (NCT, 2015).

How and why men and fathers may be affected by birth trauma

PTSD is an anxiety disorder that occurs after either witnessing or experiencing a life-threatening event. Common symptoms are nightmares and flashbacks, as well as anxiety, hypervigilance, re-experiencing of symptoms and physiological stress. If fathers go on to have more children, their antenatal anxiety can increase as they worry about witnessing the trauma once again.

Sometimes fathers or birthing partners witness more trauma than the mother or birthing person and a lack of communication and understanding in the labour ward can be a concern. Situations such as the loss of a child, birth complications and neonatal admission can increase these anxieties.

PTSD and postnatal depression symptoms can overlap, so it's important to find out what the parents' concerns were during the birth to get the right treatment. For more information, The Birth Trauma Association for partners is a really helpful organisation.

How mental health challenges may affect the experience of fatherhood

Mental health challenges can impact relationships and the father's mental health if no support is in place. Also, some research finds that when fathers are suffering they may use negative coping skills like alcohol, substance abuse, and comfort eating. All these situations can impact on children. Early prevention and support can lower rates of Adverse Childhood Experiences (ACEs). It's important that parents are fully aware of their own childhood trauma and understand what they have gone through themselves in order to break the cycle.

Many fathers have undiagnosed challenges – such as a history of anxiety, depression, and trauma before becoming a parent, which they have self-managed. The lack of sleep can negatively impact on parents' mental health, and reduce their capacity to cope. We now know testosterone levels are lower during this time and new fathers have similar experiences to mothers of feeling 'not good enough'. With fatherhood changing in recent times with more stay-at-home fathers, same-sex parents and single fathers, many services have not changed with the times – which of course can make these issues even more challenging.

How co-parents can spot mental health problems and how they can help

It's important to invite and maintain an open dialogue about each other's mental health. As men tend to suppress their feelings, mental health problems often manifest themselves in changes in their behaviour. Ask yourself if he was like this before you had children – if not, this may be a sign that he needs support.

Sometimes a father may avoid sex as he does not want his partner to conceive and have another baby, because they may go through similar trauma again. Again, having an empathic and compassionate approach can help to air these buried thoughts, find resolution, and avoid conflict in the relationship.

How men and fathers can support themselves

Education and awareness are important so that men can get the right help. There is now a lot more information available about paternal mental health and mental health awareness. Good diet, exercise, mindfulness, cognitive behaviour therapy (CBT) and connection to combat isolation are all helpful. Most importantly, men being able to be open about how they are feeling to family members and friends, and not being afraid to have a conversation with health professionals, is key to getting the right help. Being overwhelmed can lead to extreme stress and cause anxiety, so it is important to focus on what's really important. This is likely to have far better outcomes for the family and the development of the child.

Resources and sources of support

With NHS England now screening fathers to check if they have postnatal depression, more organisations are also using a family approach.

There are national mental health organisations contactable through NHS helplines.

- Hope of Hub is a database of local services in your area searchable using your postcode.
- Dad Matters UK is one the leading organisations that helps fathers gain confidence and support through antenatal groups.

Sometimes the underlying reason for conflict in certain areas such as breastfeeding or bedsharing is a lack of intimacy. The continued presence of breastfeeding in family life can unwittingly serve as a bitter reminder that all the intimacy is reserved for a child, and not a partner. This can be particularly difficult if your partner's love language is touch, and you are more than a little 'touched out'. A common scenario is where one partner is so overwhelmingly touched out that they don't even want to hug their partner, never mind have sex with them. This can be hurtful and confusing for the partner who may feel rejected, unattractive, jealous and left out. It can be hard to understand why a back rub or a shoulder squeeze is out of the question, or why they've been relegated to the spare bed, when a toddler is breastfeeding, bedsharing, cuddled and being worn in a sling a lot.

Other times the unspoken resentment is on a deeper level. Perhaps breastfeeding triggers something about your partner's own past or experience of being parented. Witnessing first-hand a close, loving relationship can spark feelings of jealousy and unresolved sadness if this wasn't your own partner's experience in childhood. Sometimes these precognitive memories are so visceral that your partner may have a very intense and angry reaction that seems hard to understand at face value. Digging a little deeper may reveal wounds that date back decades and perhaps haven't even been consciously thought.

Your partner may feel that breastfeeding is the reason they cannot get close to your child, or be more actively involved in their sleep or bedtime. Of course there are *so* many ways for partners to get involved without feeding, but sometimes, when under pressure, this feels like the most *obvious* way that they cannot be involved. Negative thinking patterns can cause people to think about what they can't do, rather than what they can do. Perhaps breastfeeding is getting the blame for why your child seems to 'prefer' you in the night.

Sometimes partners go into uber-practical fix-it mode. If breastfeeding, bedsharing, or any other parenting behaviour is perceived as the activity that is causing the sleep challenge, then the instinct of many is to argue the case for dropping that behaviour. I call this a sleep scapegoat. It may not, according to research, have any real impact on your child's sleep, but perhaps on the face of it, this might feel logical. After all, if your child wakes up five times in the night and asks to breastfeed each time, and that's the only thing that will settle them, it's fairly easy to see how breastfeeding would be blamed for 'causing' this problem. It's also easy to see that a partner not able to help by sharing the breastfeeding would respond by recommending stopping breastfeeding, in the hope that they can then be more practically involved in the night. Leaving aside the fact that breastfeeding is more than food, and stopping it is not likely to lead to an immediate reduction in night-waking, I have some sympathy for partners who, deep down, are just trying to show that they care, and want you to be less tired.

Finally, your partner may just miss you. The anger apparently directed at breastfeeding may be a smokescreen. Perhaps your partner just feels lonely and wants to connect. They may just want you back. Maybe they miss your company, your conversation. Maybe they miss how you used to laugh together. Maybe they were okay with all of this at first, but they hadn't computed that this phase might go on for as long as it has done.

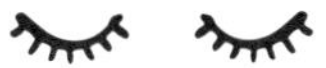

I am mindful that some people are dealing with toxic, abusive or scary relationships. Please seek support if this is you. You do not have to be beaten, hit or kicked to be abused.

Support in an abusive situation:

- Women can call the National Domestic Abuse hotline on 0808 2000 247 any time.
- Men can call the Men's Advice Line on 0808 8010 327.
- If you identify as LGBTQ+ you can call Galop on 0800 999 5428.
- For concerns and advice about forced marriage and honour crimes, you can call Karma Nirvana on 0800 5999 247.
- If you are worried that *you* are abusive, you can call Respect on 0808 802 4040.
- Amnesty www.amnesty.org.uk/domestic-abuse/how-get-help-if-youre-experiencing-domestic-abuse
- Refuge www.refuge.org.uk
- Women's Aid www.womensaid.org.uk/the-survivors-handbook/what-is-a-refuge-and-how-can-i-stay-in-one

If you do not want or need to separate from your partner then there are a range of feelings you may have – from passive tolerance and ambivalence, to sadness about the drift in your relationship, or yearning to make things right again. Fundamentally, however lost you feel in your relationship, however much the spark may feel like it has been extinguished, try to work out if you fundamentally want your partner in your life. If the conflict was stripped away, would you still want to go out for dinner with them? Go on holiday together? If the answer is yes, here is where you start. Begin with the mindset that you both want this to work, and moreover you do not want the issue that is apparently causing the conflict to be a deal-breaker.

I don't know what your situation is specifically, but I suggest you start with your relationship, rather than focus on the breastfeeding. Some practical tips I have found useful with the parents I have worked with in this situation include:

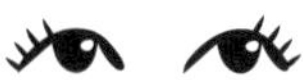

- **Be a team:** let your partner know that you and they are going to work on this together. It is not you and your baby against your partner, it is you and your partner, collectively parenting your child.
- **Focus on the relationship**: let your partner know that you *want* to make things better. This will help them to feel like you haven't rejected them, or given up on your relationship.
- **Separate the issues in your relationship from the immediate concern about breastfeeding/bedsharing or whatever the sticking point is.** Breastfeeding is likely to be a surface issue, with deeper layers of hurt underneath, if you start to look.
- **Think of solutions:** what are the solutions that you can live with? Are there any compromises that you could make that would meet both your needs and leave you both with your integrity and dignity whole?
- **Listen openly:** however much you disagree with your partner's perspective, allow them time to say what they feel.
- **Try to see the situation from your partner's point of view:** if you can leave the contentious issue aside and focus on the underlying hurt, it may help you to see why your partner feels the way they do.
- **Get practical with the love languages:** bear in mind that you or your partner's love languages may have changed. Sometimes, after a major life event, our priorities and needs change. Perhaps your partner now needs to know that you still care for them in a different way. Maybe you do too.
- **Reinstate a date night:** So often, quality time goes out the window. Make a time to sit down, connect and focus on each other. Ensure you have had these tricky conversations *before* this date, otherwise you will end up fixing problems, rather than reconnecting.

These issues are never easy to work through, but it is worth considering whether you can get to the bottom of it. Feeling squeezed into making a decision you are not happy with will leave you feeling resentful. Equally, refusing to engage in discussion may drive a wedge between you and your partner. As uncomfortable as it might be to address this head on, you may learn new things about each other, and come up with a plan to move forward that brings you closer together, rather than further apart.

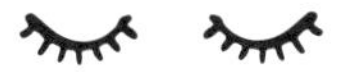

Separation, relationship difficulty and divorce

It is a fact of life that relationships sometimes struggle or break down. I am so sorry if you are going through this situation. You may be worried not only for yourself, but also for the impact on your child. While this is a hugely stressful and confusing time, there are some ways to make it easier for the children involved, to reduce distress and maintain connection. Please talk to your doctor, counsellor, or social worker (if you have one) for specific advice in your situation. Some tips that some families have found helpful include:

- Try to keep your child's routine the same, whichever home they are in.
- Try to avoid talking badly of your ex in front of your children.
- Make photo albums for your child, with pictures of both parents.
- Let your child sleep with something belonging to your ex when they are away from them, and vice versa.
- Reassure your child that this is not their fault.
- Assure your child of your (and your ex's) unconditional love.
- If at all possible and appropriate, be honest with your child – children are often very intuitive, and no matter how well we think we are hiding something, they often know that something is going on.
- Encourage your child to ask questions. Sometimes children feel they cannot ask their biggest question for fear of upsetting us. If this happens, they sometimes invent a worse reality in their mind.
- Do not stop your child from talking about your ex.
- Make your child a social story to help them understand minor nuances in routine whether they are with you or your ex.
- Sometimes children hold on to the hope that their parents will get back together. Try not to raise their hopes about this. Be honest, and assure them that no matter what happens, both of you will always love your child.

Finally, please make sure you have someone to talk to about any specific concerns. These are big, heavy issues, and you will need a village around you.

Supporting struggling relationships

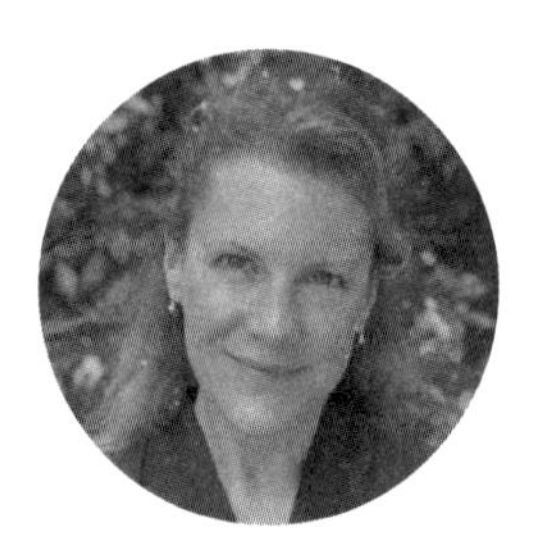

Elly Taylor, perinatal relationship specialist, author and founder of Becoming Us

Parenthood, as wonderful as it is, also comes with huge life changes and new relationship challenges that most couples are blindsided by. Unexpected issues, steep learning curves, hormonal shifts and sleep deprivation can leave even the happiest of couples in the middle of a perfect storm. In fact, over 90 percent of parents have more differences and 67 percent are less happy with their relationship in their first few years of family life: *most* couples struggle at this time!

And it's not only at the beginning. Going through rough patches is normal for long-term relationships, especially during stressful times. Relationship problems don't mean there's anything wrong with you, your partner or your partnership. Most of us need more preparation and support to get through the numerous changes and challenges that parenthood brings.

The good news is there's lots you can do to get back on track. The first step in coping with stresses or times of crisis is to look after yourself. Make sure your meals are nutritious: eating well can give you more energy. Exercise regularly – it's a great way to cope with anxiety and depression (which is suffered by around 1 in 3 new mothers and 1 in 5 new dads!). Keep it up and you may start to feel better about yourself and maybe more positive about your situation too. Good sleep can also make a huge difference. Have something to look forward to once a week. Lean on your friends.

All relationships have their ups and downs – and children can tolerate parents' arguments when they know they'll be followed by happy-again parents' hugs, but ongoing conflicts can erode a family. If you do happen to be separated there are ways to move forward and positively co-parent your child.

If you can, take a fresh look at your relationship. Is it possible your partner was also blindsided by the changes and challenges of parenthood? Might they have needed more preparation and support too? Could their words or behaviour have been signs of them struggling and not coping? A counsellor can help you to work through these questions. New perspectives may reduce negative feelings, whereas blame and resentment can keep you, your ex-partner, and your child all stuck in the mud.

Parents' separation can be challenging for children, both at the time and longer term, but it may be unavoidable, especially where there is ongoing conflict or abuse or safety issues. Children are likely to be stressed if their parents aren't talking or still fighting. A 'cold war' is still a war. So, as hard as it can be to do, your efforts to be supportive of and communicate respectfully with your child's other parent help your child's mental and emotional wellbeing as well as their future relationships. And this applies whether you're together or not.

No matter where you are now in your family's journey, your healing and growth, along with your partner's healing and growth, support your child to be happy and healthy.

For more on coping with difficult times in your relationship, check out my book *Becoming Us: the Couples' Guide to Surviving Parenthood and Growing a Family that Thrives.*

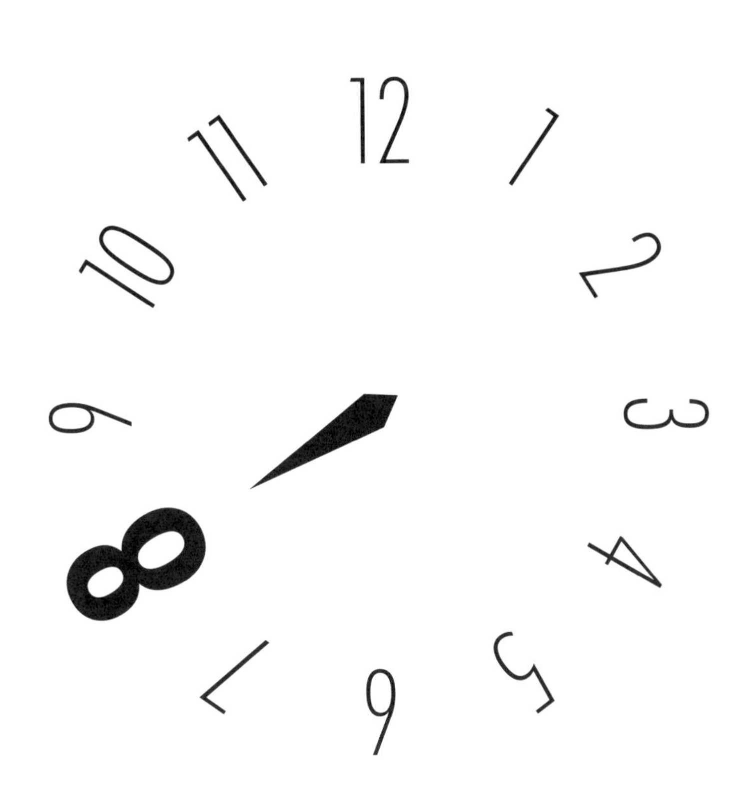

CHAPTER EIGHT

CHILDREN WITH DISABILITY AND COMPLEX NEEDS

Parents of children with disability and complex needs often feel sidelined by mainstream parenting advice and support which may make certain assumptions about what a child can do. Mainstream parenting support may feel irrelevant. You may feel invisible or your child's strengths and challenges overlooked. Being a parent of a child with complex needs has some of the same challenges that all parents face, and yet, you may also feel that you have bigger mountains to climb.

Your exceptional child should not be defined by what they can or cannot do, but by *who they are*. They are a child with a disability, not a disabled child. You are a parent of a child, who happens to have a disability. You are not defined by your child's condition. I remember being called a 'cancer mum' – which upset me at the time, because I am actually called Lyndsey. You are a person too, and your experiences as a parent should not be erased and seen as inconsequential in the face of your child's condition. You matter. Your needs matter. In this chapter, imagine standing beside the parents who have also walked a different path, and made it work.

Some children with disabilities may be more at risk of certain challenges to their sleep – such as sleep apnoea, nighttime seizures, sensory challenges and physical discomforts. Your first port of call should always be your own child's medical team, who know your child and can put in place services and professionals to support your child's unique needs. This chapter is intended to share positive and practical suggestions for some of these challenges, drawing from many parents'

Parenting a child with complex needs at night

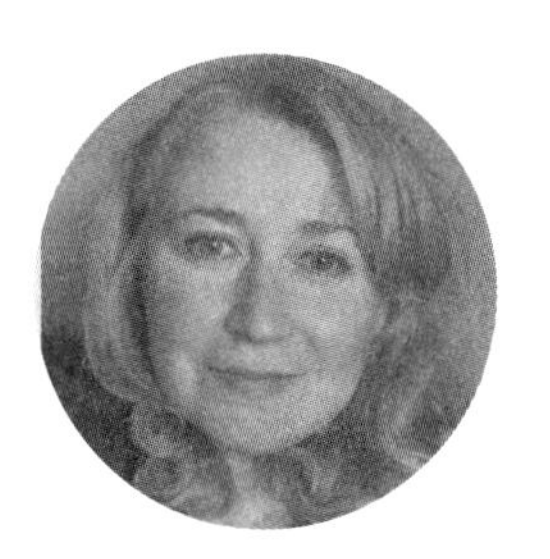

Sarah Collins, disability campaigner and charity director of First Touch Neonatal Charity

My children fall outside the 'norm', so I found myself relying on instinct when it came to sleep. My eldest daughter was born three months prematurely and spent her first four months in the care of a neonatal unit. A catastrophic brain haemorrhage has led to a wide range of disabilities and medical needs. My younger daughter was adopted at 14 months. With both girls I was desperate to compensate for their difficult early months when they couldn't be with me overnight, and I found my parenting focused on being a very strong physical presence.

Isabel, my eldest, has diagnoses that include cerebral palsy, drug-resistant epilepsy, learning disability, hydrocephalus, ADHD and autism. Isabel was always keen to be close to us when she came home from hospital and I have fond memories of watching her dad wash up at the sink with Izzy attached to him in a baby sling. Isabel could be difficult to settle in her cot, and we spent a lot of time reassuring her and ensuring she was comfortable. As she grew older it was clear that her physical disabilities meant that her left arm and leg could become stuck, so we had to make sure she was free to move. When we learned that Izzy had epilepsy, which we discovered over the course of many years was a rare drug-resistant type, my husband and I found ourselves holding vigils over her during the night as we were terrified she would have a seizure while we slept. (We now know there are alarms available for children likely to experience a seizure overnight. Additionally time has shown that Izzy's seizures tend to occur during the daytime).

I know that many of my friends with neurotypical children felt we should leave Isabel to settle herself at night, but we wanted to do all we could to convince ourselves she was safe and she would feel as loved as she possibly could be.

Isabel has never had a specialist, medical bed like some of her friends with complex needs. As she grew older Izzy enjoyed having the same 'ordinary' bed as her younger sister, although her bed was always closer to the floor so that she could get into it herself (with help) as this seemed important to her sense of independence. She had a soft mat at the side of the bed in case there was a disaster and she fell out of bed (she never did). In her teens Isabel was diagnosed with thyroid issues which, coupled with her epilepsy, left her much more tired than her peers. Izzy needs a lot of restorative sleep, and her special needs school has been very accommodating; they've provided a bean bag for afternoon naps in the corner of the classroom when she needs them.

Isabel teaches me so much about love, resilience, overcoming obstacles, the ability in disability, and how to find new strategies to live a full life. It is a privilege to be her mum.

Website: www.first-touch.org.uk

experiences of how they have overcome struggles and made sleep easier.

'Eddie (age four), has acute lymphoblastic leukaemia. While in hospital for chemotherapy induction, he had a seizure. Just before his diagnosis, we were ready to begin transitioning him to his own room from co-sleeping with us as I was pregnant. Having him in bed with us up until his brother was born was the right thing for us so we could be aware if he had any further seizures. Luckily he didn't and come March, when his brother arrived, we knew then we would have to change our sleeping arrangements to accommodate the new arrival who would be co-sleeping and feel secure enough to do so. I didn't want Eddie to feel pushed out, so we brought his mattress into our room and made a floor bed right next to where I slept. We made it fun, with a dream tent, lights, stories and had snuggles until he fell to sleep and then I could get back into my own bed.

We've started transitioning Eddie into his own room this week, again using the dream tent and having stories before bed. We've never made bed a punishment and have tried to be as gentle and positive as possible about any changes made. We've had minimal fuss with moving into his own room and no resentment with his new baby brother. I still listen at the door when I walk past at night to check he's okay, but I think I would probably do that without his illness!' **Stephanie**

'We couldn't co-sleep with my son (who had a complex cardiac problem) because he had to have an apnoea mattress when he was asleep. However breastfeeding all night with a wakeful baby and not co-sleeping made for really long nights and I hate to admit I fell asleep often with him in my arms. I always had us wedged with firm pillows so neither of us went anywhere and desperately tried to stay awake by being on my phone and stuff but sometimes it was impossible and I'd wake in a panic with him peacefully snoozing in my arms. It's hard when co-sleeping is so instinctual, but you know you just can't do it. I didn't drop any night needs until he was two because he was so tiny and I always felt those extra calories would help, and we never entertained any form of sleep-training that involved crying - not only because that's not our style, but also any strain on his heart from crying wouldn't have been good. Other than that we had a fairly standard four years of not sleeping through the night. **Rebecca**

A fairly common theme is that the strategies that might have been chosen if your child had not had a complex problem or disability are not suitable. In some situations, like Stephanie and Rebecca, adapting to the new normal may mean accommodating children for longer than you thought in your own room, feeding them for longer than you thought you would, or adapting ways of sleeping to facilitate proximity but also manage equipment.

Neurodiversity

Children with sensory processing differences or neurodevelopmental conditions such as autism spectrum disorder and attention deficit hyperactivity disorder (ADHD) often have some sleep challenges. Many children with neurodiversity have associated sensory needs, anxiety, and may need different communication strategies to explain bedtime boundaries. Children with ADHD are known to have a higher incidence of insomnia, nocturnal enuresis, restless legs and night-waking.

The mainstay of sleep support for children with neurodiversity

Sleep solutions and Down's syndrome

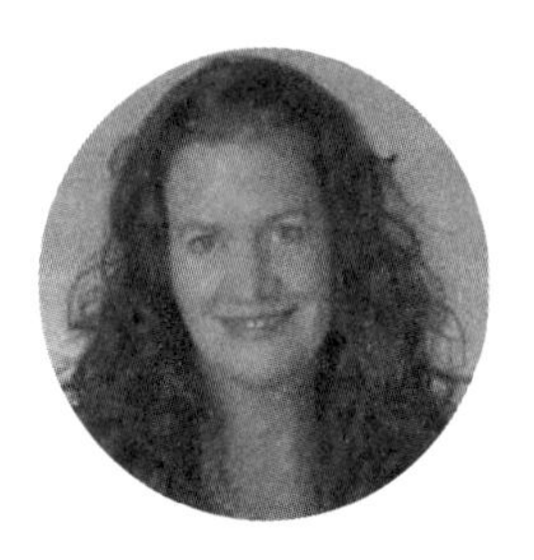

Rozanne Hay, family and child sleep specialist, founder of Baby Sleep Rescue

I'm thrilled to share my unique journey as mother to a son aged 12 with Down's syndrome. As a family and child sleep specialist and campaigner for those disadvantaged and without a voice I had a fair understanding of the challenges we were about to face.

After a turbulent journey to grow our family, my values changed. When our son arrived, I faced commiserations at a time I and his siblings were excited to be welcoming James, a viable and healthy baby, into our lives.

Medicine has advanced rapidly, but our psychological and emotional welfare often aren't in line with this advancement. I realise today that we know too much too soon. We don't trust nature enough as a way of easing parents into walking a different parenting path. The choices around 'informed choice' are themselves life-challenging. Labels are readily used, but they don't define our son, or our family life. James is our son, he just happens to have Down's syndrome. Our parenting journey has been smooth and doesn't necessarily reflect other narratives associated with parenting a child with additional and special needs.

After a routine blood test, James's red blood cells were found to be enlarged, suggesting low blood oxygen. I'd already noticed he had hyperactive moments, which I associated with sensory overload. His nights became increasingly broken and disturbed, with restless sleep sitting upright with his chin to the ceiling or sleeping on his belly on the floor with arms out in front. After a sleep study he presented with both central and obstructive sleep apnoea and retains higher levels of CO_2. Gamma aminobutyric acid (GABA) dysfunctions are also common in children with Down's syndrome and may contribute to sleep difficulties, although I don't believe this is a significant component for James.

However, James was born with nail-bed clubbing, which is often associated with low oxygen levels. It was suggested this could be linked to an arteriovenous malformation (AVM) on the bridge of James's nose, which coincidently disappeared after a tonsillectomy and adenoidectomy that took place before he was two years old. We're grateful this was offered to us, as it's not common practice to offer it to young children. We suspect James may have other AVMs as these rarely present alone and they may be the cause of his difficulties.

Once oxygen at night was introduced James gained weight quickly, calmed down and slept longer. He receives this via wafting, a non-contact oxygen delivery method, and we see the benefits clearly. Without oxygen supplementation his nights are short – no more than five or six hours long – whereas with oxygen support he can manage a 10 or 11-hour sleep. His sleep, our sleep, and our son's quality of life all improved. I want to point out that James is otherwise healthy and strong: he swims and snorkels and is a fierce tennis player!

Currently we're experimenting with continuous positive airway pressure (CPAP), but his tolerance varies.[1] Understandably, when James is well, he tolerates the CPAP headgear well. When he's unwell he is sensitive and intolerant of the headset – paradoxically, this is when he most needs this kind of support.

A recent international paediatric sleep conference in Florida explored the success of a trial using a hypoglossal nerve stimulator within the Down's syndrome community. The findings are promising and I'm hoping that this will be introduced into the UK Down's Syndrome community. A recent campaign involved a young teenager who was removed from a loving home life due to not maintaining CPAP adherence and in turn gaining weight. There's a huge need for better understanding – and support – for the group of Down's syndrome individuals who struggle with tolerance and adherence to such systems. Interventions include offering greater desensitising activities alongside titration. It's a concern to think about how many other families will have to endure the heartbreak of having a child removed, before better choice in management options is introduced.

For more help and solidarity, there are good online support groups.

is to manage their sensory needs, reduce anxiety, provide age and developmentally appropriate boundaries and treat any underlying organic causes of poor sleep.

One of the first strategies to review is managing a child's regulation.

'My 10-year-old has ASD and we've had real difficulty over the years with anxiety-causing difficulties, particularly settling down to sleep. For many years he shared my bed as that's what worked for me to be able to get him to settle at a reasonable time (much to the horror of many)! Obviously sleepless nights due to anxiety heighten difficult behaviours and anxiety into the next day so it is important that he gets as much sleep as he requires.' **Jenny**

Melatonin and other medications

Melatonin is a hormone that triggers a feeling of sleepiness. It is made by the body in a complex metabolic pathway. Tryptophan is converted to serotonin, which is then converted into melatonin. Some research has found that people with autism have an abnormal melatonin pathway, leading to lower production of melatonin. A recent meta-analysis found that lower levels of melatonin corresponded with increased difficulties with their autism.[2]

If a child is struggling to fall asleep, stay asleep or achieve enough sleep, and the simple strategies are not working, then for some children melatonin may be prescribed. In the United States, melatonin can be bought over the counter. In the United Kingdom and Australia, it requires a prescription. Melatonin is usually not prescribed for a child who has a simple sleep problem, but it is commonly prescribed for children[3] with:

- Autistic spectrum disorder
- Attention deficit hyperactivity disorder
- Neurodevelopmental disorders
- Severe insomnia
- Visually impaired children
- Children with an on-going sleep problem that has not responded to behavioural treatments
- Teenagers with delayed phase circadian rhythm disorder

Supporting children with neurodiversity and/or sensory differences to regulate

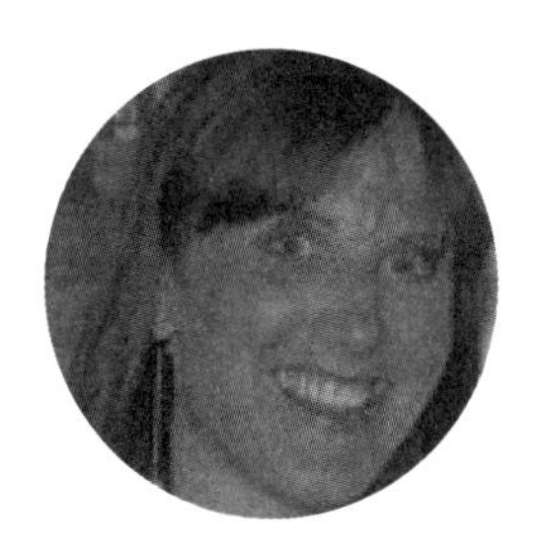

Anna Richardson, paediatric occupational therapist and founder of Brain Sense

Children who have neurodevelopmental conditions such as autism spectrum disorder (ASD), attention deficit hyperactivity disorder (ADHD) and sensory processing dysfunction (SPD) often have a range of difficulties which can impact on their ability to respond to and learn from their caregiver during early childhood. Sensory differences, social anxieties and emotional reactivity can lead to difficulties accepting the support of a caregiver in order to attain and maintain a regulated state across the day. Children with such presentations can present as passive, rarely achieving a regulated, pro-social state where they can function optimally, or as being highly active, anxious or distressed, often with a nervous system that is primed for defence, rather than approach (pro-social) behaviours. Alternatively some children can attain a calm, regulated state but lack the ability to regulate or reset their nervous system to recover from stressful events throughout the day. This means that they can often 'hold it together' during the day or in school but become explosive in their behavioural responses at home at the end of the day, as their stress levels have increased beyond their capacity to cope. These different but complex presenting difficulties can have a range of impacts on the child's ability to regulate, participate and engage actively in areas such as sleep, self-care, play and learning. Difficulties with sleep are more prevalent in children with neurodiversity and are often more challenging to manage, further impacting the life of that child and their family.

When attempting to address sleep issues in children with neurodiversity we need to consider regulation across the day, particularly with children who are highly active and/or anxious, or for those who become highly dysregulated at the end of the day. It can be difficult for parents and carers to find a simple way of understanding their child's presentation and to respond successfully with appropriate strategies, but they are often best placed to make the biggest impact when strategies are used effectively. It can be useful to create an 'emotions' profile, using the common language of emotions to more effectively co- and mutually regulate your child. Try a range of strategies and monitor whether the strategy generally works to help your child manage each emotion effectively in order to maintain or return to a more regulated state. Consider the following:

- **Use of self** the way you behave and respond and how this impacts the child e.g. position/proximity (move towards or away, crouching down, sitting with your child), tone of voice, use of breath (e.g. exaggerated exhale), giving your child space or providing spatial boundaries (e.g. a beanbag to sit on), body language, use of eye contact, empathy (recognising and responding to your child's emotions), physical support (hugs, guidance), use of language, predicting and pre-empting behaviours. If you have other people to support you, also consider change of face. Often having a few, highly effective strategies that work consistently is what is needed.
- **Physical and sensory strategies** giving more or less sensory input (sound, vision, taste, touch, movement, deep pressure/resistance, smell). This includes use of flexion postures (this means when the body is curled inwards – a powerful tool that often children with regulation difficulties do not use as a calming strategy, so encourage curling into a ball, sitting in a bean bag, playing in side-lying positions), change of position, physical activity (just walking or running can help, or star jumps with more able and older children), weighted equipment, deep pressure (through compression vests or massage), movement (trampoline, swing, jumping and rolling games). Therapeutic listening is an intervention using specifically designed audio tracks to shift the arousal state. They are often recommended by specialist occupational therapists. You can read more about them (and purchase) from vitallinks.com/therapeutic-listening/parents. Also consider calming music, use of compression, fidget and feely toys, tactile/messy play, visual toys, vibration, and theraputty.
- **Calming strategies** these are strategies that are innately calming for your child. This includes having access to liked or preferred activities (this may be time limited), alone or free time when they can choose their own activities (even if these may be unconventional), use of breathing techniques, yoga, relaxation, mindfulness.

- **Environmental strategies and transactional supports** – including changing/adapting the environment and providing strategies that support a child's understanding. This includes change of space (moving to a different room – setting up quiet spaces, sensory spaces, outdoor spaces), the use of symbols/visuals including visual timetables, pictures, 'now and next', schedules, go-to boards, emotion keyrings, timers. The use of transactional supports is essential even if your child is verbal as they will regulate your child through building in structure, routine and providing predictability.
- **Communication strategies** – building the capacity for conventional and adaptive communication is essential as this provides an alternative to using physical and sensory behaviours to communicate. Knowing when to communicate with words and when to communicate with body language is key: use of words when your child is highly distressed often fuels the intensive emotions. Support your child's understanding and ability to communicate through reading and responding to their body language, use of gesture, sign, objects of reference or augmentative and alternative communication systems (low tech and high tech).
- **Cognitive strategies** – when a child is able to achieve and maintain a regulated state and they have developed a level of language, they can then use cognitive strategies to regulate their emotions. This includes the use of the zones of regulation curriculum, the social thinking curriculum, social stories, comic strip conversations, talking mats and the 5-Point Scale.

Remember that what your child enjoys is often different from what your child finds regulating. For example, watching favourite things on an iPad or tablet can initially be regulating, but if left for too long this can become too stimulating for the child to cope with if they have a narrow band of positive arousal. Also the most regulating activities may often be initially rejected by a child, as they are yet to learn that it is what they need. For example, children who seek movement but don't regulate with it often need to learn to be still. We therefore need to support them over time to learn what calm really feels like in their bodies through relaxation.

Melatonin is usually prescribed for a short time – usually six months to one year – then reviewed. However, it is occasionally taken long term by children with neurodevelopmental disorders and visual impairments (blindness).

Not many studies have examined the long-term safety or impacts of melatonin. The studies that have been done seem to suggest no adverse effects. Melatonin seems to work well, and be safe.[4]

Specifics of the medication

The dose of melatonin varies, and if your child is prescribed it, your doctor will work out the best dose or whether it needs to be changed. Melatonin is available in tablet, capsule and liquid form.

The manufacturers usually recommend giving children their medication about 30–60 minutes before the intended bedtime. However, this does not work for all children, and can make the medication more difficult to come off. This is because children can become used to the *hypnotic* effect of the drug this way, and then find it very difficult to go to sleep without their medication.

Another way of using the drug is to give it 2–4 hours before the intended bedtime. It is then not a hypnotic, but a *chronobiotic* – that is, something which works to regulate the circadian rhythm. It's best to check with your doctor to see which approach may work best for your child.

Some children are also prescribed other medications to help them sleep, but there is less research on these. Drugs such as sedating antihistamines are commonly prescribed, as well as anti-anxiety medication.

Many parents find melatonin to be a godsend, but it's important to say that it is not a magic bullet. If you think it's not working for your child, then please do ask for more help – remember that you are the world expert on your child.

Profound and multiple learning disability

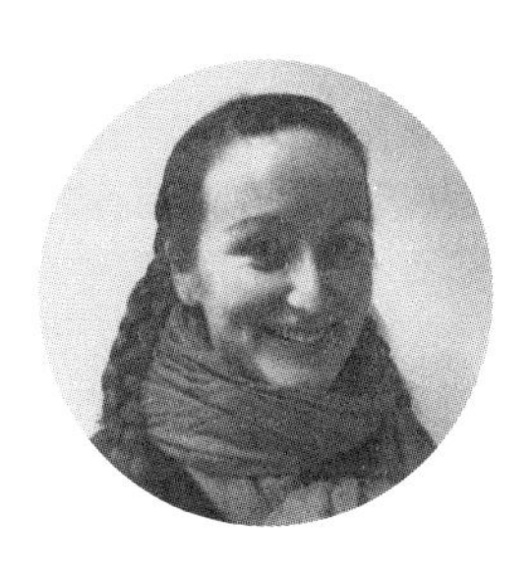

Joanna Grace, sensory engagement and inclusion specialist, author, trainer, TEDx speaker and founder of The Sensory Projects

Sleep can be a distant memory for parents of children with profound and multiple learning disabilities because often, complex medical healthcare needs mean that they need attending to multiple times through the night.

Lives often start with weeks, months, and in some cases even years in hospital. In a highly medicalised environment the natural process of drifting off to sleep can be confused by medications, bright lights and bleeps.

Parents of children with complex disabilities often find themselves disabled by the professionals they come into contact with. The message can seem to be 'only an expert can know what to do with your child.' It can be very powerful to reclaim some of the 'ordinariness' of childhood sleep rituals, for example the bedtime story.

I received a message from a parent of a six-year-old asking me if I thought they were capable of reading their own child a bedtime story. I was inspired to write *Dream: a sensory story for children with complex disabilities* (and children without complex disabilities.)

Sensory stories combine concise text with rich and relevant sensory experiences so that meaning can be shared in a sensory way as well as through words. I am a sensory engagement specialist, so I choose the sensations accompanying my stories very carefully and of course *Dream* is resourced with soothing, soporific sensations (all of which can be easily created from things around the home).

Another difference for children with complex disabilities with regards to sleep is that it is often important for them to use a sleep system to hold their body in place through the night. Poor postural care is a slow killer. It is especially tragic as it often needlessly steals the lives of people who have survived all manner of medical emergencies. Essentially, if their bodies are not held in healthy positions they slowly bend over time and this contortion impairs the function of internal organs.

The problem is that the position one is required to sleep in within a sleep system can be counter to that which you might otherwise choose to fall asleep in. Getting used to this position, and feeling safe and comfortable within it, is very important. Working with Simple Stuff Works – an organisation dedicated to improving postural care management – I created three sleepy sensory stories, written around principles of guided meditation which support people through their postural care routines. You can find these and other sensory stories on my website and I am always open to conversations that support provision for people with complex disabilities.

Websites: www.TheSensoryProjects.co.uk, www.simplestuffworks.com
Twitter: @Jo3Grace
Facebook: www.Facebook.com/JoannaGraceTheSensoryProjects

What might help children with complex needs to sleep

If you're the parent of a child with complex needs or disability, there are lots of avenues to explore for your child. Not all mainstream sleep tools are irrelevant, but since I do not know your child's specific strengths and challenges, you will have to read through these and pick out the ones you feel might be worth trying, and ignore those that are irrelevant in your situation.

I will cover overarching strategies that focus on:

- Proximity
- Safety
- Underlying factors
- Aids to sleep
- Comfort
- Sleep hygiene
- Sensory diet and tools
- Respite care

1. Proximity

Sometimes a pragmatic decision is to keep your child close. This might be because they need you, or because you feel less uneasy with them nearby. Some parents know they will need to attend to their child in the night, so it makes sense to plan for that – making it as easy as possible to quickly deal with the inevitable wake-ups. I have met many families who found that everyone slept better when they kept their children close. This might be in the same bed, or you might choose to sleep on a mattress on the floor in your child's room. Your decisions about who sleeps where and on what surface may be dictated somewhat by your child's condition – for example, if your child is ventilated, has an overnight gastrostomy feed, or needs to be at a sensible height for safety reasons, you may need to make sure they are in a bed off the floor. Other children may have limited mobility and require special mattresses, which might make bedsharing impractical. For some children, there may be more options for flexibility. If you're not sure, please check with your usual medical team.

'My daughter has complex needs. I sit by her bed until she falls asleep. We have a monitor on her still (she's four) because she often wakes. One of us often sleeps on her floor at some point in the night so she can see us if she wakes. She slept in with us for a good few years.' **Becky**

'While F was on oxygen at night (up to being around 3.5 years old) she was still in our room. It made it so much easier to keep an eye on her on normal nights, and was much needed on nights where she was ill or doing sleep studies. I know a lot of people can't wait to move baby/ toddler out of their room, but I think it would have caused me more stress and led to a much poorer quality of sleep for everyone. In fact, F and her twin sister still share our room (and mostly our bed) at almost four and a half years old.' **Shelley**

2. Safety

For some children, helping them sleep is bound up with ensuring their safety during sleep. If your child has seizures or struggles with breathing, then you may find it easier to sleep close to them so that you are more likely to be aware if there is a problem. Many parents also end up keeping their monitor for longer than they thought. Other children need a CPAP machine, feeding pump, oxygen, apnoea monitor or medication to keep them safe and well.

'My son has a complex airway disorder. He has a monitor and I sleep

on the camp bed! In the first few hours of the night he tends to have way more apnoeas so once he is more settled about 2am I will go into my own bed.' **Ellie**

3. Underlying factors

Other times, children with complex needs have underlying issues or conditions which exacerbate their sleeping difficulties. It's worth ruling out the red flags. Just because a child has complex needs, doesn't necessarily mean that their sleep issue is complex, or even related to their disability. It is important to rule out the usual red flags, check your sleep hygiene, maintain as many usual boundaries as possible, and also consider the more unusual problems that might crop up overnight.

'My son is four and has never slept through the night. He wakes on average four times a night, sometimes more, sometimes less. Never less than twice. He has ASD and some associated mental health issues. We are still working on the medical issues. He had his tonsils and adenoids removed but it hasn't really helped sleep. We've tried everything and the only things that have helped him are medication (melatonin) from his GP and an anti-anxiety medicine from his psychiatrist. I was so worried about medicating him as he's so young but it's truly helped him with everyday functioning as well as helping him sleep. He still wakes but he has told me that since starting his medicine his dreams are less scary. I also have a 20-month-old who has hypotonia of unknown origin at this point. We will be looking for a diagnosis for a while I suspect. He sleeps as babies do... I just take it one day at a time and sleep when I can. I've learned to exist on less sleep and accept that some days everyone being alive and fed is all that I'm capable of. I wish more people knew that not everyone's child sleeps by 2–3 years. Personally, I have found that if you keep pushing you can find providers who are supportive and won't just push sleep-training and the like but will actually take you seriously and listen to your concerns.' **Lucy**

4. Aids to sleep

You can't always buy a product that will instantly fix sleep! But just sometimes, if a product meets a specific need that your child has, it may

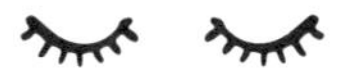

work to quickly improve sleep. These may be aids to comfort, sensory differences or preferences, regulation, or to manage a problem. Some products that some families I have worked with have found useful include:

- **Sensory toys** – to support regulation during the day.
- **Wedges** – to maintain a comfortable position in the night, or to prevent heads being knocked into pieces of equipment.
- **Cushions and special pillows** – to prevent pressure sores and maintain a safe and comfortable position.
- **Posture supports** – to prevent slumping, muscle-wasting and discomfort during the day, which can be one reason why a child is unsettled at night.
- **Weighted blankets** – to provide deep proprioceptive input, and can be very calming. They need to be the right weight for your child though, for safety reasons, so check with your occupational therapist.
- **Waterproof sheets** – if your child is not dry at night, or their nappy/pull-up/pyjama pants sometimes leak, then waterproof sheets are essential. Try layering the sheets if this is a regular problem: waterproof sheet, normal bedsheet, waterproof sheet, normal bedsheet. This way, if your child wets the bed, their nappy leaks or they have any other kind of spillage in the night, you just need to strip off the wet sheets and the bed is ready for you underneath.
- **Duvet clips** – these are simple little clips that fasten on to your child's duvet or cover on an elastic strip that goes under the mattress. They stop your child kicking the covers off and getting cold.
- **Sound machine** – some children find background noise really soothing. You don't have to use white noise if you don't like it. There are other types of noise, such as pink or brown noise, or your child might prefer nature sounds, running water, or the sound of a breeze. Experiment to see what you like. I often suggest downloading a track from YouTube or iTunes first, to see if it's a good fit, before investing in a more expensive sound machine.
- **Red light nightlights** – these can be really helpful if your child is afraid of the dark. Many people are aware that blue light inhibits melatonin production, whereas red light does not. Be cautious about some lights and projectors, as some of them use blue light.

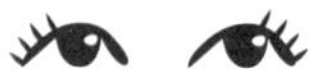

'My son has autism, and has always struggled to sleep. Last year, I bought a projector, a bubble tube, a lava lamp, some LED lights and a weighted blanket and things have been much better since.' **Jenny**

5. Comfort

I have met many children who are unwell or in some degree of discomfort. The priority for some children is providing comfort. This may be in the form of physical reassurance – such as cuddles. Other times it may be in the form of food and drink. Or it may be related to pain-relief provision. Many parents find that they have to provide multiple forms of comfort and reassurance, and may also have to be creative about their approach to providing comfort.

'My daughter, Esther, was diagnosed with acute lymphoblastic leukaemia at 12 months; she was breastfeeding on demand and co-sleeping already. We haven't changed anything. She just turned three a few days ago, and has about nine months of treatment left. She nurses through the night a lot of the time. While it's hard on my body sometimes, the excessive day and night breastfeeding (and clinginess) is, I know, her way of coping. She's pretty well adjusted otherwise. I let her nurse just about whenever she wants, and it seems to keep her feeling safe as well as healthy. If the situation was different, I might be trying to limit her nursing a bit more.' **Abigail**

'My son Teddi has a life-threatening swallowing condition which wasn't picked up until he was 12 months when he had to be resuscitated and ventilated for the second time after aspirating. We started out with an NG (nasogastric) tube which I had to pass most days because he just loved to pull it out! His feeding regime initially required quite a few night feeds as he would be sick if he had too much at once so I had to spread them out. I would set an alarm and stay awake through his feeds because the worst thing was if you left it for two or three hours and found it was pulled out and had been pumping milk all over his cot and then you have to try and fit in extra hours which weren't there over 24 hours. I also worried he would tangle himself in the tubing. I would lie next to him and rest my hand on him or even hold him through most of the feeds. Gradually his solid

food increased until he only needed water through his tube and he had an operation to give it straight into his stomach. He's now four and goes to SEN school as he is globally delayed but we still enjoy our cuddles and he comes on my lap when it's time for his fluids. He no longer requires the pump as much so he 'helps' me push the syringe. I'm very proud of him and how he's such a happy little boy even after everything he's been through.' **Terri**

6. Sleep hygiene

There are many aspects of sleep hygiene that work for all children, regardless of whether they have a condition or not: communicating a bedtime routine in an age and developmentally appropriate way, having a predictable and soothing end to the day, and ring-fencing your bedtime routine with boundaries. You can also choose some of the love bombing and connection strategies that work for all children. Finally, making sure that your child's bedroom environment is geared for sleep and calm will help optimise sleep. Check chapter 3 for more ideas and a sleep hygiene overview.

'We have always ensured that there was no screen time in the lead up to bed and focused on a calming routine before bedtime, including colouring or reading, however this didn't always help. One thing that has really made a difference is 10 minutes of golden time with a parent before settling down to sleep where we do something of his choosing (he has traits of pathological demand avoidance so allowing him to choose keeps it in his control).' **Jenny**

'My son was diagnosed with cerebral palsy from nearly 16 weeks old. Sleep has always been a big problem for him and me. It was not a problem to get him to sleep, it was the issue of him staying asleep throughout the night or getting a reasonable length of time for rest. This resulted in me having anxiety when I saw that the evening was coming because I knew what the night would bring. This lasted for four and a half years. Throughout this time I had looked into many different approaches to solving our sleep problem. I tried going to sleep classes which gave me lots of information on ways I could get him to sleep. The nights, weeks, months that turned into years of no

sleep continued until February 2019 when I introduced the '3B's'. This method for me was bath-bottle-bed. At 8pm every evening I started the process of giving him a bath, then warm milk in his bottle and tucked him into bed. Now, this process was not easy as he tested his boundaries. There were days when I was tired and did not want to do the routine but I knew deep down if I did not persevere there was room to break the pattern. He now sleeps from approximately 8:30 until about 5am. For me, coming from no sleep I can appreciate approximately eight hours of sleep. I would recommend that when you decide to create a bedtime routine for your child you are mentally ready and if there is a partner involved you both are prepared to work as a team to ensure that the routine is kept. I always used my son's disability as an excuse as to why some things are an exception.' **Naiya**

7. Sensory diet and tools

All of us have sensory needs and preferences. Some of us fidget when we are trying to sit still. Some of us twirl hair, tap our foot, chew gum, hate the sensation of pure wool, or find auditory distractions impossible to concentrate with. But for some children, their sensory needs begin to impede their everyday activities, or make family life really difficult. Managing a child's sensory needs can stop them from feeling like they're on high alert all day, and begin to calm down. As you know, sleep is a function of the rest and digest state, not the fight/flight response. So anything that causes your child anxiety, discomfort or dysregulation is likely to have a negative impact on sleep. If your child has an occupational therapist, they would be best placed to suggest whether any of the following tools that many parents find helpful might be a good fit for your child:

- **Therapeutic listening** – certain audio tracks are specifically designed to down-regulate the stress response and calm a child. See vitallinks.com/quickshifts/for-parents for more details.
- **Flopping over a yoga ball and rocking slowly** can be very calming for some children.
- **Deep pressure** – this may be a deep massage, wrapping or some of the sensory play ideas in chapter 3.
- **Weighted vest** – these can help to literally 'weigh' a child down and

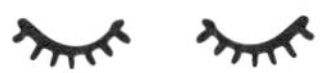

help them feel calmer and more grounded. Weighted lap blankets sometimes help with sitting down to eat or focus as well. You can improvise with a couple of water bottles inside a little backpack worn on your child's back as well.

- **Chewellery (chewable jewellery)** – this can be a brilliant investment for a child who chews their hair, clothing, or fingers.
- **Bouncing on a space hopper or sitting on a wobble cushion** – these tools can help to provide an outlet for children who are wriggly and have trouble sitting still.

8. Respite

Finally, although this may not solve your child's sleep problem as such, one option for some is to organise some respite care. You may be eligible for some additional support from your child's medical team, or via your social worker. It is sometimes hard to find someone you trust enough to care for your child if they have complex needs. You may be able to have a nurse if your child has significant needs to allow you to rest easy overnight knowing that someone will attend to your child in the night if they need attention. Other people have close family members who are capable of helping, or you could tag team with your co-parent.

Caring for children with complex or medical needs overnight can be very tiring. Please don't wait until you're on your knees to ask for help. I know you're wonderful at managing and coping. You are also the absolute best person to take care of your amazing child, but saying that you need help is not a sign of failure. Your needs matter too.

Summary of tools that may help

There are many tools that may help discussed throughout this book. I appreciate that as a parent of a child with a disability of complex needs you may have come to this chapter first. You'll find some of the topics mentioned briefly in this chapter discussed in more detail elsewhere in the book. On the next page is your quick start guide so you can quickly navigate to where you need to go. Please do also discuss any of these ideas with your child's multi-disciplinary team.

Tool, strategy, or more information	Where you can find more information
Sensory play ideas	71–76
Fading	234–236
Sleep hygiene	53–56
Sleep disordered breathing	59
Floor beds	236–238
Social stories	251–252
Love languages and love bombing	126–127
Red flags	58–60
Nocturnal enuresis	145–147
Regulation and self-soothing	30–50
Bedtime routine	64–69
Nighttime sleep tools	52–82

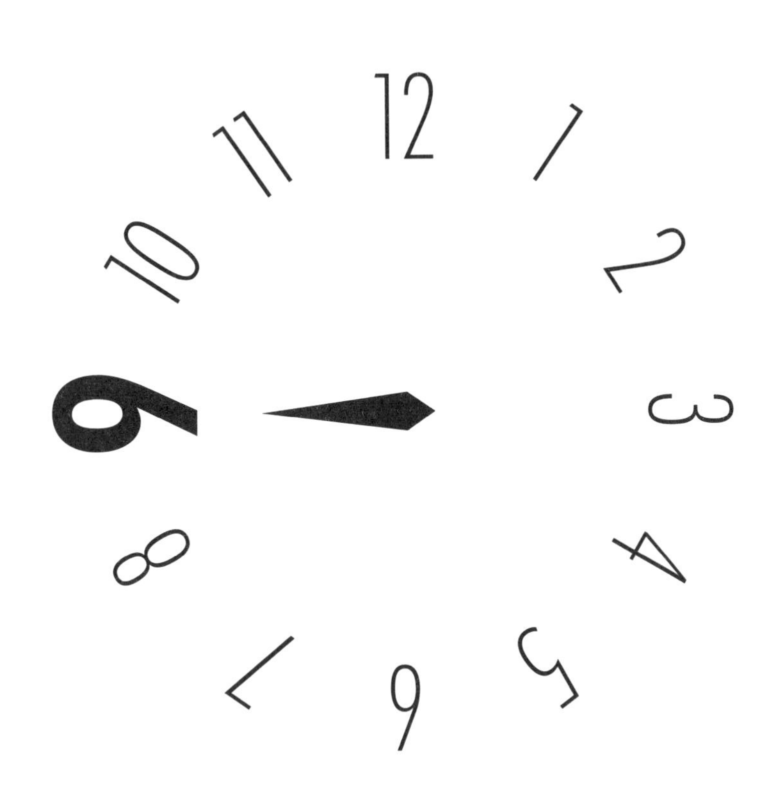

CHAPTER NINE

ALL ABOUT NAPS

Naps are a different animal to nights, in terms of purpose, regulation, and consistency. Robust literature explaining what to expect with naps is sparse, and it seems there is considerable variability of napping patterns around the world, and depending on different studies.[1] Naps in children are mostly influenced by sleep pressure, which will build as children spend time awake. Because of the variability of sleep needs, and how quickly children build up sleep pressure, the amount of sleep a child needs in the day, and for how long, is also variable. By contrast, nighttime sleep is partly driven by sleep pressure, but also by the circadian rhythm. During the day, melatonin levels are extremely low, so this is not a factor that influences your child's napping pattern. Finally, whereas bedtime and total sleep duration at night may be fairly consistent, naps evolve and change. The timings need to be adjusted, and that's okay.

Naps are sometimes needed by children up to about the age of four or five years. Dropping them is not always a linear and simple process, and it can be hard to know when the right time is to drop them. Just like all children have different nap needs – in terms of timing, length, location and organisation – they also drop them at different times too. In fact, academic literature is pretty unspecific about when children drop naps. Most articles suggest that napping after the age of two years reduces the quality and quantity of sleep at night[2] – but have you met many two-year-olds who can make it (tantrum-free) through the day

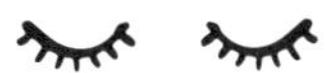

without a nap? Sure, it sometimes happens, but it's unusual. As with so many other aspects of toddler to tween sleep, keep an open mind about naps.

Normal napping

Naps are sometimes sold as the answer to a bad night. You have probably come across the concept of 'sleep breeding sleep' – meaning the better a child sleeps in the day, the better they sleep at night. This is actually a real stretch. I've said this many times, but it is worth repeating that you can only get so much sleep in 24 hours.

What makes understanding naps confusing to figure out is that you'll need to remember the three elements of children's sleep:

1. Your child's circadian rhythm
2. Your child's sleep pressure
3. Your child's total sleep needs

The circadian rhythm, if you remember from chapter 1, should be well established by the age of two years and beyond. The circadian rhythm is in control of when a child's sleepy and alerting hormones are released. Putting your child to bed too early may mean they are simply not ready for bed.

Sleep pressure builds during waking hours, and there is some evidence that it builds more when our brain is busier.[3] Therefore sleep pressure may be a little more variable on a day-to-day basis than the circadian rhythm. Some days are just more tiring than others. Sometimes parents see the evidence of sleep pressure, or physical fatigue, and respond to it by initiating a nap, only to find that bedtime goes awry. It's not easy to balance your child's needs, be responsive, and also take a longer-term view and consider the impact of a nap on the rest of the 24 hours. This is where we need to remember part three of the puzzle.

Your child's total sleep needs have to be factored into the overall picture of whether a nap is sensible.

Let's take the scenario of a child who gets multiple or long naps in the day. The child with high sleep needs may get away with this and still sleep well at night. We could even go so far as to say that this 'proves' the 'sleep

breeds sleep' theory. Yet for a child who needs more sleep, this is just a happy coincidence.

Let's take the same sleep pattern of napping for a low sleep child, and what will happen is nap and bedtime resistance and fragmented or split nights. Think of your child needing to fill their sleep tank over 24 hours. Imagine that your child needs 12 hours of total sleep in 24 hours. If they get a two-hour nap, they have filled up their tank with two hours' worth of sleep. There is only room in the tank for another 10 hours. This either means you will need to put them to bed later, put up with an early start, or they may throw a curve ball and have a fragmented night.

We have to start by understanding a child's overall sleep needs in context. It's all in the individuality of a child. What works for one child will be a disaster for another.

In a very general sense, napping after the age of two, according to most research,[4] results in shorter total nighttime sleep as well as a longer, drawn-out bedtime. However, some children have higher sleep needs, and become unbearably cranky and miserable if they do not nap.[5] You may decide that on balance, you'd rather have a later bedtime and a more cheerful child!

Here are some loose guidelines:

- It's common to drop down to just one nap at about 16–18 months
- It's common to drop the nap entirely anywhere between 2–5 years
- It is also common to think a child needs to drop a nap if bedtime battles arise, or naps are more difficult to achieve
- Frustrations often occur at developmental phases
- True readiness to drop a nap is not always linear
- Nap lengths are highly variable

Nap timings

Toddlers often need a longer stretch of awake time between their nap and bedtime than younger babies. If your toddler or preschooler naps too long, you may pay for this at night.

> *Jonah (30 months) attended preschool every morning and when he got home, he was exhausted. He slept for 2.5 hours after a quick lunch, and was full of beans after he woke. But he then didn't fall*

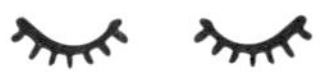

asleep until 9.30pm, and had to be woken for preschool at 7am.

In this scenario, Jonah is achieving 9.5 hours of sleep overnight, and 2.5 hours in the day, totalling 12 hours. This is totally normal for a child of this age. But the distribution of the sleep isn't working for this family. While this sleep pattern is very common in many cultures, it is not right for everyone. The solution here would be to cap Jonah's nap – some experimenting with how short to make it would be a good idea, to find out what is a good compromise.

If the nap is too early, your child may not be able to last till bedtime, and then you can end up in a cycle of early rising and early bedtimes.

Maya (24 months) had a two-hour nap from 10–12 every morning, but then couldn't make it past 6pm, and had fallen into a pattern of waking at 5am.

For this child, sleeping 11 hours overnight and two hours in the day adds up to a normal amount of sleep at her age, but her nap is early, which means that her sleep pressure is very high by early in the evening. However, she has filled up her sleep tank by 5am. The cycle is perpetuated because the early start means she is tired by mid-morning. The only way around this is to gradually make the nap later. Another option would be to make this a very short nap and try for another nap after lunch, followed by a later bedtime.

Some children cannot seem to make it past about 6–7pm, but can only achieve 10–11 hours of overnight sleep. The problem with this is that you will have an early start on your hands. Sometimes the way to make this work is to maintain a nap – even if it's just 20 minutes – so that your child can make it to an 8pm bedtime and then sleep till a more sensible time in the morning.

If the nap is too late, you may not get your toddler down till much later than you'd like. Every child is different, but as a loose rule of thumb, aim for a nap right in the middle of the awake time. So if they wake at 6am and go to bed at 8pm, aim for a nap at around 12.30–1pm, for 1–2 hours at the most. Naps longer than two hours may well come back to bite you in the evening. Many parents find that by trial and error they find the length of nap that seems to work well to alleviate their child's daytime sleep

pressure, without upsetting bedtime. Your child may need 90 minutes, or 45 may be too long. Rest assured, there is very little literature, so you will have to play around with it.

Many books and apps suggest lengths of time for naps. These work well for some toddlers, but may be very unrealistic for others. Not all toddlers are capable of a two-hour nap. Furthermore, some toddlers might have a long nap, but then aren't able to consolidate sleep in the night. Be careful what you wish for – there is only so much sleep you can get in 24 hours!

Check your toddler's overall sleep needs on this table to see if there's an obvious sleep deficit. If there isn't, and your toddler generally seems happy, then it is likely that this is normal for them. I am often asked for something approximate. I stress that there is really no evidence beyond total sleep times, but in case it is helpful, as a rough guide, you can expect:

Your child's age	Total sleep in 24 hours	Nap length	Your child may need up to this amount of awake time between nap ending and bedtime
18–24 months	11–14 hours	Up to two hours	Up to six hours awake before bed
2–2.5 years	10–13 hours	1.5-2 hours max	Up to seven hours awake before bed
2.5–3 years	10–13 hours	1–1.5 hours	May manage the whole day
3+ years	10–13 hours	Up to one hour	May manage the whole day

You might find that your child gets to a certain age and you will know that if they sleep after a certain time, you can write off the evening. The best person to work this out is you, so if this table bears no resemblance to your child, that's totally fine.

If your toddler wakes up cranky from their nap, there are two main reasons you could consider. If this just happens occasionally, I wouldn't overthink it. After all, sometimes we *all* wake up on the wrong side of bed! But the main reasons for this are:

1. Your toddler has slept a little too long, and has woken from a deep sleep. Waking from light sleep is much easier than deep sleep (you know this too!). If you are waking your toddler at a set time, try leaving them to wake spontaneously, or wait until you see them moving around a bit more in a light sleep. If they wake up by themselves in this state, then try waking them a bit earlier, to see if you can wake them in a light sleep, which might be easier for them.
2. Your toddler is still tired and woke up too soon. Refer to the average sleep need table to figure out if this is likely. If your toddler woke up after just a short nap, and this is common, then try getting to them before they usually wake up. For instance, if they often wake up after 30 minutes of sleep, try getting to them at around 25 minutes, and lay a hand on them, softly shush, or nurse them again to see if you can prolong the sleep a little longer. Sometimes just an extra 15 minutes make a big difference to their mood!

Dropping naps

Naps do not last forever. If you find that your child's nap is causing considerable stress and frustration – either at nap or bedtime – then on balance it may be better to scrap it. Be prepared for an adjustment period though. Sometimes, if I'm being really honest with you, there are no perfect options. In reality, you may have to choose between persevering with a nap, and accepting a much later bedtime, or having no nap, and an easy bedtime, but a slightly cranky child in the afternoon. Like I said – neither option is perfect, but this is sometimes the reality for a few months. One rule of thumb is that if it is very difficult to keep your child awake at their usual nap time, or you have to avoid all car journeys between 2pm and 6pm, then it is likely that your child is not quite ready to drop their nap.

If your child seems to do better with a nap, but it makes for a drawn out and stressful bedtime, then try capping the nap. Play around with how much daytime sleep is a good compromise. It may be that you need to cap it at 45 minutes, 30 minutes, or even 15 minutes.

You could think about changing the time of your child's nap. If you

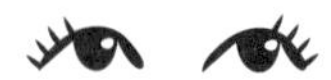

find that they seem to need eight hours of awake time before bed in order to sleep, for instance, then you may need to try an earlier nap, to allow enough time for your child's sleep pressure to build up again.

Consider being flexible – is it possible that on more active days you opt for keeping the nap, and on more sedentary and relaxed days you don't have it?

If the nap seems to lead to a frustrating bedtime, and you feel it's best to drop it, it's often best to avoid sitting and snuggling on the sofa during the 'danger zone' of 3–5pm when an accidental nap might occur and derail your evening!

The dropped nap, early bedtime, early rising triple whammy

The triple whammy is a situation that crops up from time to time. Often when a nap gets dropped, in the short term, this makes bedtime super easy and early (because the child's sleep pressure increases). Your child may then sleep well (or better) at night for a day or two. But what can sometimes happen is that this early bedtime leads to early rising.

But here's where it gets confusing. A child who wakes at 5am may initially be happy about it, but they often get cranky soon after waking. Why would this be when they've had a full night's sleep? Well, the answer is that their circadian rhythm and sleep pressure are misaligned.

Your child's circadian rhythm is responsible for releasing either alerting or sleepy hormones at the right time. If they wake at 5am, they have woken because they have had enough sleep, and their sleep pressure is low, but their circadian rhythm is shouting – 'Hey! It's not time to wake up yet'.

You probably won't have the same circadian misalignment problem at bedtime, as their sleep pressure will be high, so you'll get away with it. But the early bedtime is going to perpetuate that early rising.

So, here's what you could do:

- Try a catnap instead of a full nap, so your child can make it to a later bedtime that seems to be consistent with how much sleep they need overnight.
- Try to inch their bedtime later in small increments.
- Put them to bed at their usual early time, but wake them up after 45 minutes and get them back up for an hour. I call this a bedtime

nap. This isn't always easy. If your child is happy with this, then by all means carry on, but if they are unhappy and seem like they're desperate to go back to bed, abandon this tactic.

- Get your child outside in broad spectrum daylight in the late afternoon, to try to help their circadian signalling.
- Try to keep your child in the dark when they wake up, and use the early rising tools on pages 284–285 to help.

Reluctant nappers

We've all met those toddlers who are convinced they're not tired, don't need a nap, or think sleep is a dirty word! Working out when your child is truly ready to drop a nap, or all naps, as opposed to a being a reluctant napper, can be a game-changer. You'll need to review your little one's behaviour, bedtime, nighttime sleep and daytime fatigue to try to figure this out.

Often naps get refused during a time of acute developmental change or progress. You might have remembered that when your child was a baby, their sleep may have gone a little wonky when they were learning to crawl, walk, roll or babble.

Another common time for nap mayhem is during or after illness. Illness can make our little ones uncomfortable and grouchy. You might think that when they are ill children would sleep more. However, it's often been my experience, both as a children's nurse and mother, that when children are *really* unwell, they sleep a lot. If they are at that grouchy, uncomfortable, recovering stage, they tend to sleep a lot less. You may find that they nap more in the day, only to then be wide awake and ready to party at night. Or you might find that they nap less, and wake in the night as well. There may be nothing you can do about this besides trying to keep them hydrated, comfortable and manage their fever if they have one.

Toddlers are also very susceptible to FOMO (fear of missing out), and the thought of lying down for a nap when there are exciting activities happening (even if this is just laundry) can be unbearable. They can have another wave of separation anxiety that can mess up sleep, and, if they are under-exercised they tend to have too much excess energy to calm down and sleep.

Finally, total sleep needs do reduce over time, so if you are finding

that your child is getting later and later to bed, or waking early, you could consider capping or dropping their nap.

Creative nap hacks

If your child really seems to need a nap, but is reluctant to have one, try to not call it a nap. I call this the nap 'rebrand'! Snuggle time, story time, or a rest can be used instead. You could try sitting with them on the sofa, or on their bed, and listening to an audiobook, music or a guided meditation, and see if they 'accidentally' fall asleep without you trying.

Some little ones only nap well if they are physically tired. I've lost count of the number of toddlers who sleep best after going swimming! Consider whether you could squeeze some more exercise into your day – cycling, riding a scooter, walking, jumping, dancing and climbing all help toddlers to feel more physical fatigue, which might help them sleep.

You could also consider a change in location. An inside pop-up tent or teepee can be a great place for a nap. There's something about crawling into a cosy, small, child-sized space that is often irresistible for a toddler or preschooler. Another idea for children who need some quiet, dark space is to make a den under a table by throwing a blanket over it and putting a yoga mat inside so they can lie down in a 'cave' like a bear.

Some children need some motion or close contact to fall asleep. Just as this is understandable for infants, it's normal for toddlers as well. A tactical car-ride, walk in the pushchair, or a sling/carrier nap can help a reluctant napper to get the sleep you know they will benefit from.

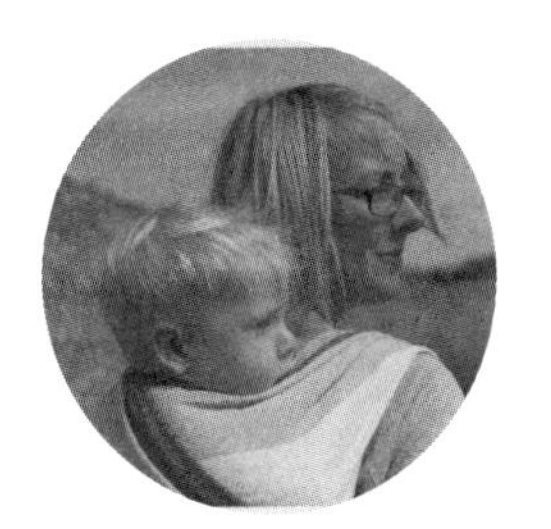

Carrying: babies, toddlers and beyond

Zoë Woodman, carrying consultant

The term 'babywearing' describes the act of using an aid to carry your child. It is something that humans have done for millennia. Up until industrialisation and the invention of the pram in the 1700s, carrying was the main way infants were cared for. It just didn't have a name.

The positive impact of carrying or holding infants is well documented:

- Reduces crying, through increased responsiveness
- Improves regulation of nervous system
- Improves sleep
- Improves regulation of heartrate
- Increase in and maintaining of body temperature
- A secure attachment (bond)
- Reduces stress hormones supporting brain development
- More quiet alert time, aiding learning and exploration of the world
- Improved social development and communication

What about as your baby gets older, into toddlerhood and beyond? Carrying can be a useful tool at any age. How?

- **Accessibility** – you can visit places or do things that might be challenging otherwise. Busy places, steps, narrow spaces and uneven ground can be navigated with ease. Using a sling/carrier gives you your hands free to hold onto rails etc.
- **Convenience** – it can be quick to pop a toddler in a sling/carrier to nip into the shops or when travelling for example. Slings/carriers fold up to quite a small size, so it is easy to stuff them in a bag or hang on the door for storage. They are reasonably priced compared to other transportation methods, and are more environmentally friendly. Toddlers can be fickle, wanting to walk and then not, and this can mean you can help support them when they need it!
- **Connection** – tired, sad or over-stimulated children can benefit from a hug to help them to calm down and to help regulate their nervous system. It can also be a useful way to reconnect with your child. Being closer to you also

means more chatting about the world and what is going on. This is positive for language and social development. Research shows that speech develops when a caregiver holds, smiles at, and talks to a child, engaging with them about the world. Having your child close exposes them to more language, interactions and social experiences.

Carrying older ones often encompasses all of these.

Practical tips

Having a sling/carrier that fits well is key to comfortable carrying, as typically older children are heavier to carry than a newborn. Most standard slings/carriers are marketed up to 2+yrs old or 15kg for example and yet in reality this doesn't mean it will always be comfy even under these limits. They may not fit older ones very well and for quick ups this may be fine. Listen to your body: it may be hard physically to carry but it should not cause pain, in the moment or after.

Back carrying can be more comfortable as your child gets bigger. Using buckle carriers you can do this from around six months of age. If the carrier is fitting knee-to-knee from the base of the carrier width wise and supporting their back up to the base of their neck height wise, this will typically be more comfortable to use. However, if you are using a sling/carrier that is not knee-to-knee or up to their neck but is comfortable for you, then carry on. If you have an adjustable carrier then ensure this is on the largest/widest settings.

You don't always need a sling/carrier. Piggy backs can be helpful! Although if you can carry on your body, in-arms, a well-fitting sling/carrier can provide support and make things easier, giving you use of your hands.

If you are finding carrying uncomfortable seek trained support. Often there are adjustments that can help or other options to try. There are slings/carriers specifically designed for older children, as well as those who have conditions that limit mobility, or low muscle tone. These are typically wider and taller than standard slings/carriers. It doesn't mean you have to stop carrying if it is something that you and your child enjoy or find useful.

- To find your local sling library or consultant: www.carryingmatters.co.uk/sling-pages
- Online sling hire: www.itsaslingthing.com
- www.carryingmatters.co.uk/why-carrying-children-matters
- www.theslingconsultancy.co.uk/blog

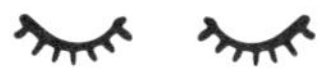

Children who may nap for longer

There are some children who may need to nap for longer than you might expect. They include children who have a chronic illness or disability that affects their energy levels. Children who have sleep apnoea or another sleep pathology that reduces the quality of their sleep overnight may experience daytime fatigue. In some cultures, it is normal for *everyone* to nap, and in these cases, the child will probably just follow the pattern of the family.

When it's really over

You may mourn the finality of the dropped nap, but most people can rationalise that when the nap starts to cause more problems than it solves, it is pragmatically the right thing to drop it. One of the main reasons people feel lost without the nap in the day is that having the day split into two can help to give some structure. It also allows a period of rest for parents. Having no nap means there is a risk the day can feel long and a little daunting, if we're honest. It's absolutely normal to feel like this, and to need some adult time. Parenting is hard work, and we all need some time away from the chatter, playing and caring. Stick with me, there may be a way.

Once your child has dropped their nap, try to model a quiet time, to allow you both an opportunity for some recharging. This time can either be for you to be quiet and restful together, or some children may be able to have a quiet time independently, depending on their age, temperament, and the activity you choose. This can be particularly important if you have a younger child who still naps (especially if they need your help to nap). Engage your older non-napping child in quiet activities that might give you a chance to have a break. I can't promise these will mean no interruptions, but at least it's a change of pace. Ideas that can work include:

- Puzzles
- Playing with scarves
- Threading cotton reels
- Looking at picture books
- Let them snuggle under a blanket and listen to an audio book or guided meditation

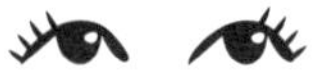

- Dolls and teddies
- Lego or Duplo, blocks or magnetic construction toys
- Colouring books
- Sewing with a large, safe plastic needle
- Sorting buttons into colours
- A selection of dried pasta, mixing bowls and kitchen utensils can keep some children happy for a good thirty minutes.

Remember as well that when your child first drops their nap, they may temporarily need an earlier bedtime. Keep an eye on how this strategy affects their morning wake-up time though – if you notice their wake-up getting earlier, you may need to inch their bedtime later, to avoid the triple whammy. Now, there isn't always much you can do about this. After all, some children are natural early risers, and 6am is not usually considered 'early'. But if your child used to sleep later in the morning when they had a nap and had a later bedtime, then it is possible you can get that later wake-up time back.

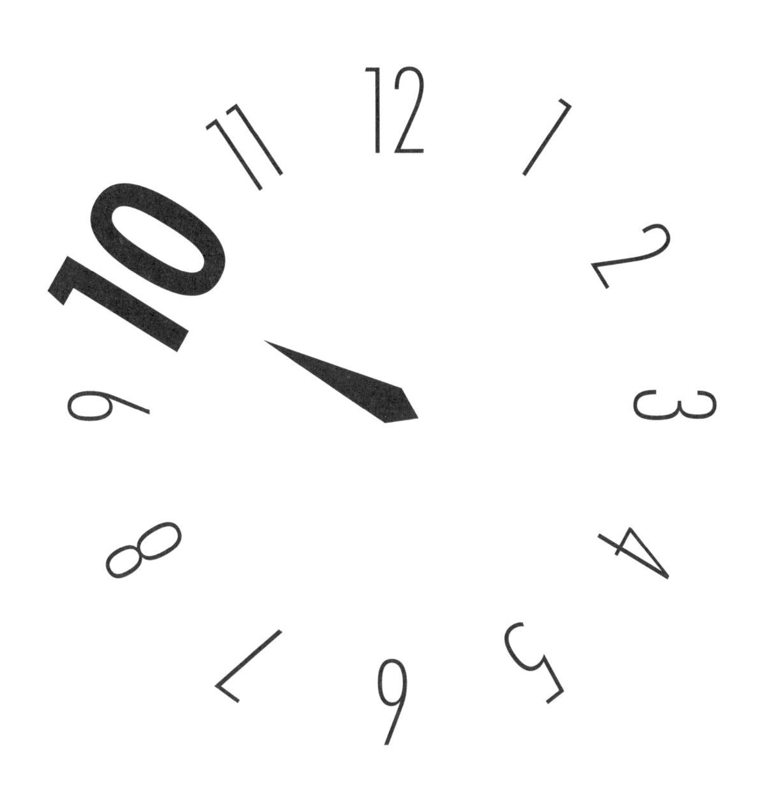

CHAPTER TEN

ALL ABOUT NIGHTS

Night-waking is not just a part of infancy. A large systematic review studied normal sleep patterns across a global sample of children aged 0–12 and found that in the 1–2-year-old group children woke up to 2.5 times in the night. Unfortunately there was not enough data in this particular sample to provide night-waking data for older children, which is a shame, because it is highly unlikely that a child stops waking twice a night the second they reach their third year.[1] A more recent study found that 2.5–3.5-year-old children wake on average four times per night. Many of these wake-ups last for more than 30 minutes.[2] I'm not sure whether that information makes you feel depressed, relieved or validated, but at least you know the truth! For many people, knowing that they are not the only one with an older child who still doesn't sleep through makes them feel less alone.

Night-waking in older children is a different ball game compared to babies though, isn't it? If you're parenting a three, four, five, or six-year-old, you have several years now of sleep fragmentation and the chances are you have heard many ideas and theories about why they wake up. Perhaps you have tried the simple solutions already. Maybe the only solutions that seem to be on offer are the ones that don't work. I don't have a single method, mnemonic to remember, or a three-step plan because every situation is different. However, many sleep challenges can be grouped into clusters of behaviour. Your child may not have the exact same scenario, but if it broadly fits into that cluster, you could try

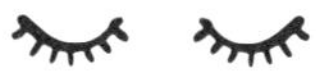

some of the suggestions and see if they work. The tools in this chapter are grouped into clusters based on their aim:

1. Strategies based on sleep biology
2. Managing anxiety, including fear of being alone
3. Maintaining connection
4. Building trust, not testing endurance
5. Ideas that help with limits and boundaries

As parents, we are instinctively drawn to stories that fit our exact scenario. It is highly unlikely that I will describe exactly what is going on in your home, with your family. While examples are useful to a point, it is natural to think that because an example does not perfectly match ours, it will not apply. I assure you that there is plenty of room for flexibility, adaptation, mashing up a combination of many tools, using these tools to inspire a completely creative new approach, or making something up as you go along.

While I have used all of the tools in this chapter hundreds of times, different tools work for different children and families, and you are the best person to decide which one is likely to be a good fit. If you're not sure which tool might work, have at look at this table to help you decide. Obviously, because life isn't neatly compartmentalised into little boxes, it is likely that you may need to use more than one tool. That's totally fine – you cannot overdose on any of these tools. You will find more tips and ideas in chapter 12.

Your main sleep drama	Possible reasons	Tools that may work	Page(s)
Early rising	• Early bedtime • Low sleep need • Lark child • Stressful evening	• Later bedtime • Early rising tools	67 284–285
Split nights	• Bedtime too early • Low sleep need • Night discomfort • Triple whammy (page 220)	• Later bedtime • Eliminate underlying causes • Reinstate brief nap to facilitate later bedtime	295 58–60 216–219

Waking in the middle of the night	• Shift from predominantly deep to predominantly light sleep • Discomfort • Full bladder • Nightmare • Habitual	• Background noise • Rule out underlying factors including itching, pain and gas • Reduce fluids, or try a dream-wee • Scheduled awakening	207 58–60 146 233
Very long bedtime/ bedtime battles	• Circadian rhythm/ sleep pressure misalignment • Limit testing • Anxiety/sensitivity	• Fading • Daytime limits • Meditations • Managing anxiety	234–236 121–125 240 244–249
Multiple night wakes	• Sensitive child • Developmental phase • Hunger • Discomfort • Low sleep pressure • Low sleep needs	• Floor bed • Eliminate under-lying causes • Later bedtime • Drop the nap	236–238 58–60 67 219–220
Negotiating and procrastinating	• Boundary testing • Developmental • Seeking more control	• Social story • Magic sleep cush-ion • Sleep ribbon • Daytime limits	251–252 249–251 245–246 121–125
Coming into your bed	• Sensitive child • Major changes in home • Developmental • Nightmares • Anxiety	• Camp bed in your room • Floor bed • Sibling bed	297 236–238 238–240
Strange noises or movements in the night	• Underlying causes need to be ruled out • Could be normal • Parasomnias	• Video the behaviour/noise • Rule out underly-ing causes	149 58–60
Anxiety about bedtime	• Sensitive child • Situational stress • Major changes in home • Separation anxiety	• Bad dream spray • Meditations • Sleep ribbon • Transference	140 240 245–246 243–244

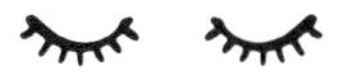

Needing you to stay with them at bedtime	• Normal • Developmental • Sensitive child • Limit testing • Anxiety	• Magic sleep cushion • Pop outs • Acceptance • Social story	249–251 249–249 232–233 251–252
Bedsharing no longer working	• Wriggly child • New pregnancy/ baby • Touched out parent • Child wants to move	• Floor bed • Sibling bed • Toddler/single bed	236–238 238–240 237
Night feeding	• Normal • Habitual • Hunger • Thirsty (check for mouth breathing/ snoring)	• Limiting feeds • Night weaning • Acceptance • Review daytime intake	263–265 259–263 255–256 260–261

You will probably need to start by making sure you have exhausted all the other aspects of your child's sleep. Use your background sleep checklist, and create your own action plan if you need to, before you think about whether you need a sleep tool overnight.

Background sleep checklist:

Have I ruled out or addressed:	x	Action needed?
Underlying causes and red flags		
Sleep hygiene		
My child's total sleep needs (low-average-high)		
Does my child need to reinstate, cap or drop a nap?		
Lifestyle factors (food, love, exercise, mental stimulation, fun)		
Bedtime routine		
Loving limits and boundaries		

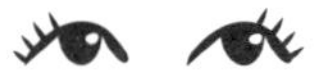

Suitable age ranges

You may be wanting to zero in on a strategy that is suitable for your child and the age they are now. I have not provided age ranges for these strategies because in my experience when an age range is given people tend to think these are inflexible. The reality is that a strategy that works for a two-year-old may also work beautifully for an 11-year-old, with some adaptations, different language or modifying the timing. The strategies also depend on your child's cognitive ability, language, developmental stage, strengths, challenges, interests, anxieties and energy levels. For all these reasons, I suggest you read through and try to imagine implementing the tool with your child. Trust your gut instinct here – if you intuitively feel that something will not work, you're probably right. Mentally scrap that tool and move on to the next. Eventually something will feel like it has potential.

One final tip – try any strategy for at least a week before reviewing and deciding whether this is worth sticking with or changing for a different tool. Sometimes older children need a little time to adjust to a new way of falling asleep or settling, so try not to abandon a tool after one or two nights – it probably won't have had enough time to work. When you review your situation, try to be objective and positive. Is *anything* better? Even a little bit? Older children sometimes make progress quite slowly, so managing your expectations is really important. Of course we all love it when there is a dramatic U-turn, but more often, there are small, subtle and distinct improvements that build over time. After a week, if you are genuinely not seeing any progress at all, or the situation is worse, then press pause. Consider whether there is an underlying problem, or a major developmental stage or anxiety is preventing progress. It's fine to try a different strategy if the first one is not working. Just repeat the process of trying for a week and evaluating honestly.

Acceptance

I want to make it clear that acceptance is an option you can frame as a positive choice at any time, and with any scenario that isn't a medical problem. Acceptance does not need to feel like defeat. Acceptance means to quietly sit with whatever situation you are facing, knowing that it will pass. Acceptance means that you are choosing to accommodate for and adapt to a situation, rather than address it head-on. Sometimes it is right

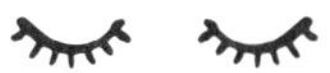

to choose acceptance at the outset. Other times you might start to use a particular strategy, and then choose to press pause. This is not giving up. It is a conscious choice that whatever place you are in right now, change is not something that is right for your family. This might be because you simply don't have the capacity to change, you lack the resources, you're too exhausted or it might be that a new circumstance makes change inappropriate. Whatever the reason, part of responsive parenting is to be willing to be flexible according to the current status quo.

1. Ideas based on sleep biology

Some strategies simply use an understanding and awareness of how sleep works, and how the body responds to factors that we can manipulate with timings. The following tools are not about changing behaviour or response at all, but simply involve altering timings.

Scheduled awakening

This is a tried and tested method of stopping a predictable wake-up. It is especially good for children who always get up around the same time every night, whether that is to come into your bed, or call out. It is also good for children who are having a recurring nightmare or terror. What you do is go to your child *before* you think they usually wake up, and 'stir' them a little. You are not trying to fully wake them up, you just want to see some evidence that their sleep state has shifted slightly. You may see some changes in their breathing, movements, or they may make a little noise. I sometimes explain that this is a little like restarting or rebooting a computer. You're essentially trying to interrupt their sleep cycle, but help them stay asleep through it. There is a fair amount of evidence for this technique, even in mainstream sleep-training literature[3,4] and it is definitely worth a try for a couple of weeks if you'd like to give it a go.

Consistent wake up and bedtimes

It might be an obvious point, but because an older child usually has a fairly well established circadian rhythm, it may be worth checking whether there is room for more consistency in your wake up and bedtimes. This is especially relevant for tweens who may be starting to sleep later in the morning, and may get into the trap of sleeping later on weekends, only to then struggle to get up in time for school on Monday.

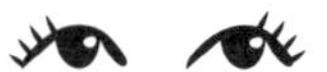

Try to tighten up the timings, which may mean waking your child at a consistent time and shooting for a more predictable bedtime. This doesn't remove the importance of being child-led and responsive – of course you should be reactive when your child is particularly tired for whatever reason. But in a general sense, if bedtime is very loose, and the wake up time is variable, for a child with a more sensitive chronotype, this may not be helpful for the sleep rhythms.

Fading

Fading is a technique that is used for insomnia in adults, and may help you too if this is something your child struggles with.[5] Insomnia causes difficulty with falling asleep or staying asleep, and results in inefficient sleep – essentially, the amount of time spent in bed awake is proportionally high compared to the time actually asleep in bed. Taking more than 30 minutes is common with insomnia, and while this could also be associated with putting a child to bed too early, before they are actually tired, insomnia may also have a behavioural cause. Going to bed should be associated with a rapid onset of sleep, and if being in bed, the bedtime routine and the sleep space are associated with wakefulness, then this can have a negative impact on sleep.

First of all, you may need to adjust the nap, bed and food timings. You could also adjust the bedtime routine, eliminating activities that don't seem conducive to calming down, and try more activity in the day. You may need to consider whether the bedroom environment is a hindrance – for example, are there scary shadows or distractions from lots of decorations?

Finally, you could try fading, which is similar to a technique used in adult insomnia called sleep restriction. The idea is to not to go to bed until the sleep pressure is very high and sleep is inevitable. Once going to bed is associated with a rapid onset of sleep, then you will have successfully corrected the negative association of wakefulness with bedtime, and can begin making the bedtime earlier in very small increments, taking care not to bring it forward by too much, or too quickly.

There are two main ways that this technique can backfire. Firstly, if your child compensates for a later bedtime by sleeping later. So you'll need to wake them at a consistent time for this to work. Secondly, if you do not make the bedtime late enough (I find this is usually due to anxiety about depriving a child of sleep) then your child still won't have enough sleep pressure, and all that happens is an even later bedtime than usual. I know it sounds counter-intuitive, but sometimes you have to be fairly bold with fading.

> *Xavier (aged six) took at least two hours to go to bed. His parents started bedtime at 7pm, and by 7.30 he was in bed. But he was up and down the stairs, procrastinating and not able to fall asleep until around 9.30–10pm. He woke up at 7am for school the next day but seemed tired when he woke up. Most of Xavier's friends go to sleep at 7–7.30pm and his parents were getting increasingly anxious that he was chronically sleep deprived. Most evenings would end with Xavier's parents getting frustrated, and everyone had begun to dread bedtime.*

In this situation, it seems sensible to first check the total sleep time. Xavier is getting nine hours' overnight sleep. This is actually within the normal range of 9–11 hours, so it could be that he does not need any more sleep than this. He seems tired in the morning, which may be because he is a natural owl, and waking early does not suit his particular circadian rhythm. Or it may be that he does indeed need a little more sleep. Fading is a good option to test whether Xavier could benefit from improved sleep hygiene to condense the falling asleep process, take the stress out of the situation, and then begin to make bedtime earlier. If, when they bring bedtime earlier, Xavier begins to wake even earlier, or falling asleep seems to take longer again, then his parents may need to accept that either his circadian rhythm is just built this way, or he really is a lower sleep need child. To test the theory, his parents started bedtime at 9.15, and Xavier was in bed by 9.30. He fell asleep within 15 minutes without any fussing or fighting. After two weeks of consistently easier bedtimes, they began bringing bedtime forward by 15 minutes, keeping a close eye on how long it took Xavier to go to sleep. Once it started to take 30 minutes, they stopped making bedtime any earlier, and accepted that this was the earliest possible bedtime. Ultimately, Xavier ended up having a bedtime of 8pm, and was asleep by 8.30. Not the 7.30 bedtime of his peers, but on the other hand there was much less stress, and an understanding that he just didn't need as much sleep as his friends.

Many parents are nervous about whether their child will get really tired with this approach. They may not want to try it due to anxiety over

the fact that their child is already sleep deprived. I usually explain to parents that there are two problems with a child who procrastinates so much at bedtime that they don't fall asleep until late:

1. The association of wakefulness with the bedtime routine
2. Not enough sleep

The tricky thing with this scenario is that parents are usually equally anxious about both problems. But you cannot tackle problem number two, until you have first corrected problem number one. So, you will need to be bold, make that bedtime later, and only when your child is consistently falling asleep within 30 minutes do you inch bedtime earlier to begin to correct problem number two. Ultimately, if your child is falling asleep late anyway, you are not depriving them of any *more* sleep, you're just cutting out the stressful, drawn-out part of bedtime. If nothing else, it will make the evening less frustrating.

Finally, you may be wondering what to do with all that extra time in the evening. Since you will be starting the bedtime later, you will have more space at the end of the day. This may be a good time to rethink how your evening flows. Perhaps this is a new window of opportunity for family time. Or maybe, depending on the age of your child, they can play quietly, or read a book. Perhaps you can both do some yoga or Pilates together, or go for an evening walk.

2. Managing anxiety, including fear of being alone

It is perfectly normal for children to have some reservations about being alone. We are social and relational beings, and from a logical point of view, 9–12 hours is a long time to be away from the person you love and trust most in the world. The next few tools are designed to manage and alleviate the anxiety of being alone at night.

Floor beds

I am a big fan of floor beds. They can work really well for children who wake in the night, need lots of parental reassurance, come into your bed in the night, or are transitioning away from bedsharing. They can also work well for children who are in the process of being night-weaned. Here are the main reasons why I like them:

- They make it easier for a parent to lie next to their child and then sneak away. If your child needs your physical presence to fall asleep, it can be a lot easier to lie on a floor bed rather than a toddler bed.
- They can make a transition from bedsharing to solo sleeping easier. For a child who has had your physical proximity, it can be hard to be completely separate. Giving them a floor bed and lying beside them so that they are in their room, on their sleep surface, but still with your reassuring presence, may be an easier bridge.
- They are low down, and feel safe for toddlers (plus – no monsters under the bed!)
- If your child has recently moved from a crib/cot and you're worried they may roll out of bed, especially if they are a wriggler – the floor bed avoids this problem.
- The air near the floor is cooler, which can be more comfortable and may be useful for children who seem to have a little internal hot water bottle.
- It's cheaper to buy a single bed mattress than a special toddler bed with mattress, and you can use the mattress for longer.
- It promotes independence (when the child is ready).

Sometimes a family floor bed works well. This is actually completely normal in many cultures. You could put your own mattress on the floor, and then have your child's mattress next to yours. This way, everyone gets more space, but your child's need for closeness is met. You may need to clear a bit of space, and of course, there may not physically be room for your child's mattress, but if you can make it work, this might be a solution that gets everyone the rest they need.

If you choose to have the floor bed in your child's bedroom, I recommend having the floor bed in the corner of a room, so it feels nice and contained and safe. Again, you will need to make sure their environment is safe, and take any toys out of their room that you would rather they didn't play with unattended. I recommend the removal of paint, marker pens, putty, slime, and nail varnish. From personal experience I can confirm that these items will leave a permanent record of your child's artwork in places not designed for that purpose...

You can also consider a canopy if your child is very sensitive – sometime this 'den-like' environment makes children feel a bit safer. You can buy mosquito nets, as well as purpose-designed canopies, that make the space feel smaller and cosier.

Put mirrors or artwork low down, at your child's eye level, and it will feel like their space. The more your child feels ownership of their sleep space, and finds it a relaxing and pleasant place to be, the more likely they are to associate it with a feeling of safety and calm, which helps sleep.

Floor beds aren't for everyone, and you'll need to make sure the environment is safe and kid-proof. You'll also need to have some boundaries in place, but apart from that, this could be a winner for your little one.

Sibling bed

An alternative to a solo floor bed or family floor bed is a sibling bed. This is exactly what it sounds like. It could be a mattress on the floor, but equally, it could be a double bed, or two twin beds pushed close together. Admittedly not all siblings will go for this idea, but you would be surprised how many siblings adore cuddling up to each other to fall asleep. We are, after all, mammals. All young (and many adult) mammals like cuddling up to someone to sleep. When we brought home our second pup, she immediately decided that our older dog was going to be her surrogate sister, and the pair quickly fell into a pattern of sleeping in the same bed, despite having their own beds. It's just normal. If you have more than one child, and they are both over the age of one, have a think about whether this might be a viable option for your family. Some helpful tips if you decide to try this arrangement:

- Consider making sure each of your sharing children has a private space of their own, with a special place to store favourite toys and precious things. Children love to keep their bits and pieces in a safe place.
- Make sure there are no gaps or hazards where little fingers, toes and other body parts can become trapped or pinched.
- Consider giving each child a duvet or cover of their own, rather than expecting them to share a double duvet. Many children can be duvet hogs which can leave one sibling literally out in the cold.
- If one child tends to wake up before their sibling, set out the expectations for what they can do, so they do not wake their sibling up. Have a look at the early rising tools on page 284–285 for ideas of how to manage this.

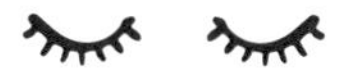

Sibling beds work best for children who are able to go to bed at the same time, but you might be able to make it work for children who have staggered bedtimes. For example, your later-to-bed child could read a book in another location, or perhaps they could both have a snuggle and a story together with you, and then your later-to-bed child could leave the room once the lights are turned off, until it is time for their bed.

Here are some stories from parents who have embraced sibling beds:

'My twins would get into bed together as soon as they could. It was so lovely. They had such a close bond and slept really well when they were sharing a bed. When we introduced a bunk bed when they were older they chose to share the top bunk to begin with. Once my third baby was born, one of my twins loved to sleep with him once he was a toddler.' **Kathryn**

'We have a sibling bed set up for two of our boys who are four and six. Although they both have their own bedrooms, they go to bed together in either of the rooms. We bought everyone double beds when we moved house in order to facilitate comfortable sleep in any combination of child/adult as our children were waking frequently at that point. They get comfort from being close to each other and it means bedtime goes more smoothly. When we tried to do bedtimes separately, whichever child was waiting would get scared on their own or cause a riot and run about the house so this was a logical solution to make bedtimes quicker and easier for us.' **Adele**

'I have definitely found that my kids sleep better together in the same bed than in their own beds. It's very cute to see them sleeping in the same posture or cuddled up to each other. Of course they will sometimes roll all over each other or wake each other but I think overall the experience is more positive. Sometimes the older ones will pat or cuddle the younger ones when they see them being distressed and even help them find us or bring us to the baby. It's just an extension of their daytime relationship with each other and it's lovely to experience the moments of them taking care of each other overnight as well.' **Katie**

'There are never any problems going to bed. The girls are happy to go to bed and fall asleep easily and happily. Of course they do, it's a nice experience. We all get into bed, read a story or two and I stay there till they fall asleep. No battles. We also go to bed when they are tired. No bedtimes just working on feel: if one is tired then that's fine for bed. If they have a bad dream and wake, because I'm right there, it's a simple matter of a cuddle as I'm right there and then everyone is straight back to sleep. Same when they're ill. It's all very easy. And it's lovely. For all of us. That's a big factor and one I've managed to feel proud of now rather than hiding away from for fear of what other people say or think.' **Katharine**

Meditations and yoga

Another tool I'm a huge fan of is meditations and guided relaxations. Toddlers can have a wild imagination and some are prone to overthinking. Listening to a guided relaxation or meditation can be a great tool to help your little people calm down, settle and sleep.

Children who are anxious also benefit from meditations. Children's meditations are essentially a sweet story. They usually incorporate some aspect of progressive muscle relaxation, or slow breathing. They often have some soothing music in the background, and most of them are designed to last about the length of time that is common to fall asleep – about 15–20 minutes. Some of them are designed for specific age groups, so check whether the one you have found is suitable before trying it out. Some of my favourites include:

- Jason Stephenson – he has lots of meditations for adults and children. I love the hot air balloon ride, but check out the rest here: www.youtube.com/channel/UCqPYhcdFgrlUXiGmPRAej1w
- Christiane Kerr – a yoga and mindfulness instructor. I've loved every single one of the meditation CDs we have used for our children: calmforkids.com
- New Horizons – their YouTube channel has hundreds of themed meditations for children: www.youtube.com/channel/UCjW-3doUmNsyY5aLQHLiNXg

The power of breath

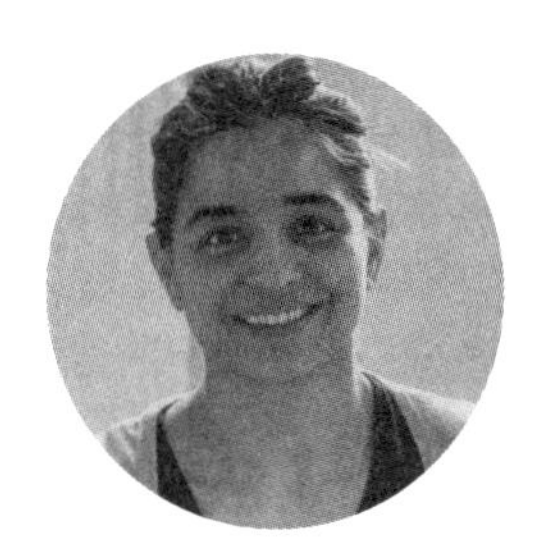

Dr Rehana Jawadwala, exercise physiologist, author and founder of MummyYoga, a specialist perinatal yoga service

Think about all the 'systems' we have in our body... our circulatory, respiratory, nervous, endocrine, reproductive, digestive, lymph, immune... among others. How many of these are under our voluntary control? Possibly only a fraction of the respiratory system! But this little window of control we have over our breathing affects all the other involuntary systems, impacting our health and wellbeing in ways that can be profound.

Most often, our breathing changes involuntarily depending on the way our body and mind perceive our environment. If we feel threatened, we activate a fast and shallow breath that in turn signals our brain and body to prepare for flight or fight. When we feel calm and relaxed our breathing rate slows down, activating the part of our nervous system responsible for the rest and digest state. However, this is a two-way street. We can change our breathing pattern to simulate the state of being that we wish to be in. So, if we voluntarily activate our deep and relaxed breathing pattern our brains perceive our environment to be calm despite what the reality may be.

This way of affecting our minds via controlling our breathing is a simple and powerful method of navigating the world on our terms. We don't need to *react* to everything that is happening around us, we can choose to *respond* in a considered way to the experiences that matter to us and let go of the ones that are either trivial or out of our control. This is the crux in stress, anger and anxiety management.

Despite popular media mentioning the many benefits of yoga for kids, the reality is that kids will not want to engage in an activity simply because you think it is beneficial for them. Most kids by now have heard that yoga is good for them, so they will either go along if they wish to please you or rebel against what you think is cool.

If you want your child to embrace the transformational practice of yoga and meditation, you will need to experience its power first. Once you are a convert, then simply employ a breath-based response to *your* high-stress situations and demonstrate for your children the kind of behaviour that will transform their relationship with stressful external stimuli. Our brains are primed to learn by watching and mimicking. From the moment we are born, the mirror neurons in our brains are growing at an exponential rate allowing for this form of learning to be the predominant way our children will learn, make sense of and accumulate knowledge and behaviour patterns.

Personally, I would not recommend emulating a traditional yoga class for an at-home yoga practice. Your practice at home should be intimate, personal and unique to you and your family. You need to create a ritual that is meaningful to you and your children. You don't have to close your eyes, sit cross-legged or even sit for that matter. You know your kids best: use an activity that is important to them to include some breath awareness practice. This could be as basic as counting their breaths! You could even start with just counting aloud in a rhythmic tone, ignoring your breath in the beginning. Just the repeated practice of counting or breath counting every time they feel stress mounting around them will show them the subtle yet important nature of what you are trying to achieve.

There are some cool jingles on the internet such as 'countdown to calm down' in the cartoon series Daniel Tiger and others worth looking at. All these are non-serious ways of bringing in a deep yoga practice into your children's lives very early on without making them feel like they are engaging in this new fad that everyone is telling them about. This way of incorporating yoga will be personal to them and will not feel like they are in school doing yet another activity on schedule.

Kids have a far more intuitive and experiential side to their learning that we adults have lost. Appeal to that way of learning by helping them experience how simple breath-based practices make them feel. Initially, as you are incorporating these into their lives, do not talk about the benefits or even how they may be feeling when doing the breath awareness practice. We parents tend to intellectualise things so we can extract the 'lessons' from activities. Try to give your kids the space to breathe, metaphorically and literally! Once their internal space changes with the breath awareness practice, they will employ these powerful strategies even when you are not around and that's true learning. My three-year-old at times reminds me, 'Mumma just breathe now...!', that's when I know my job is done.

Some simple breath-based practice to try:

1. Counting – count up or down in a monotone, low-pitched voice with a slow rhythm after stories at bedtime.
2. Breath counts – keep your hand on your belly and you can ask the kids to do the same and count your full breaths, both inhale and exhale.
3. Breath elongation – as you get used to breath counting, slowly start to elongate your exhalations and build this practice of activating your parasympathetic nervous system, which will help in managing stressful situations over time.

Website: www.MummyYoga.com
Social: @MummyYoga
Videos: vimeo.com/MummyYoga
Podcast: anchor.fm/MummyYoga

Transference
This is a nice technique for sensitive and empathic children who need lots of support at bedtime, or feel anxious or nervous about being alone. You encourage your child to be concerned for someone or something else, and what often happens is that their own anxiety melts away. You can of course use this technique alongside many others suggested in this book.

You can help transfer your child's caring and empathic concerns on to any object that they care about. It could be a doll, teddy, or other toy. Children are both naturally caring and kind, and also have vivid imaginations. Toys and teddies become animate objects with feelings and emotions in the mind of a child, and you can use this to help not only their sleep, but also develop the caring and empathic side of your child's personality.

Sometimes you can reinforce this concept by going out to buy a new toy or teddy. What I recommend is that you suggest to your child that the new toy/doll/teddy might feel a little lonely away from all the other teddies/toys, or on their first night in a new home. Ask for your child's help to care for the toy and make sure they feel super loved and cared about, to help the toy settle in. Many parents find that when their child is on board with this concept, they discover their child murmuring words of reassurance to the toy, and eventually fall asleep snuggled close to it.

My youngest daughter always used to be more anxious at bedtime after one of her many hospital admissions. On the first few nights back home, I would let her have my very special (and expensive!) breastfeeding/teaching doll – 'Jennifer'. The baby doll is not a plaything and my daughter knew that the baby had to be especially well looked after. It was a *privilege* to care for Jennifer and her eyes would light up with the honour of being trusted to put Jennifer to sleep. She always used to fall asleep cuddled up to the baby – interestingly in the classic safer bedsharing position – and was more concerned for the baby (being away from me – her actual 'mummy') than for herself.

3. Maintaining connection

Because sleep is a time of separation, maintaining connection can be the key to settled bedtimes and consolidated nights. Helping children to be calm, regulated and relaxed helps them stay in their 'rest and digest' autonomic state. If they feel stressed because of the looming separation that they know is coming, they may become more alert and find it harder to wind down. For this reason, choosing some strategies that may lessen the worry about separation could be a back door route to easier and more peaceful bedtimes. The following tools are all based on the idea of maintaining connection.

Give them an object to 'look after'

This is a sweet, but simple idea to help children feel connected to a parent. Having something that belongs to their parent to 'keep safe' can maintain the feeling of connectedness. These are a few things you could try:

- Draw a kiss, heart, or flower on your child's hand, and show them how they can kiss it if they feel they need some extra love.
- Give your child something of yours to keep safe under their pillow – this has to be a smooth object that poses no strangulation, choking or injury risk. Try a watch, bracelet, or other safely sized item.
- Give your child an item of your clothing to sleep with. They could even wear your top as a supersized nightshirt! Something that smells of a parent can be hugely comforting, which is why clothing is often a good idea.

- Try a special blanket, or other comfort object.

While a common recommendation is to give a child a comfort blanket or special lovey or teddy, some children don't seem to develop a strong attachment to one toy. For these children, having a basket of available toys and asking them every night to choose which one they would like to keep safe and look after might work better. This strategy also seems to work well for children who seem to develop some fatigue or boredom with the same toy, and need change. It also works well for children who like to feel a sense of ownership or control over a situation.

Ribbon trick
This is a good tool to maintain connection, and it helps with separation anxiety. It works well for children who are anxious about being left alone, and need a parent to stay with them. It helps children understand concepts that are difficult to imagine or intangible. The idea with the ribbon is to create a physical reminder that you and your child are still connected even when you are not physically present. There is an invisible and permanent connection between you, but your younger child may not be able to imagine that, so you can use a tangible object to help them understand this concept first.

Here's how you do it:

- Go out with your child to choose a ribbon together. It needs to be about five metres long. Your child may choose a silky one, a sparkly one or a patterned one.
- At bedtime, give one end of the ribbon to your child, and you hold the other end.
- At your child's pace, let out the ribbon so that they are further away, yet still holding the ribbon. Keep the tension on the ribbon firm so your little one can feel you still holding on.
- Eventually, the ribbon tension can go slack, and you are out of sight.
- Once your child is asleep, obviously you must return to your child's room and remove the ribbon from their hand for safety reasons.

Your little one will still feel connected to you. I love this strategy for children who are anxious about being alone. Children love the physical imagery with the ribbon, and even when the ribbon is no longer needed, children can imagine in their mind's eye a ribbon or thread running from themselves to their parent in another room. This strategy works particularly well alongside a story called 'The Invisible String' by Patrice Karst.

Photos of special people

One more idea to help children feel connected is to surround them with images of the people they love. Ask your child for ideas of who they would like to feel close to at night, and put photos around their sleep space of these people, places or objects. Your child may choose random things – I would just go with it, because children who feel they are part of the decision-making are usually more on board with the strategy. If they want a photo of a Lego model they made, a friend they haven't seen for six months, or the next-door neighbours' cat, that's fine. You can also suggest special people if this feels appropriate. Print these images out and ask your child where they would like to stick them up. Your child may choose to kiss the images goodnight at bedtime, or wave goodnight to them, or they might just be happy knowing that their favourite toy truck is watching over them as they sleep. Kids are funny like this sometimes – we might not always understand what is going on in those wonderful minds, but honestly, just embrace the weirdness and see if it works.

4. Building trust, not testing endurance

Often, mainstream sleep strategies are founded on the principle of behavioural training. They assume that children are delaying or procrastinating at bedtime because the 'reward' is more time with a parent. I frequently like to turn that on its head and challenge this. After all, if children need more time with an adult, then if we meet the need, they will not crave it. Rather than thinking of behaviour as an undesirable thing to be extinguished through denying parental presence, I prefer to think of it as a symptom that may be better managed through careful and therapeutic relationships. The next few strategies are designed to *build* trust, not test how far we can push children's' confidence. You will find that they work with many ages of children, but I have made suggestions for modifications and adaptations that you could consider depending on your child's cognitive and language abilities. As with all the tools in the book, you can use them alongside other strategies if you like.

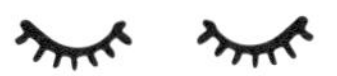

Pop-outs

One of my favourite tools for children is the pop-out. This is a great tool for eventually moving your child towards being able to fall asleep alone (when they are ready). As you read this, you might think it sounds like controlled crying. It is the *opposite* of controlled crying. So let me preemptively explain!

Controlled crying (which I never, ever recommend) goes like this: you put your child down awake, in their crib/bed, and leave the room. You do not re-enter the room, irrespective of crying, until it has been a certain number of minutes – perhaps five minutes, or perhaps 20. You briefly reassure, and then leave the room again. The child's crying makes no difference to your behaviour or how frequently you return.

Okay, breathe gentle people. Don't worry. I'm not about to suggest anything that stressful. Pop-outs are the psychological opposite of controlled crying. In fact, *pop-outs do not involve* any *crying at all*. If your child starts to cry – this is the wrong tool. I cannot stress enough that leaving your child to cry is *not* the aim here.

With a pop-out, you stay with your little one until they are settled, and then you briefly leave their side, for the shortest amount of time possible – perhaps just 5–10 seconds. You immediately return.

The idea is to get back before they can even *think* about getting upset. You then stay with them a while longer, and repeat. You can stay by your child's side as long as you like, and you can leave the room as often as you like. You go at your child's pace, staying out of the room for longer, and more frequently leaving as they are ready.

The idea with the pop-out is that your child learns through multiple repetitions that you *always come back*. You never leave them long enough for them to worry or get upset, and you show them with your behaviour that they do not need to cry to get you back in the room.

You ultimately want your child to get *bored* of you leaving. They are so confident and relaxed about you always coming back (because you've demonstrated this with the pop outs) that they don't fret or flinch when you leave. They expect you to return and you have never let them down on this front.

Eventually, you'll be able to leave the room frequently, and stay out for longer. And at some point, because your child is so confident you'll come back, they will fall asleep without you even being there. It may

take a long time, but it is a zero stress and no crying technique.

Baby pop out

If you are at the stage where your child will fall asleep with you lying beside them, but they get upset as soon as you are out of sight, then you could try the baby pop-out. With this tool, you will not be leaving their room at all. You will stay beside them, and then perhaps walk to the end of their bed, pretend to tidy something, or bend to pick an imaginary item off the floor, fold laundry or whatever. They may need you to do this for a while, until their confidence that you *always* return is built. This is good for more anxious or sensitive children. Once they are falling asleep and not batting an eyelid, then you could start proper pop-outs, and go very slowly.

First minute alone

This is a slight variation on the pop-out that may work well for older children. Instead of coming in and out frequently, you give your child the first minute on their own after you've said goodnight. After the first minute, come and stay with your child until they are asleep. This works well for anxious children who need your presence, but easily get over-excited by you coming and going. Again, the idea isn't to make them upset, so if they do get upset, you may need to wait with them a while longer, filling their love tank, making sure you're speaking their love language, and dealing with any underlying anxiety before trying again.

Once the first minute has gone well, give it a few days staying at the one-minute mark, and then stay out for two minutes. Go very slowly, so your child doesn't notice that the time is extending. The idea once again is to build their confidence that you *always* come back, and they begin to relax during that alone time. Go more slowly at first, as they get used to the idea, and then you may find you can move on to staying out of the room for longer once their confidence is built. Given that it takes about 15–20 minutes to fall asleep, you're working up to being able to stay out while they fall asleep independently.

If you actually *like* sitting with your child while they fall asleep (lots of people do!) then you could stay with them for the first few minutes, and then just pop out for one minute, building the time up as their confidence increases. The idea with this is that you both get the best of both worlds.

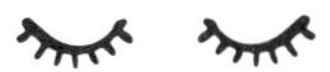

You get to sit with your child during that peaceful time of falling asleep, quietly connecting with them, thinking of them, or praying for them while they relax into sleep, but you also build in the option to leave and get some time for yourself.

'Oops I forgot'/I'll be right back

This is a verbal variation on the pop-out theme. You sit and stay with your child, and then calmly leave the room, promising to come right back. There are a couple of ways to try it, and each way works better for different temperaments:

1. Simply say, I'll be right back, *or*
2. For more curious children who want to know *where* you're going, you could give them a reason:
   - 'Oops, I forgot to turn the bath water off'
   - 'I just need to go the bathroom'
   - 'I'll be right back, after I go and put the oven on for my dinner'

You will know instinctively which approach will work best for your child.

5. Ideas that help with limits and boundaries

Some children's sleep issue is around limit-testing. You may fall into the vortex of language loopholes, or your child may be exploiting inconsistencies between the limits you and your co-parent set. These challenges nearly always respond to more connection, one-to-one time, or a more specific type of connection in the day – by using the love languages. These sleep challenges also respond to kind and firm age-appropriate limits and boundaries, providing a limited range of choices, and clear and consistent communication about what to expect at bedtime.

Magic sleep cushion

This is a good trick for children who seem to have a need to control elements of the bedtime. You'll know immediately if this is your child! Some children like to know exactly what's going on, ask where you will be, or demand that you do certain things at bedtime. If this sounds like your child's style, then this technique might be worth a try.

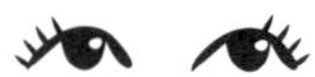

The magic sleep cushion works well for children who need a parent to sit with them in their room while they fall asleep. They are not distressed if you leave, but keep coming out to find you, or asking for repeat items after lights out. It's not a great tool for multiple middle of the night wake-ups, as you are likely to find it frustrating and exhausting. However, sometimes the way you support your child to sleep at bedtime seems to set the tone for the rest of the night – so it may still be worth a try.

You explain to your child that after the bedtime routine and saying goodnight, you will sit on the magic sleep cushion until they are asleep. You can designate a cushion you already have, or go out together and buy a special cushion just for this purpose. Sounds simple enough right? The rules are:

1. The cushion cannot be in their room.
2. The cushion can be anywhere in the house (you can set some boundaries here – i.e. the cushion will not be in the garden, or somewhere you can't hear).
3. They may come out and check that you are where they asked you to be, once.
4. If they come out to 'check' again, they lose the freedom to dictate where the cushion will be, and *you* get to say where the cushion is going – which might be on to the sofa in the living room.

The idea is that you give your child some control, with boundaries over the extent of the control. If they misuse the privilege of the control, then they lose it. There is no punishment for coming out, but the child loses the chance to dictate the location.

In my experience, children often pick somewhere silly for the cushion to be – like the toilet seat for instance, or the bath. That's fine. Calmly put the cushion on the closed toilet lid and be prepared to stay there for 20 minutes or so (bring a book!). Your child will come out to 'check' you are where they asked you to be, and you calmly smile and tell them goodnight.

If they come back again (for non-urgent reasons) then you could just say 'Oh no, you came back out. Oops! I guess it's my turn to choose where the cushion is going to be now. Never mind, we can try this again tomorrow.'

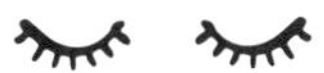

If this happens more than 2–3 times, this is probably not the right tool for your child! Don't worry – there are plenty of others to try.

Bedtime books and social stories

The bedtime book is a simple strategy that you can use alongside any other strategy. The idea is to involve your child as much as possible in the process of deciding how bedtime will flow, and also to show them the steps involved. Even very verbal and bright children are often able to articulate more than they can actually understand. Bedtime and going to sleep are quite abstract concepts in many ways, and it can help to break down what will happen. This may sound like madness – after all, you possibly do the same steps every single night, but believe me, some children over-think and worry about this significant time of separation from you.

What you do is to sit down with your child and work out what should be included in the bedtime routine. You can act forgetful and say to them, 'I've forgotten what we need to do before bed!'. They will probably forget one or two elements – such as cleaning teeth. You can act like you suddenly remember if something essential gets missed off the list. Just write down all the parts of the bedtime routine, in any order for now.

Next, you could ask your child, 'What do you think we should do first?' and take their suggestions seriously. Obviously if they suggest teeth before a bedtime snack, then you might have to act like you've just realised that might be in the wrong order, but the point of this exercise is to get them as involved as possible. Let's face it, it doesn't actually matter what order most of the steps happen in. Even if your child suggests the steps in exactly the order that they currently occur in, don't worry, they will still feel more involved. This is called co-creation, and everyone feels better when they have been consulted about an activity that concerns them.

You could then take photos of your child at each distinct stage of their bedtime, or if that is too much work right now, you could print pictures off the internet. Make a book out of the pictures, and invite your child to decorate it if they like.

You could also incorporate a social story. This is an idea borrowed from resources to help children with neurodiversity, including autism spectrum disorder and social communication difficulties. They are used to create a story about an activity or behaviour that is difficult

or challenging. I actually recommend social stories a lot – for both neurotypical children as well as children with neurodiversity. Why? Because they are about enhancing and making communication better. Anything that is about improving communication sounds like a good idea to me! If you'd like to try this, the social story about bedtime would go something like this:

Page 1: This is George. George is four.
Page 2: George lives with his Mummy and baby sister Annie, and Max the dog.
Page 3: When the day is over, it is time for George to go to bed.
Page 4: George sleeps in a bed with his toy dinosaurs, in his cosy room right next to Mummy. Max sleeps in his dog bed. Annie sleeps in her crib.
Page 5: First, George has a bath with his sister and cleans his teeth.
Page 6: After his bath, Mummy gives George a back rub, and next, he puts his pyjamas on.
Page 7: George chooses three stories, and Mummy reads to George while he sits in his bed.
Page 8: After his stories, George chooses two toys to go to bed with, and he tucks them in.
Page 9: Mummy turns off the light and sits with George to sing his special goodnight song.
Page 10: Mummy draws a heart on George's hand. If George needs to feel Mummy's love, he can kiss the heart on his hand.
Page 11: Mummy sits beside George until he is ready to go to sleep.
Page 12: While George sleeps, everybody else sleeps safely in their beds.
Page 13: After a lovely sleep, everyone can have another good day.

Obviously, you can use the social story to address any fears, such as the dark – explaining that you will leave a light on, or whatever their specific concern is. Most children love reading a story about themselves, and I suggest you read this before the start of the bedtime routine so that your child knows what to expect at the outset.

Nearly all children will respond to a combination of the strategies in your background sleep checklist, alongside one or two of the tools here. Good luck with them.

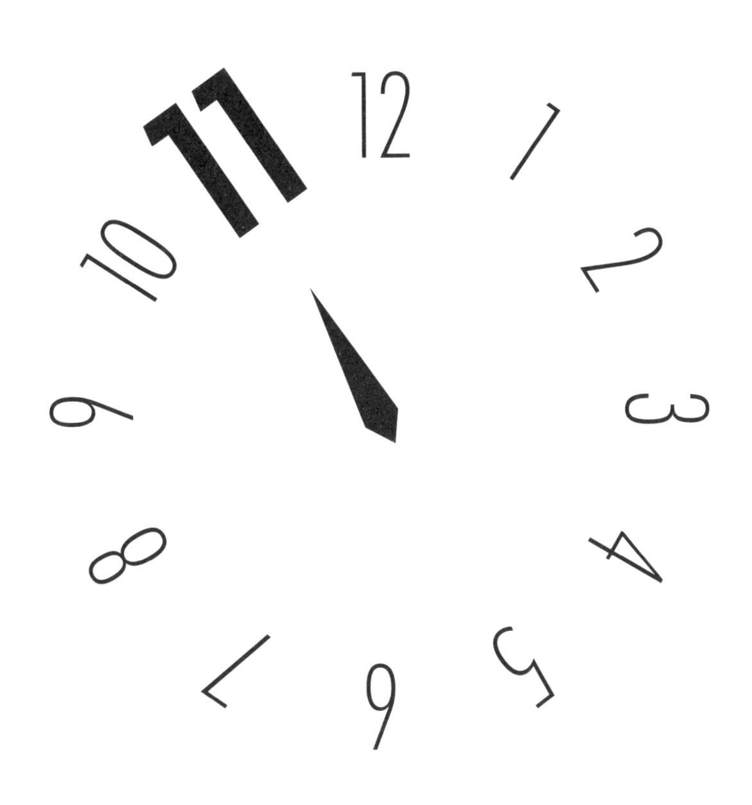

CHAPTER ELEVEN

NIGHT FEEDING

I don't know whether your child is or was breast or chest fed, formula fed, or given a combination. I don't know your feeding history – what went well, what was difficult, your disappointments, struggles and triumphs. This section is in no way intended to be judgemental or upsetting, but the nature of infant feeding is that families often receive very little support and do not always meet their own personal feeding goals.[1] This means that parents can be unintentionally triggered by references to something that has or continues to cause emotional pain. If this is you, firstly, I'm so sorry, and secondly I urge you to seek emotional support. Breastfeeding counsellors and IBCLCs are trained to provide debriefing after a disappointing feeding experience, and will be happy to listen as you talk about what happened. Professor Amy Brown's book: *Why Breastfeeding Grief and Trauma Matter* is another excellent resource you might find validating and affirming.

This chapter will mainly cover breastfeeding toddlers and older children, but there is also some information about bottle-feeding from page 272 onwards if this is more relevant for your family.

How you feel about night feeding

If you are still feeding your toddler, 'threenager' or even older child, the chances are that by this point that you have given some thought as to whether you will wait for your child to spontaneously wean, or initiate a more parent-led weaning. All children will eventually wean from the breast – though the average age range is rather wide, and may be anything from two to seven years.[2]

The decision about what to do with night feeding may depend a little on your own thoughts and feelings about it. Do you feel trapped and fed up? Or do you feel connected and in-tune? Do night feeds feel poignant and peaceful? Or do they feel like an imposition? If I was to paint a future reality for you, and offer two parallel visions: one is a vision of your child falling asleep without feeding. Perhaps they still wake in the night, but you have a gentle and responsive alternative tool that works to get them back to sleep. The second is a vision of you continuing to feed your child to sleep, knowing that one day it will pass, and if at any time you change your mind, you can stop. Which vision is the one that you feel most aligned with? Do either of them make you feel sad? Do either of them make you feel expectant, liberated or relieved?

Continuing to breastfeed beyond infancy is something that many parents feel is quite a lonely business. You may feel like you are the only person in your circle of acquaintances who is nursing past babyhood. I assure you that you are not. Some research suggests that parents go 'underground', keeping their nursing relationship private.[3] They may not even choose to tell healthcare professionals, fearing that they will be advised to stop, or given inaccurate and insensitive information,[4] which can mean that many parents feel they have nobody to talk to about some of the challenges of nursing an older child.

The choices you make about night feeding are intensely personal, and can only be made by you. There will always be people who have deeply held opinions about when it is right to stop feeding to sleep, or breastfeeding in general. There are also people who believe it is never right to impose weaning on a child. Certainly, the World Health Organization recommends breastfeeding for two years and beyond,[5] and breastfeeding can provide a significant proportion of a toddler's daily nutrients. A recent study found that breastmilk can provide 28 percent of a toddler's daily energy and 16 percent of their total protein requirements.[6] Human milk never 'turns to water', and always responds to the needs of your child.

But this is just factual information, and has perhaps very little to do with your emotional decision-making process. My take on this is a compassionate, balanced and pragmatic one: it's your body. You, and you

alone get to decide who uses it, for what, how often, and for how long. End of story. But rest assured, whether you choose to wean, or adopt a child-led weaning approach, you can make an informed choice and prioritise your child's emotional needs in the process.

Breastfeeding at night

Perhaps we should start by saying here that it is okay if you want to breastfeed at night. It's also okay if you don't. You can stop breastfeeding at night and it may make no difference to your child's night waking. Equally, you can continue to feed your child to sleep and make improvements in their nighttime sleep.

Stories from families

I have the privilege of working with hundreds of inspirational families. When I started to write this chapter, I realised that what would make it complete would be to have some examples from families who have made feeding to sleep work. What follows is a collection of their stories.

> *'With breastfeeding to sleep, I learned an important lesson the hard way. When I discovered I was pregnant with my second baby, my firstborn was just past two years. I figured that he was ready to move on, so I bribed him to stop breastfeeding. I quickly realised that I'd made a very foolish trade-off. In the time that it had previously taken to breastfeed him to sleep, it took four times longer using other comfort methods. Same for soothing him when he fell down, or was upset. For that reason, with baby #2 and #3, I didn't look at feeding to sleep as anything less than an amazing bit of magic. It was my 'superpower' and no one could convince me otherwise. Sure, it meant that I was the one who put the baby to sleep, but my husband was in charge of the big kids. We each had a part to play.'* **Theresa**

> *'My first daughter and I fed to sleep until she was four and a half. She didn't share a bed with me until after we moved away from her father as he had several risk factors that I wasn't prepared to take, and the NHS was staunchly anti-bedsharing at that point. She went into her own room at six months old, but I was responsively feeding.*

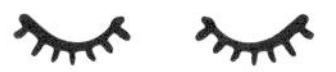

We bedshared a lot of the time later on. It was a way of escaping a lot of the things that were going on around us that were beyond our control. We fled domestic abuse when she was age one, but our circumstances didn't really settle until she was three because of court proceedings and emergency housing. She is now nine, and occasionally comes into bed with me and her stepdad and little sister. She is independent, funny and caring. We are still each other's safe spaces, but she hasn't fed for a long time.' **Laura**

'Feeding to sleep worked a treat and was far easier and quicker than any other way of settling him. Eventually my breastfeeding aversion got the better of me, so I started timing the feeds and getting him to settle the last bit with a cuddle. Then we night weaned. Without the aversion I would have continued longer.' **Kathryn**

'Feeding to sleep beyond infancy took the stress out of bedtime. I night weaned at one, but will carry on feeding to sleep for as long as we feel like it. She chose when she didn't want to feed to sleep. She still needs that booby cuddle before story and sleep. It's mainly the routine she likes. She is three and a half now, and has a 5–10 minute feed before bedtime.' **Danielle**

'Having my second baby was a turning point in my parenting. Often out of necessity I had to do things a certain way, or couldn't find the time to do what I thought I should do. For example, she had a dummy until 12 months because I couldn't cope with her crying if I had to do something with my two-year-old. I feared she'd have it until her teen years, such is the propaganda! But we stopped it at 12 months and it was seamless. I realised I should just stop worrying and go with the flow. Similarly I breastfed her until she was three. Not only did people think this was 'odd', but I also wondered if she'd be on the boob till her teens! But I grew in my own confidence that things could and should be allowed to happen organically. And just before she was three she self-weaned. And this was a baby who had fed to sleep every single day! I think I learned to have confidence in what felt right and nice for our family. Feeding a baby to sleep, feeding a baby when she cries etc just felt right. I can't see how it can't be. And it stopped when it

was right, organically. The barrier for me at the start of my parenting journey was fear of other people's judgement. Nowadays I like that we're a bit different and feel proud of it. I just wish more people felt able to do it!' **Katharine**

'I'm currently feeding my little boy who is two years and two months old. I have left him overnight with my husband/friends/grandparents but any time I am with him we feed to sleep/bedshare. I really love seeing his little face after he has drifted off and he turns back from 'big boy' into a baby again. For us bedsharing has worked as it was my expectation going into parenting. I come from a breastfeeding and co-sleeping family and I have some friends who parent that way too. We bought the biggest mattress we could find (continental superking 2m x 2m) and put it on the floor.

My husband sleeps in the spare room so he's rested for work. I am at home full time and take a night off in the spare room once a week to get an undisturbed 8 hours. During a regular night my son can sometimes sleep 10pm–5am.

It's a mixed bag but any time we discuss making changes my husband and I come back to the fact that this is a fleeting time in our life. My hope is that by providing this support to Naoise when he is small, we are raising an empathetic and compassionate person who will support others around him. That perhaps a time will come when he really needs help for some big issue, and he will feel able to ask us as there is a baseline of trust and availability.

I have no idea how we will transition away from this style of sleeping but I know 100 percent there are very few teenagers who choose to sleep with their parents!' **Sian**

'I am tandem feeding a three-and-a-half-year old and a 15-month-old and breastsleeping is by far the easiest way of getting everyone to lie down at the same time to go to sleep. Thanks to your work Lyndsey, and the work of James McKenna, Helen Ball and Amy Brown, my eyes are opened to normal young human nocturnal feeding and sleeping behaviours so I'm free to do what is easiest for me and my family. Having the ability to feed a child to sleep has been so helpful in different situations. I can get my toddler to sleep with a boobie

and a cuddle even under very unlikely sleeping conditions like in the middle of those indoor playground places full of squealing children running around with all the noise bouncing off all the surfaces and in the middle of parties/activities. Restaurants, airports, flights. The other thing is not having to work too hard to create conditions for sleeping or reading pre-sleep cues. It probably also has to do with my children's personalities as well. But I have noticed that both of them will seek me out for a boobie when they feel tired and will just go off to sleep and they have very different personalities. Whereas with my six-year-old who I didn't breastfeed to sleep I had to be more intentional around putting her down for naps and sleep. It allows me to get on with my days, which are very busy!' **Katie**

My daughter was breastfed till 32 months. I always fed her to sleep as it was easiest, but my husband could cuddle her to sleep from about the age of one. After she weaned I cuddled her to sleep and she was fine with that. We bedshared till she was three. We had a double and single mattress on the floor next to each other, so my husband could join us too. At age three she asked for her own bed in her own bedroom. As I was pregnant and needed to sleep, my husband had a mattress on the floor of my three-year-old's room so if she woke I wouldn't. There was no crying or upset in this transition. Now I'm bedsharing with my one-year-old and my husband still room-shares with our now four-year-old. They wake up around 6am and me and my one-year-old sleep in till about 8.' **Alice**

Night-weaning (or full weaning)

As an IBCLC, I spend a lot of my time supporting parents to start breast or chest-feeding. But I believe that the way we slow down, reduce or stop feeding our little ones in many ways is just as important as how we start. It's another change in the relationship, that we can manage with compassion and understanding.

There are so many reasons why you might be thinking about night weaning. Perhaps you've wanted to do this for many months and you were holding on until you feel your toddler is old enough. Perhaps you're hoping that this might improve nighttime sleep? These are the most common reasons people ask me for support with night-weaning a toddler:

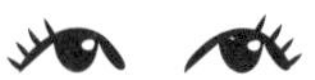

- They are feeling touched out
- They are unwell, and urgently need to stop feeding
- They want someone else to be able to settle their child
- They want their fertility to return
- They are pregnant and not keen on the idea of tandem feeding
- They are experiencing nursing aversion

For toddlers, stopping breastfeeding can be an emotional task! This is really best handled with a lot of time, patience and compassion. I often recommend setting limits in the daytime first. This might sound strange if it is only the nighttime feeds that are bothersome, but setting limits in the day is easier. Just like boundaries for any other type of behaviour, if the only limits your child encounters are in the nighttime, this is hard for them. It's actually easier if there are limits in the day as well. Here are some ideas – you do not have to use all of these, of course.

1. First, consider which of your toddler's feeds seem to be the least significant – start by trying to cut these ones! Strategies I like to use include offering a snack instead, or a cuddle, or simply being busy and offering a really fun alternative.
2. Consider which of the feeds you find the most difficult. Sometimes, if you eliminate this/these feed(s) then you find you don't actually want to give up all of the others.
3. Try setting a timer or feed for only a specified amount of time. Reduce the time on the timer by a minute (or 30 seconds if it's very short!) every couple of days. Keep your toddler close and offer cuddles, stroking, and soothing instead while they fall back to sleep in your arms. For older toddlers who can comprehend the concept, I love the book *Nursies when the Sun Shines* which aims to prepare your toddler for stopping feeding at night.
4. You could try using role play, with teddies, dolls or puppets, to show your child how bedtime will go, or what will happen in the middle of the night.
5. Consider the countdown approach – you start off feeding and after a while, you tell your child that you will count down from five to zero, and when you get to zero, the milk is going away. I suggest you don't say the milk is 'all gone' because many bright and astute toddlers

will confidently declare that the milk is *not* all gone, and will continue feeding to prove it!

6. Try being less flexible about where you will breastfeed. So, pick only one location. Make it somewhere you don't already feel very used to breastfeeding in, so it has less of a cosy feel! Do not restrict breastfeeds at this point, just the location. So, no breastfeeds when out and about, only at home, in the chair. If you go away for a few days, find a temporary location, and explain that this will be the feeding chair while you stay there.
7. Once your toddler has accepted that level of restriction in their breastfeeding habits, you could start to place limits on *when* you will breastfeed. It's up to you how you do this, and it might depend on how many feeds there are. Perhaps just morning, lunchtime and evening? Or only after meals? Just at bedtime? It is your choice.
8. Then, start to plan to be *out* during those designated times. Your toddler will probably just 'forget'. When you return home, if they ask for a feed, patiently say when the next feed will be, and offer an alternative.
9. It really helps if you can be somewhere *super* fun during the expected feed times – swimming, or the playground, or soft play, or with friends in the park – or whatever.
10. Try not to be out for more than one of the feeds per day, but consider changing around which feed you will miss, so your toddler doesn't always miss the same one.
11. When you get down to one or two feeds per day, offer a snack instead, and a cuddle. See if they will accept a cup of water, or a fruit smoothie, or a milkshake. It may have to be a fairly rewarding drink to compensate for the fact that it's not milk.
12. You may find it useful to express if you become full. It will feel much harder to do if you're uncomfortable, and your little one will know that you have plenty of milk. It's more authentic if you're well-drained.

Setting limits on daytime weaning is sometimes hard on both parents and children, but be kind to yourself, and patient and gentle with your little one – you will both get there. Allow yourself the opportunity to grieve the loss of the breastfeeding relationship – it's normal to feel quite sad about it. Celebrate your wonderful achievement in some way – get a

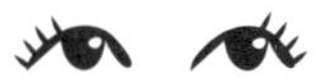

photo of you breastfeeding your child; they will love to see it in years to come. Or consider a charm bracelet, breastmilk pendant, or some other way of remembering the closeness and special memories.

Night-weaning to improve sleep?

One of the primary motivators for many to night-wean is the hope of a sleep upgrade. It is important for you to know that night-weaning does not always lead to an immediate improvement in sleep, so make sure you know what you're getting into if this is the only reason you are thinking of night-weaning. Remember that we all wake in the night and some children are natural self-soothers, and some are born signallers. Children will gradually sleep longer stretches with age and developmental maturity, though the self-soothers may get there sooner. If your child is a signaller and they wake in the night for a feed, in many ways it's logical to assume that stopping the feed will stop the night-waking.

But remember: children wake in the night for comfort. Breastfeeding may meet a child's nutritional and hunger needs, but it is wrapped up with comfort and relationship as well. You are not just meeting a need for food when you feed them. If you remove food as an option (i.e. stop breastfeeding) they will almost certainly still wake for comfort. You'll just have to find *other* ways to comfort them. I am not trying to put you off – merely to help you make an informed decision and go into this with your eyes open. Night-weaning is absolutely the right thing for many families, but it may not be the right option if your *primary* reason is more sleep quickly. Night-weaning may eventually be part of the reason your little one sleeps longer, but it may be some weeks before you get those consolidated stretches.

Okay, warning over. Let's talk about how you *actually* manage night-weaning.

You can use some of the tools in the night-waking chapter, as well as cuddling and holding your toddler while you set limits on night feeds. Some tips for night weaning:

- Try setting limits in the day first, so not all the limits are in the night.
- Make sure your toddler has other ways of finding comfort.
- Enlist help from a non-lactating partner.
- Choose which feeds are meaningful and keep these a while longer if

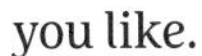

you like.
- Keep your toddler in your bed while you night-wean – it is sometimes easier.
- Be prepared for a few sleepless nights.

Tonight is the night

You will need to make the decision about how night-weaning or reducing night feeds will go for you. I'll share five main options:

1. You could continue to feed to sleep, and still offer one or two night feeds, at times that work for you – basically, you're setting limits that feel reasonable, but still accepting that your little one needs some milk at night. This can be a good option for a younger toddler who feeds frequently and eats poorly. You may feel like you want to cut feeds down more gradually. You might decide that you will pick a couple of tactical times when you will feed your child, but at every other feed you will cuddle, love and hug them back to sleep. You do not have to keep to rigid times – just choose an approximate time and decide that any wake-ups within about half an hour of that target time will mean you feed back to sleep. This also guarantees a relatively easy return to sleep at least twice in the night, which can preserve your sleep and maintain sanity.
2. Establish one stretch of sleep, by not feeding at the first few times they wake up. This means that you might decide that you will not feed your child for a solid 4–6 hours at the start of the night. Sometimes this can work to establish a longer break between feeds. It also means that you are doing the hard part at a time of the night when you or your co-parent are more likely to be awake. You then decide that you will change the rules after a certain time – it might be when *you* go to bed, or you might pick a time. Either way, after that time, you just feed your child back to sleep. With this approach, you are reserving your feed to sleep tool as a kind of 'trump' card, maximising everyone's sleep.
3. You could continue to feed to sleep, but then not feed in the night, at all. The next feed is in the morning. Sometimes the feed as part of the bedtime routine is the one that many parents and children feel the most attached to. Keeping this one often feels like the best of both worlds. There are many children who feed to sleep, but then sleep all

night long, so if you feel strongly about the bedtime feed, there is no reason why you can't keep this one.

4. You could choose to stop feeding to sleep, and hope that this sets the tone for the rest of the night, and see what happens in the night. Perhaps the bedtime section of the night is the most valuable time for you, and you are happy to let someone else take care of bedtime, and then you'll continue to night feed. You could still feed your child in the evening, but just not feed to sleep. This may feel like a good option to test out how your child responds to some limits. Many parents are surprised by how well their child handles a change.
5. Or finally, you could not feed to sleep, and also not feed in the night, offering comfort in other ways when your toddler wakes up in the night. There is some evidence that feeding to sleep and back to sleep is associated with more night-waking – however, although this was a large study of 10,000 children, they were under the age of one, so how applicable this is to the older age group is hard to say.[7]

Which option you choose is very personal. Sometimes people choose to start very gently and slowly, and work up the steps until they get to somewhere they feel comfortable. It might depend how old your child is, or how persistent their personality.

I often find very strong-willed toddlers need a really clear and black and white strategy. Sometimes they get upset and confused by the mixed messages of being able to feed at some times, but not others. Other toddlers who are more sensitive need a very gradual reduction. You'll instinctively feel that your toddler fits best into one or other of these camps.

Obviously, when you are not feeding your little one, you will need to offer them other forms of comfort – such as cuddles, stroking, shushing, patting, or holding. Don't worry about what you have to do to settle them. You and your child are settling in and adjusting to another way of responsive parenting. Change can be hard for little people, so they'll need lots of reassurance. Remember that there are many ways of being responsive – feeding has worked for you for a long time, but it doesn't mean that there are no other ways.

It's also important to say that if at any time it doesn't feel right, or you change your mind, you can stop, abandon it completely, and do what feels right. These strategies will still be open to you at whatever point if and when you choose to try again.

How *you* feel about stopping breastfeeding

Stopping breastfeeding can be a really emotional time for parents too. While you may earnestly desire more sleep or to have your body to yourself again, there may be, deep down, a little bit of sadness, or even ambivalence about stopping. Perhaps, although you desperately long for more sleep, you secretly treasure those quiet night feeds, just you and your child. It's a funny thing, but sometimes the thing we long for also makes us sad. There is a certain poignancy about those night feeds. They are inextricably linked to our child's infancy, and the way we were born into the relationship of parenthood and nurturance. Stopping the behaviour that is bound up with all that can feel like a monumental step not only for our children, but also for us.

All this doesn't necessarily mean it's not the right time, but just be kind to yourself. It's normal to have some mixed feelings about stopping or reducing breastfeeding. Most very gentle parents hate denying their children what they ask for, so it can feel a bit counterintuitive to place limits. While limits and boundaries are essential for children, if you're not used to feeding being an area of parenting with limits, then this can take some getting used to. You will possibly also feel like this is the end of an era. As your child's needs change, you may feel both joy and also sadness. It's good to acknowledge your feelings and allow them. Perhaps write a letter to your little one about how you felt during this time, or keep a journal to remember this as a meaningful time.

Finally, it's worth knowing that breastfeeding can help you return to sleep faster. Without it, you may find it harder to fall asleep – though this is temporary. There is a clever relationship between prolactin, and another chemical called dopamine. Prolactin downregulates dopamine.[8] What happens when you stop breastfeeding is that as prolactin levels decrease, dopamine levels start to rise again, and dopamine can make you feel really alert. You might find that it's harder to drop off to sleep than it was before. Rest assured these effects are temporary, but it sometimes helps to know what to expect so you're not alarmed or disappointed.

If you decide to wean, be prepared for some other hormonal changes,

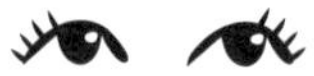

and the return of your periods if they haven't already.[9] Make sure you sort out your contraception, because you may have a surprise otherwise! Also, many women find that they feel quite teary, and emotional – elevated breastfeeding hormones provide some protection against anxiety and depression, and some people feel a bit low when they stop.[10] Some also find that they are more vulnerable to illnesses after they stop breastfeeding. Look after yourself. Take a good multivitamin, plan some lovely activities, get your favourite food in the house ready for those wobbly moments, and have someone you can talk to honestly on speed-dial.

Is this a good time for your child?

You may also need to consider whether this is a good time for your little one. You can't always be flexible around the needs of your child. I have worked with many families who are forced to night-wean or completely wean due to medical emergencies that genuinely necessitate cessation of breastfeeding. But often there is a degree of flexibility about exactly when you wean.

Do they have a lot going on right now? Are they about to start daycare? Are you about to move, or go on holiday? Are you starting work? Are they unwell? While there is never a perfect time, some moments are better or worse than others in the grand scheme of things! So, have a look at your diary, and work out whether this is a moment of relative calm. Factor in whether your toddler is having a major developmental phase right now, or whether they have just got over a nasty illness. Whether you wean this week or in three months is not likely to make a huge difference to your overall breastfeeding journey when you look back, but it may affect the acute experience of weaning. If delaying a few weeks reduces the stress, it's probably worth it, but you will have to weigh up your situation, considering all the variables and pressures on you.

Who should be the one to set the limits?

A common piece of advice is that someone other than the lactating parent should settle the child. The idea behind this is that if the child smells milk, or is in the arms of the parent who normally feeds them, they will want milk more and get distressed or very persistent about wanting milk. While this advice may work for many older toddlers, I honestly think that this tip works best for younger infants. Once a child develops a definite primary attachment figure, certainly by about 6–8 months, if they become upset, they are likely to want to be with that person – who is likely to be their mother.

I know that if you are the mother and you're tired, you may be desperate for someone else to give you a break. I know you're longing to share the load at night. That day will come. But during the hard part, which is usually the first 3–4 nights, you may find that both for your child's sake, as well as your own, it may be better for you to hold, love and hug your little one through their wake-ups without feeding.

I also know that often, your co-parent desires a closer and more involved relationship with your child, and may want to play a more active role in bedtime. It can come to feel like your child 'prefers' one parent over the other. This can feel demoralising.

What I have found is that if it is not the mother (or lactating parent) who holds their child, the child may get very angry, and desire their mother even more, pushing their other parent away. This is not necessarily what you want if you're trying to get your co-parent involved more.

Finally, you do not want to create the association that one parent equals milk, and the other parent equals no milk. While you may be able to change your child's habits with the non-lactating parent, you may have to then repeat the process with their mother. So, one tip is to night-wean in the mother's arms – giving your child the clear message that whichever parent settles them, milk is not an option. It's often faster this way, which is better for everyone.

The exception of course is in an emergency. You may decide, on balance, that you will send the child's father, or your co-parent, in for a few nights while you have some respite sleep, or receive treatment, or go to work – whatever the scenario is. Ultimately, this is your choice, but there is so little information around to support parents of older nurslings that people often give advice that seems to be tailored to children far younger. When the context is different, sometimes the strategy has to change as well.

Setting the scene for night-weaning

You may have some apprehension going into night weaning. That's totally normal. If you have decided that this is the right decision for you and your family, then you have nothing to feel guilty for, but you might want to make some preparations, and also go into it knowing what to expect.

Prepare your child, prepare yourself

You may have been reading a personalised social story about night-weaning with your child, or perhaps a book about weaning. You may have tried to role play how this will go with toys, or talked to your child about night-weaning. None of this guarantees a quiet night, but you will at least know you have done all you can to communicate the change to your child kindly. You also need to prepare yourself – both mentally and practically. Wrapping your head around this includes choosing how to respond if and when your child asks for milk, and gets upset, frustrated, angry and confused about wanting milk. You can choose to validate and hold space for those feelings, without getting sucked into your child's drama yourself. That's not easy. It's natural to feel sorry for our little ones when they are sad. But while you need to acknowledge their emotions, you do not need to feel sorry for them. As the parent, you can choose to be calm, confident and compassionate. I suggest you also prepare practically too. Whether you have chosen to feed to sleep but then not feed all night, or not feed to sleep and also not in the night, will affect how bedtime is likely to go. If you mentally write off your evening, and expect more disruption than usual, you are likely to be less surprised. Get ready for bed early yourself, and make sure you have eaten, and prepared where you will sleep, ahead of time.

What to expect

I would be lying if I said night-weaning was likely to be quick, easy and free from drama. Some little ones do surprise their parents, but it's sensible to expect several disrupted nights. Your child may plead, beg, negotiate, tug at your clothing, demand, cry and get angry. There may be ugly crying with snot. At any time you feel this is not the right moment, it's okay to stop, but try not to start this process and stop it many times – this can feel unsettling. A lot of parents want to know how long to expect this process to last. Usually, if you are going for full night-weaning it will be about 3–5 days of your child asking and protesting about not having a feed. Often the first night is the worst, and then it gets rapidly better. I feel I should also warn you of two phenomena. Firstly, after some

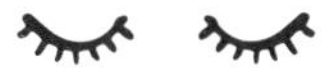

improvement around night 4–5, you may see a bit of a backslide. This is really normal. Stay calm, and don't lose hope. Secondly, for one last time, while your child may settle calmly without milk after this process, they may still continue to wake and need comfort in other ways. It will gradually get better, and at least you may be able to involve others, but it is unlikely to immediately improve your nighttime sleep.

Some tips:

- If you are not going to feed to sleep, consider a temporarily later bedtime. It's much easier for some children to accept a big change if they are really fatigued. Try putting them to bed 30–60 minutes later than usual, and they may be so tired they crash out without being too sad about the loss of milk. Once your child seems to be accepting the change, you can bring bedtime earlier in small increments again.
- It is often a lot easier to night-wean with your child in your bed, or on a floor bed that you plan to sleep in. You are likely to have some disrupted nights, and settling your child in a cot or another room is likely to be very difficult and exhausting. Night-weaning *before* moving on from bedsharing is often a pragmatic choice. This is not to suggest that you *have* to move away from bedsharing – you may just want to night-wean and continue the family bed. However, if moving on from the family bed is part of your plan, I do often suggest making this a later change.
- When your little one wakes and asks for milk, decide on a gentle soothing phrase you will say – something like: 'Not now sweetheart, we'll have milk in the morning'.
- Validate your child's feelings: 'I know it's hard. I'm here'.
- Practise emotion coaching in the day, and use the same language at night.
- Offer lots of reassurance and comfort – it's fine to do whatever feels natural; cuddles, stroking, kisses, singing songs, holding, rocking, walking...
- Try not to use distractions like TV or iPads in the night.
- You don't need to make the tears go away. Expressing emotion about this change is normal and understandable. It's not your job to erase the emotion, or distract your child out of it, but to acknowledge that it's hard for your child and provide emotional scaffolding through it.

- It's absolutely fine to offer your child sips of water in a cup. They may not want it, but it is absolutely appropriate to make water available.
- You may want to plan for your co-parent to sleep somewhere else, and arrange a tactical sleepover for older siblings if you are worried their sleep will also be disrupted.

Building in flexibility with your trump card

If you decide to cut out all night feeds, you might find that some of the night wakes are easier to deal with than others. The dreaded scenario is the one where it is 4am, and your child has accepted the limits on night feeding up until now. By this time in the morning, you have biology against you. Your child's melatonin levels are falling, and their alerting cortisol levels are rising in preparation for morning. Their body is getting ready to start the day, so if they wake up now, it may be a choice between getting them back to sleep very quickly, or risk them starting the day at this ungodly hour. Of course, only you will be able to say what the right play is. Maybe it's right to persevere and be totally consistent. But you may decide to play the sun/star visual as your emergency 'get-out-of-jail-free' card.

What you do is create a drawing (or print one out) of a sun, and another drawing on a separate piece of paper of stars. Write the words 'sun' or 'stars' on the reverse side of the paper so you can see which is which when they are face down. Leave the sheets of paper face down on a table in the room where your child sleeps. You can familiarise your child with the concept that if you pick up the star card, it is still nighttime and there is no milk. If you pick up the sun card, it is okay to have a feed. This way, you have a little bit of flexible autonomy over whether your child gets a night feed. You can play the star card (and not feed) if you're pretty convinced that you can persuade your child to go back to sleep. If you think you're in danger of your child ramping up and not going back to sleep, you can play the tactical sun card, hopefully get them promptly back to sleep before they get loud and wide awake, and hopefully catch a bit more sleep before you start the day.

If this seems to work, but you find that you're stuck with that 4am fear-feed, at some point you may decide that you're going to tough it out and play the star card for that feed. If you do this, you could always try to make the feed fractionally later every few days in the hope that this

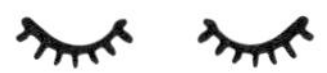

may delay the morning wake-up. Try holding and cuddling your child, and then making a point of going over to check the cards, pick up the sun card, then offer your child a feed to see if they will go back to sleep for a while.

Night feeding and daytime eating

Many people blame night feeding for a child's small appetite in the daytime. In fact, this can be one reason why parents may be interested in night-weaning. Perhaps you have been told by a professional that the reason your child doesn't eat much is because they feed in the night. Maybe this is your own suspicion. It is probable that there is an element of chicken and egg in this theory. Does your child feed in the night *because* they are not a big eater, or does feeding in the night *cause* a reduced appetite in the day?

But besides this question, the more practical questions are:

1. Would stopping feeding at night encourage them to eat more in the day?
2. Are they just a grazer, and therefore night-weaning may be unlikely to alter their daytime eating habits?

You may not know for sure which camp your child falls into. Some children do seem to drink a lot of milk in the night, which certainly seems to reduce their appetite for breakfast, but if we remember that breastmilk provides about 28 percent of the daily energy needs for a toddler, it is not very plausible that they would simply not eat at all in the day due to their nursing habits. Even if their appetite for breakfast was low, by lunchtime – or possibly even earlier – they would be hungry if this rationale were true. If you find your child has a very small appetite all day long, it is highly unlikely that night feeding is the cause. It is more likely that night feeding is an extension of their daytime grazing behaviour, coupled of course with the fact that breastfeeding is not just about food.

By all means night-wean if it is right for you, but be aware that doing so may not suddenly turn your snacking and grazing child into a three-chunky-meals-per-day kind of child.

Bottle-feeding at night

We must also think about bottle-feeding at night. Feeding is a relational and nurturing activity, and parents who bottle-feed their little ones at night do so to meet both their children's' nutritional and also their emotional needs. If your toddler or preschooler still wakes in the night and wants a bottle, you are not alone.

These are some of the main reasons I hear from parents whose children wake in the night for a bottle.

1. Giving bottles in the night due to concerns over poor eating habits in the day

Many parents give their children milk in bottles overnight, as well as during the day, because they feel this is a safety net for children who eat very little or do not eat a huge variety of food. Toddler milks are often marketed for fussy eaters and capitalise on parental anxiety about nutrient intake. I totally understand the logic in getting your child to drink calories if they won't eat calories, but toddler milks are an unregulated product that get around a lot of legal loopholes. They are often far higher in sugar than regular cows' milk or non-dairy alternatives.[11]

2. Giving bottles in the night because of low milk intake during the day

Another reason parents give their children milk in the night is because they may be concerned that their child isn't drinking enough milk in the day. Remember though, that by age one, most calories and nutrients will come from food, not milk. This is the same for breastfed children as well. At least 70 percent of their energy should be from food, not milk, which means their milk intake will naturally drop. It can feel scary to go from a large bottle of milk to a plate of carrot sticks and pitta bread fingers, but children's growth rates slow down in toddlerhood, so they don't need all the extra calories from milk.[12] Your child technically doesn't actually *have* to have milk. What they need is calcium. We are culturally predisposed to think that the best source of calcium is milk and dairy products, but in fact there are many good sources of calcium – just ask any vegan! Try nuts, oranges, and dark green vegetables. If your child does like dairy products, remember that all dairy counts, not just milk – including cheese, yoghurt, milk-based sauces, and milk on cereal. When you add all this up, they may be getting more milk in their diet than you think.

3. Giving bottles in the night because it is the quickest and easiest (or only) way to get your child back to sleep

Many parents give their toddler a bottle to go back to sleep because, quite simply, it works. Feeding has a naturally soporific effect, and so I quite understand why parents would do this. As well as this, your child did not become a toddler overnight. One day you were responsively feeding your baby back to sleep, and the next day you're feeding your two-year-old. I understand this. In fact, in one study, the main reason parents fed their children bottles of milk in the night was to get them back to sleep.[13]

4. Giving a bottle in the night due to concerns about your child's growth or weight

Many parents are concerned about their child's weight. Toddlers are very busy little people and sometimes seem to thrive on very little food. They can also sometimes appear leaner than they did as infants, causing some parents to worry that they are losing weight. In the vast majority of children, there is no cause for concern, but some children do struggle with weight gain. Children who have underlying health problems, such as cardiac and respiratory problems, metabolic problems, chronic conditions such as cystic fibrosis and other problems may struggle to gain weight. In these cases, your child should be under the care of a paediatrician and dietician. For other children, if you have concerns, please ask your child's usual doctor or health visitor. Formula is not usually recommended as a way of managing faltering growth in toddlers.[14]

5. Giving a bottle in the night because the cuddles and nurturing experience of feeding your child is lovely

Finally, sometimes parents give a bottle in the night just because they want to and it's a close, nurturing time with their little one. Many people feel like the night feeds are a poignant time-limited activity with their child, and in some ways, it is the last remnant of babyhood. Moving on from bottles is an acknowledgement of the passing of infancy which can feel both exciting, but also a little sad.

Whether you relate to one or more of these reasons, or yours is entirely different, you will have personal feelings about this and reasons for continuing to bottle-feed at night that are important to you. I don't judge you for any of them, but I will support you to make a change when the time is right for your family.

What is in the bottle – cows' milk, non-dairy milk or formula

By the age of one, all guidelines around the world recommend stopping infant formula and moving onto whole cows' milk instead. There is nothing very magic about being one. It's just that by this age, we would reasonably expect a child to be eating a variety of family foods. The main problem with whole cows' milk for babies under one is that firstly it has too much protein, and not enough lactose. Formula is modified cows' milk, with the main difference being that the proportions of fat, protein and carbohydrates, as well as calorie content, are altered to mimic those of human breast milk. Cows' milk also has very little iron, so formula has to have iron added to it. By the time your child is one, we would hope that they are eating foods that contain iron, so they do not need extra iron.

Growing-up milks, toddler milks and follow-on formula are actually not recommended by the World Health Organization. They are unregulated products, and often contain too much sugar. This is quite a naughty trick by the formula milk companies to make your child prefer the formula over unsweetened cows' milk. So if your child prefers formula, it might be worth mixing it with cows' milk so it is half formula, half cows' milk, to try to wean them off the sweet taste of the formula.

Other children, especially those with cows' milk allergy, or children from families where dairy products are avoided for dietary, cultural or health reasons, may be drinking one of the many non-dairy drinks. These include soy, oat milk, almond, coconut, rice and hazelnut milk. As long as your child is eating a varied diet and you have no growth or nutritional concerns for your child, it is fine for you to use a non-dairy milk/drink.

For more brilliant advice and unbiased tips about milk, formula, toddler feeding and more, see: www.firststepsnutrition.org

Whatever you have in your child's bottle, it is probably a good idea to try to wean them on to a cup instead, and in fairness, if you're reading this section, the chances are you are keen to do this – presumably because your child is waking in the night for a bottle and you'd like to be able to settle them in other ways, or for them to sleep in longer stretches. In case you're not sure whether or not to try to cut down the bottles, here is why bottles are not recommended for toddlers.

Why not to give a bottle

I know it might feel unfair or confusing that the guidelines for bottle-feeding are different to those for breastfeeding. The differences are mainly due to the mechanism of feeding – it's not the same action, and therefore longer-term bottle use is generally not recommended by paediatric and dentistry guidelines.[15] The recommendations are that your child should not have a bottle beyond 12–18 months, and that they should not feed to sleep, feed in the night, or have a bottle propped up for them. Children tend to drink more from a bottle than they would from a breast (irrespective of whether it is cows' milk, formula or breastmilk in the bottle), so one concern is that there is a higher risk of being overweight if children continue to drink from bottles. Milk also flows passively from a bottle, which means children are more at risk of choking, and also of fluid build-up in the inner ear.[16] Milk can also pool in the mouth because of the mechanism of feeding, so children are at higher risk of dental caries.[17] Finally, there is good evidence that sucking on a bottle, especially after 18 months, is associated with greater risk of dental malocclusion – or teeth overlap/crossbite. This is also true of prolonged dummy/pacifier/soother use.[18]

You are probably aware of many of these reasons, and perhaps you are keen to wean from the bottle-feeding at night, but you're not sure how to go about this kindly and gently. The following is a collection of tips that have worked over the years with various families.

How to wean off the bottle

Your child will probably respond best to being prepared for this change with kindness and clear, age-appropriate communication. Change is really hard for little people, and not only that, but if your child has been used to drinking quite large volumes of milk in the night, they may have developed a bit of an appetite for it. This means that they may be genuinely hungry in the night, which can be hard. You don't have to do everything at once, but here are a few ideas:

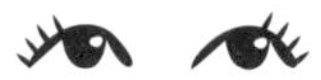

- Prepare your child by making them a social story about stopping nighttime milk.
- Establish boundaries for bottles in the daytime. It may be easier for your child to accept limits on bottle feeds at night if you limit or stop bottles in the daytime.
- Show your child pictures of when they were much younger having a bottle. This may lead into a conversation where you can honestly point out how much they've grown.
- Try not to tell your child that they are a 'baby' if they have a bottle. Some children may resist even more if they sense they are being forced to 'grow up'. This can be especially hard if they have a younger sibling. It is normal for children to have regressive play behaviours at times, and if they feel they are being pushed along, this can backfire.
- Consider which bottle-feed your child seems most attached to, and perhaps leave that one till last.
- Try doing the bedtime routine without a bottle, perhaps by moving it to the beginning of the bedtime routine.
- If you think your child is hungry, and you have been relying on your bedtime bottle to fill them up before bed, consider an evening snack, perhaps with some milk in a cup.
- Consider making your child's bedtime temporarily later. If their sleep pressure is higher, they may be less resistant to a big change. Once they are settling quietly and calmly without milk, you could make bedtime earlier again in small increments.
- If your child has been having large volumes of milk, you may decide to reduce the volume first, before taking the milk away. Consider reducing the volume every 2–3 days, to slowly reduce the overall volume.
- Once you get to a minimal amount of milk, you may feel that it is easier to just not offer milk at all.
- If your child has several feeds in the night, you could decide to leave one night feed in place while you eliminate the others completely. This may mean that during at least one wake-up, you have a way to return your child to sleep promptly.
- You might decide, based on your child's personality, that a very clear, black-and-white strategy of 'no more milk in the night' is the best way to avoid mixed messages.

At any point, if you decide to eliminate the bottles completely, you will obviously need to provide comfort and reassurance to your child in other ways. Milk is not just about food and calories, as you know. It's absolutely appropriate to hold, cuddle, rock, stroke, kiss and love your little one back to sleep. They may need more physical presence and reassurance, so consider lying next to them at night for a few days. A floor bed or bedsharing arrangement can work well to make this process easier and less tiring. You will also need to validate and acknowledge their feelings during the process: 'I know this is hard, I'm here'.

Finally, while it is recommended to wean your little one from a bottle by the age of 12–18 months, whether you do this today, next week, or in three weeks makes very little difference in the grand scheme of things. If now is not a great time – the arrival of a new baby, starting preschool, illness, molars – it's fine to wait a while. You are the expert on your child, and only you know whether night-weaning is something your little one can handle right now. You also have needs – so if for some reason you know you will find it hard to stay consistent or patient at the moment, then that's another good reason to delay. Good luck!

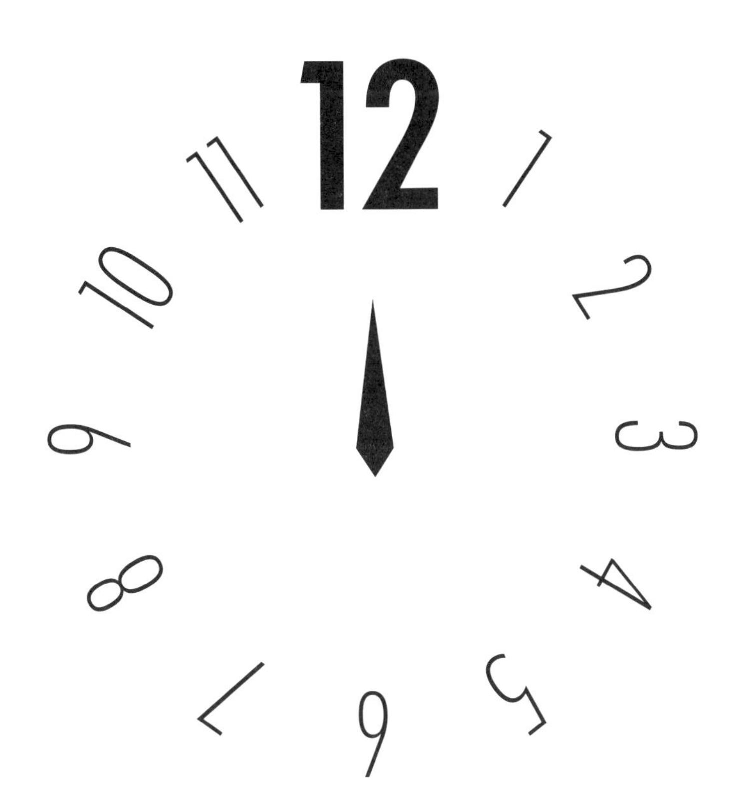

CHAPTER TWELVE

TROUBLESHOOTING

Sometimes when you are in the thick of sleep deprivation it is hard to think widely. This chapter is organised into some of the most common issues that crop up for families. Whether your child goes to bed like a dream but wakes up early, or the other way around, you should find some ideas to try. Don't forget to go back to chapters 10 and 11 to review your nighttime tools and night-feeding strategies if you need to.

Bedtime 'battling'

If bedtimes have become really stressful, they may have come to be the part of the day that you dread, rather than a gentle and calm transition to sleep. Review chapter 3 on bedtimes and look for the obvious causes of bedtime drama:

- Are you trying to put your child to bed when they're not tired?
- Check the bedtime boundaries.
- Has your child had enough exercise and silly time?
- Has your child had a chance to connect with you in a way that meets their needs and speaks their love language?
- Has your child had a chance to calm down after silly time?
- Is there something in your child's bedroom or sleep environment that they are scared of?
- Does your child get plenty of control over other parts of their day? If they don't have enough opportunity to exercise their own free will, independence and make their own choices, sometimes they try to

claw back power by resisting the bedtime boundaries.
- Has bedtime become full of drama? I absolutely know that bedtime battles can be draining and exhausting, but children love drama, and sometimes forcing yourself to stay calm will make it less fun and rewarding to act up at bedtime.
- Has your child got something on their mind?
- Is there a sleep red flag?

It is worth trying to understand the underlying reason for your child procrastinating, because then you can target the solution to address the cause, like this:

- **Are you trying to put your child to bed when they're not tired?** Try observing the time your child *actually* falls asleep for a week. Then start bedtime 30 minutes before this time. This should make bedtime more succinct in most cases.
- **Check the bedtime boundaries.** Review what the expectations are for bedtime, and communicate these to your child with a visual bedtime book.
- **Has your child had enough exercise and silly time?** I'm not suggesting your child doesn't exercise. It's just that most children benefit from *even more* exercise. Is there room for a little more? Does your child seem to have lots of pent-up frustration and energy at the end of the day? If so, how could you help them expend it?
- **Has your child had a chance to connect with you in a way that meets their needs and speaks their love language?** Again – I'm not suggesting that you don't love your child! But sometimes we default to showing our loved ones that we love them in *our* love language, rather than theirs. Try to build in some time to super-charge your child's love tank before bedtime.
- **Has your child had a chance to calm down after silly time?** Silly time is great, and it often helps to allow children to release that pent up energy and frustration. But if you try to go from bouncing on the trampoline or a big tickle fight to bed, it may backfire. Build in 10–20 minutes of calm-down time depending on how easily your child decelerates.
- **Is there something in your child's bedroom or sleep environment**

that they are scared of? You may want to overhaul the bedroom – think temperature, light, noise, shadows, clutter and toys, and the purpose and association of the space.

- **Does your child get plenty of control over other parts of their day?** Children need to have some power, or they will often try to claw this back. There is relatively little they are in ultimate control of, but sleep and eating are big areas that children can control. If they are not given the opportunity to exercise their choices, you may find they exercise a little too much free will at bedtime.
- **Has bedtime become full of drama?** It might help to turn down the theatrics at bedtime. Sometimes this can take the patience of a saint, but keeping bedtime free from raised voices and drama can really help to make bedtime calm, peaceful and succinct.
- **Has your child got something on their mind?** Ask the big questions earlier in the day so your child can get whatever is troubling them off their chest. Sometimes little ones ponder a seemingly insignificant event from the school playground all day and it all comes out at bedtime. Try to make space for these chats earlier. For younger children you could also get them to draw, sing or dance out how they feel.
- **Is there a sleep red flag?** Finally, just make sure there are no obvious medical causes for your child to be delaying at bedtime. If this is a new behaviour it is especially wise to be objective.

Bedtime delays, procrastination, fallouts and negotiations can really test everyone to the limit. But work through and see if you can identify what the triggers and underlying factors are. You may find, firstly, that it's not necessarily easy to work it out – that's okay, just try a few things and use your intuition to work out the most likely cause. Secondly, you may find that you can't put your finger on just one factor – it is very likely to be more than one. But as with nearly all the strategies in this book, it will not be harmful to try a few strategies at the same time.

Dummy/pacifier use

You may already have some ideas about why you want to stop your child relying on their dummy/pacifier. Do you feel they are too old for it? Is it beginning to affect their speech? Are people staring? Or is your child waking up every 30 minutes because their dummy has fallen out? Both choosing to start using a dummy and choosing when to stop using it are intensely personal decisions. I'm not here to judge any of them.

However, if you've decided that the time is right to get rid of the dummy, you may want to consider whether you do this 'cold turkey' or gradually. There are a few options you could think about.

1. First of all, only try removing a dummy when your child is well. A child with a heavy cold, earache, or with new teeth coming through is not going to be impressed with having their dummy removed. Also avoid doing this when there is something stressful going on – such as a house move, starting nursery/daycare, or the imminent arrival of a new sibling.
2. Initially, start by removing your child's dummy during wakeful times in the day. Restrict use of the dummy only to sleep times, and use emotion coaching and reassurance to help your child if they miss it during the day. It is absolutely fine to offer them an alternative comfort object such as a teddy, doll, blanket or muslin to carry and snuggle.
3. From a sleep point of view, start with removing the dummy for the nap. This is often the easiest time, but if that's not how your little one rolls, then try at the best time for them. If you want to try this very gently, consider taking the dummy out just as they are falling asleep. You'll probably need to pat or reassure them, and they may startle a bit. If it's a real disaster, then try again at bedtime, or the next day.
4. Once you have one nap going well, move on to bedtime.
5. You could try overlapping some new sleep cues at the same time as your little one falls asleep – such as a comforter, some soothing music or white noise/nature sounds, and a scent in the room which may make it easier for your child to accept ditching the dummy. I call this habit stacking, and it can work really well to help a little one accept an alternative way of being supported to sleep.
6. Tackle the nights last of all – as they are harder for everyone.
7. Some parents talk with their child about sending the dummy to the dummy fairy. It's totally up to you whether you think this approach might work. Some children will go for this, while others may get really upset.

You might find that lying beside your child while they get used to falling asleep without a dummy is the only thing that prevents a lot of crying. Don't worry that this is a 'backward step'. If your little one is learning to do without something that has been bringing them comfort for a long time, it is very understandable that they will need a lot of reassurance.

Some children don't respond well to a gradual removal of a dummy. In this case, the kindest thing to do is probably to remove the dummy and replace it with cuddles and reassurance and be prepared for 3–5 rough nights. You will probably find that your child has accepted the loss of the dummy by then.

Early rising

Early rising is usually counted as waking up before 6am. I know that many of us would like it if our day didn't start until 7.30am, but this may not be realistic for many little ones. Here are the most common reasons for early rising, and their solutions.

Let's start with the bad news. There is a genetic component to our chronotype (time type). This means that whether we tend to wake early and go to bed early or wake late and go to bed late is genetic. A particular gene for chronotype has been identified that leads an individual's tendency towards their sleep timings.[1] Most of the time, babies don't have an obvious chronotype – this tendency seems to become apparent in the preschool years.[2] If your child is genetically an early riser, then there may be very little you can do about this. Sometimes this will shift a little as your child enters puberty, but an early riser will pretty much always be an early riser.

Low sleep needs are another reason for early rising. If you suspect your child doesn't need much sleep, and has actually banked the amount of sleep they need by 5am, a later bedtime should help. This is especially likely if your child is achieving 10–11 hours of sleep, and has an early bedtime.

Sometimes, a too-late bedtime will actually make children wake earlier. I don't see this as often, but I definitely run into many children who need more sleep than they are currently managing. If your child seems to be achieving far less sleep than you might expect and appears cranky, or compensates with more naps than you would expect, then an earlier bedtime is sensible.

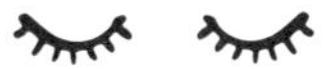

Some people are more sensitive than others to the gradual increase in light in the early hours of the morning. I know you've probably heard this before, but if the room is light, and your child wakes up with the sunrise, then blackout blinds are a good option. This trick doesn't work for all children, which is hardly surprising because, firstly, there are many reasons for early rising – this may not be the factor that is relevant for your child and, secondly, not all of us are this sensitive to light. But some people really do wake up early if there is a chink of light escaping round the side of a loosely fitting blackout blind. I sometimes recommend a little hack if you suspect this is a problem for you or your child. Get a cheap blackout blind and cut it to the same shape and size as your window. Then get a roll of Velcro, and literally stick the blackout blind to the window frame. I promise – total darkness is coming your way!

Anecdotally, some parents notice that early rising is more likely after a chaotic afternoon/evening. If the end of the day tends to be stressful, then restructuring it so that it is calmer may help.

Some children wake early because they are hungry. This may be because they ate their last meal early, have a high metabolic rate, have developed a habit of waking and eating early, or just because they are a child who is growing and needs a lot of energy. The night is a long time to last without food. If you suspect hunger, then offering a snack before bedtime might be the way forward. Try something like a bowl of porridge or a slice of wholewheat toast and peanut butter. Slow-release carbohydrates and proteins provide sustained energy release and prevent blood sugar spikes.

If your little one wakes up with a very full nappy/diaper, then consider a tactical nappy change before your own bedtime, and review how much fluid they drink in the last couple of hours before bedtime.

Finally, if you can't rule out the wake-up being habitual, you could try 'wake to sleep', where you go to your child before they normally awaken, and try to gently resettle them. This sometimes works to 'reboot' the sleep cycle and delay the waking time, even if only by a small amount.

Late to bed

I've said many times already that late bedtimes are a subjective concept. What is considered late by one family will be normal for another, and early for yet another family. At a fundamental level, if your child's sleep

patterns are meeting their needs, then there is no need to change them. There are a few reasons why you may be concerned about a late bedtime. Here are some of the most common ones I run into.

First of all, let's be honest. One reason many parents want their child to go to bed earlier is so that they can have some adult time. I don't judge you for that. You've been working or parenting (or both) all day, and need some time to decompress. I totally understand that. You'd like your child to go to bed at a reasonable hour so that you can catch up with your partner, watch TV, eat, study, work, or whatever else you need to do. It's real life. I don't necessarily have an easy answer here. I wish there was a way of everybody getting their needs met, but the reality is that we may need to compromise. It might not be possible to have your child go earlier to bed, and fall asleep promptly, and stay in bed till a reasonable hour, and sleep all the way through.

I know it sounds obvious, but as children get older, they go to bed later. I didn't really compute this when my children were very young. As bedtime creeps to 8.30pm, 9pm and later, our natural knee-jerk reaction may be to try to get them to go to bed earlier. But this is not a reasonable expectation of older children and tweens. You'll eventually end up either deciding that after a certain time your children can play quiet games, read books, and do their homework, or you'll learn to embrace this new-found time in the evening as family time. The only problem with this is that you'll need to think outside the box when it comes to having some quality time with your partner. Here are some suggestions:

- Have designated 'family time' on certain evenings, and 'couple time' on other evenings.
- Plan a date night. The only way some parents manage to go out and have some quality time is by escaping the house in the evening and leaving bedtime to a babysitter or trusted family member.
- Try lunch dates if you want to have some quality time with your partner and can't face organising a babysitter to handle the usual chaos of bedtime.
- Get organised ahead of time, so that as soon as your child is settled for the night, you're not then rushing around doing household tasks and making dinner.
- Eat as a family, rather than hoping for an 'adult' meal later on. I used

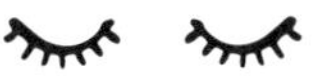

to feed my children and then try to eat with my husband later, but as bedtimes got later, this meant increasingly that we didn't eat until perhaps 9pm or later.

As your child enters the pre-pubescent years, they may suddenly start to sleep deeper and later. In fact, a change in their sleep patterns is often one of the very first signs that puberty is looming, coming even before the classic growth spurt that many tweens have. They often sleep much more deeply because, during this sleep, the brain is reorganising, pruning and paring down inefficient or unused neural pathways.[3] They also tend to fall asleep later, and naturally wake later as well. This is all well and good, but it can be a real challenge when they still need to go to school. You may want to try the following:

- Help your child have a calm-down or wind-down time before bed. Perhaps they could listen to a guided relaxation, do some yoga or Pilates, draw, read, or do something else they find calming.
- Try to make sure that your child doesn't do their homework in their room – this can make it very hard to switch off and fall asleep.
- Keep a consistent wake-up time for your child – try to avoid letting them sleep later on weekends as this tends to upset the body clock and cause a kind of jet lag every single Monday, which can then take most of the week to get over, only for it all to start over again.
- Try exposing them to bright light when they wake in the morning.
- Try sunglasses in the late afternoon and early evening – this will reduce the light levels and may help them get ready for sleep.
- Be careful of what your child is watching on TV, or what they're doing on their phone if they have one. Cyber bullying can cause stress and tension, screen use can inhibit melatonin production, and action, horror or even reality TV can increase alertness, excitement or anxiety.
- Remember to go back to basics with your bedtime routine. It is just as important for an older child as it is for an infant or toddler.

You may be concerned about your child's late bedtime because although they seem to naturally fall into this pattern, perhaps you have to wake them at a certain time to be ready for nursery or school. Perhaps your

child goes to bed at a time that is culturally normal for you, and yet it does not allow them to bank enough hours of sleep, bearing in mind the time you have to wake them up the next day. If this is the case, you may have to work towards an earlier bedtime slowly. Some children are natural owls, and for these kids it can be really hard to adjust their sleep rhythms. In an ideal world, we could have an adaptive response to this, with staggered school start times and so on, but alas – most systems do not allow for this level of flexibility.

Later bedtimes are also common in cultures where a later or longer nap is common. It may seem obvious, but if your child only needs 14 hours of sleep per day, and they manage to get three hours of sleep in the daytime, then they will only need 11 hours at night. Work around the total amount of sleep your child needs when you think about what time to put your little one to bed. Even if your child does not nap, a later bedtime may still be culturally normal for your family. If this is the case, there is no issue with it if the sleep your child achieves is meeting their individual needs. The only problem is when the logistics and societal expectations don't match the cultural norm. If you have to wake your child every single day, they seem sleepy and fatigued in the day, and cannot compensate with a nap, perhaps because they are at school, then you may need to accept an earlier bedtime to allow your child to get the sleep they need. It's an obvious point but sometimes compromises, though not ideal, have to be made.

The nighttime visitor

This is a tricky problem to manage, because on the one hand, children need to know that they can *always* seek out reassurance if they are sick, scared, or sad. But on the other hand, frequent nocturnal visits can be really exhausting, and unsustainable.

First of all, rule out underlying factors:

- Anxiety
- Recurrent nightmares
- Discomfort (stomach ache, constipation, itchy skin, allergies)
- Sleep red flags
- Full bladder
- Temperature changes (are they sweating, or freezing cold?)

Next, review your sleep hygiene. Does your child go to bed about the same time every day, and have a predictable and soothing bedtime routine incorporating the three Cs – calm, connection, containment (see chapter 3)?

How does your child feel about their sleep space? Do they feel like it is a safe, cosy space? What do they want when they come out of their room? Do they only want to be with you? Will they calmly be returned to bed, or do they refuse to settle unless they are with you? Working out what your child needs from the nighttime visits is helpful to target the best approach.

Most of the time, when children get out of their bed and come into the parental bed, it is for connection and security. The mainstream approach to deal with this is to keep consistently returning your child to their bed, without making a fuss about it. But this approach only tackles the behavioural element, and does nothing to address the underlying emotional and relational need.

In my experience, there are four main ways to change this: delay them, make it more comfortable for you, focus on keeping them in their sleep space, and address issues around boundaries.

1. Delay them

Sometimes when children get out of their bed, it's almost like they are on autopilot. These children will often return to sleep immediately when they get into the parental bed. But turning them around and leading them back to their own bedroom or sleep space can wake them up fully and make it harder to get them back to sleep. For these children, I have seen some families use a strategy that attempts to interrupt the autopilot. What you do is attach a little bell to your child's door, or your own door. You are trying to get to them before they make it all the way to your bed, to interrupt the behaviour in its tracks. This obviously works best if you hear your child immediately and can get to them before they make it all the way to your room – it's not a great strategy if you are a deep sleeper, or your child's bedroom is so close you would only have about two seconds' warning. There are other options for interrupting the pattern – for example, if you sleep with a co-parent, could you swap sides of the bed? Or could you shut your bedroom door and use a monitor? Sometimes, if it takes a little longer to get to you, you might buy yourself the extra time your need to change the behaviour.

2. Make it more comfortable for you
Because I have seen this issue more in sensitive children, my preferred strategy is to adopt an approach of acceptance that nighttime reassurance is normal. If we start from this perspective, then this changes how we manage nighttime visits. One option is to make it easier to manage the nighttime visits by setting up an emergency bed on the floor by the side of your bed. The message is – sure, if you need me in the night, I'm here for you, but these are the parameters. You can meet your child's needs while making it work for you. Place an airbed, yoga mat with sleeping bag, or mattress on the floor, and explain to your child that if they need you in the night, they can get into the special bed. You could give the bed a name, or invite your child to make up the bed. Don't worry about making the emergency bed 'appealing'. Ultimately, it needs to be appealing enough that they won't mind too much about not being in your bed. This approach works well for very habitual night-wakers, who do not respond well to being taken back to their bed, and for situations where arguing or negotiating just makes everyone more tired and stressed.

Here's how Theresa managed this:

'Our youngest stayed in our bed until after she self-weaned at two years ten months. Being quite the lark, she continued to slip silently into bed beside me early in the morning, lovingly combing her fingers through my hair until I woke up. For several years, this was the most pleasant imaginable 'alarm clock'. No better way to welcome the new day! This is the same child who, as a tween, still occasionally comes to cuddle with me on lazy Sunday mornings.

For a long time, we kept a cot-sized mattress under our bed as an 'overflow' sleeping area when thunderstorms brought all three frightened little ones into our bedroom. My husband used to joke with them that their job was to come in as quietly as possible, so as not to wake mama. They would slip in silently and cuddle close.

This was our strategy for managing bedsharing manners. They knew they were welcome in our bed. We were there for the tears and fears, but we also established boundaries. No kicking or flailing. No stealing blankets.'

3. Keep them in their sleep space

If your child wakes up, part of the habit that may be hard to change is the fact that they physically move out of their room/sleep space into yours. You may be able to change that part of the habit by temporarily moving into their room and sleeping beside them. This way, you may be able to resettle them very promptly, prevent them from fully waking up, and in time, prevent them waking at all. The idea is that if they are feeling anxious but consistently find that you are there whenever they wake in the night, their anxiety levels may reduce and they may stop waking up at all because they are confident that you are there.

4. Address boundaries

Finally, sometimes children visit the parental bedroom in the night because there are more generalised limit-setting issues. If this seems to strike a chord for your child, then work on tightening up the boundaries in the daytime, and at bedtime. Focus on what limits your child is testing at bedtime and address those. Sometimes, parents find that when their child begins to understand those loving, firm and kind boundaries, they stop pushing the boundaries at other times.

Bedsharing isn't working anymore

If I were to stand up in a room full of parents and say the word 'bedsharing', it's likely that within five minutes there would be an 'interesting' debate going on. But let's talk about bedsharing from the perspective that it is culturally normal in most of the world. Let's acknowledge that it's prevalent, and often chosen by informed parents who wish to maximise their sleep, and provide close, responsive care to their little ones. I'll also assume that if you're reading this section, you're either curious and open-minded about bedsharing, or already practise it. Bedsharing can be fabulous, and a wonderful tool to address a specific sleep concern, even if you don't plan on making bedsharing your family's long-term sleep arrangement. Some of the reasons it can be helpful include:

- Faster and easier settling during extreme fatigue. I often find that even for families who do not currently bedshare, sometimes introducing this practice temporarily (as a sideways step) helps to reduce the number of wake-ups. It 'banks' sleep ahead of making other changes to overnight sleep so that everyone is more rested. It also can establish some longer stretches of sleep so that a child only stirs minimally, finding comfort and reassurance in the close presence of a loving parent.

- A chance to reconnect overnight if you've been separated from your child in the day. Parents often find that bedsharing helps with the return to work, because babies and toddlers are able to be physically close. It's normal to miss the people we love, and many parents feel this acutely too.
- It is often easier to place limits on night feeds for a nursing toddler within the context of the family bed. Having to get out of bed to resettle a little one without a feed can be fairly brutal for everyone. If you need or want to limit night-feeding in a toddler then it's often easier to only make one change at a time. Maintaining close proximity to a parent is often a gentler and easier way to do this.
- It can calm a very sensitive child and support secure attachment. Some little ones are slower to warm up, harder to settle in general, and are sensitive to many things. Keeping them in bed beside you can help them to feel safe and connected. It's also important for parents – children who are described as sensitive, high need, or orchid are often more challenging to parent and we can feel like we're getting it 'wrong'. Bedsharing can be reassuring to parents in these situations too.
- It can be a bridge to facilitate more independent sleeping, through the use of bedsharing in your child's room (if they are old enough). I often suggest that rather than moving out of the parental room straight into their own room, that a parent bedshares with their child in the child's room first to ease them into this change. Having the familiar presence of you may help this adjustment to be smoother and calmer.

However, bedsharing is not the answer to all sleep dramas, and the best place to discuss this is somewhere where the community understands the beauty of bedsharing. Discussing this in a safe place means that the answer you get when bedsharing is no longer working, or not an option, is not a non-responsive one!

I run into all kinds of scenarios where bedsharing is *not* the answer.

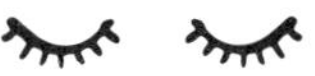

Here are the main ones for older children, and some tips to help if you identify with any of these.

You can't switch off. I know this sounds really obvious, but one of the main reasons for bedsharing is to maximise sleep. If you lie there unable to sleep because of hypervigilance about your little one, or you find yourself waking up frequently, then you may actually find that you sleep better in separate sleep spaces. Hypervigilance is sometimes associated with trauma and anxiety, so I strongly encourage you to get some help for this if you can.

Your baby or child is super wriggly. We nicknamed our second child 'Spider' as she was so wriggly. Sometimes, a new onset of nighttime movements can indicate an iron deficiency, so it's worth thinking about your child's diet, and discussing this with your doctor if you're concerned. But sometimes kids are just wriggly, and this doesn't always make for a pleasant bedfellow. You could consider a sibling bed as long as all children are over one. Siblings often love sharing a bed, and children are often more tolerant of wriggly people in their sleep.

You're expecting another baby. While you may have mixed feelings about transferring your older child to their own bed with the arrival of a new sibling, there are times when this may be the best option. It's not safe to have a newborn and a toddler next to each other in the bed. You would need to make sure there is a child on either side of you, with the baby on the lactating parent's side. If this isn't going to work, you could try having your co-parent bedshare with your older child while you bedshare with your baby. This also means you won't wake your toddler in the night when you wake to change their nappy or feed them either.

You're touched out. Sometimes it just gets to the point where you just need a bit of space. It's sometimes too much to be needed and touched all day, and then needed and touched all night too. I think we have a 'touch threshold' that, when maxed out, causes us to feel irritable and frustrated. If you're feeling touched out, make sure you have tried to think of creative ways to invest in your own self-care. I know this isn't easy if you're on your own at home with dependent children, so ask

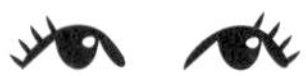

family, friends and your co-parent to watch your little one for an hour or two every week. If bedsharing is part of the problem, and not part of the solution for you, then it's okay to gently and kindly make the transition. Consider a floor bed, co-sleeper, sibling bed, or have them sleep on your co-parent's side of the bed.

Here is how these parents moved on from bedsharing:

'We used a floor bed from one. We had bedshared and then moved to co-sleeping using a cot next to the bed, then moved to their own room on an adult mattress on the floor. This meant we could co-sleep as required (and still can). We then also had a mattress in her room so we could respond quickly. As time went on, a little 'hush' would reassure her. Eventually we were able to leave her room. Some nights she sleeps through, but it takes less than five minutes for her to fall back to sleep once we put her back in bed. I think waiting for her to be cognitively able to understand has been vital'. **Danielle**

'I am a mother to four children and bedshared with all of them, more so with my youngest two aged five years (part-time bedsharer) and 18 months. I love the experience of it and the closeness you feel – both me and my children are safe, happy and comfortable and that's all that matters. My youngest was 10 weeks premature and spent the first six weeks of life in hospital so I was very keen to be close to her a lot of the time and am not in a rush to get her in her own bed. I have found that although my five-year-old still jumps in bed with us occasionally she can still successfully sleep in her own bed with no worries. With my oldest I tried to get them in their own bed by around three years old and it was a lot harder work. I just guess they were not ready. **Elisha**

'I have a 2.5 year old who I bedshared with from birth. She decided at 22 months old that she wanted to sleep in her own room. I was devastated! But it was good because I was 28 weeks pregnant. She's slept in her double bed since then with her daddy for most of the night (he joins her when she wakes). We love this arrangement and are so happy with it. I now bedshare with the baby who is six months.'
Danielle

'Partial co-sleeping was a wonderful way of moving away from bedsharing. Once he got used to his new bed, I gradually reduced the amount of time spent feeding or cuddling to sleep. He was eventually fine with being tucked in, a hug and a kiss and then he would settle. It took a long time to get from full bedsharing to none at all, probably about two years in total, but it was so lovely and gentle.' **Kathryn**

Split nights

Earlier bedtimes may also cause the dreaded split night, which is where your little one initially sleeps well for a few hours, but then wakes up for a middle of the night party. They will usually be perfectly happy, wanting to play, and show no interest at all in returning to sleep. You may roll out all your usual tricks, only for your child to remain resolutely wide awake. This can feel particularly brutal if you have not long gone to bed yourself. The split night is more likely with a very long daytime nap, especially when combined with an early night. Sometimes an early night all by itself will result in a split night.

You could try these ideas:

- Try a catnap instead of a full nap, so your child can make it to a later bedtime that seems to be consistent with how much sleep they need overnight.
- Try to inch their bedtime later in small increments.
- Put them to bed at their usual early time, but wake them up after 45 minutes and get them back up for an hour. I call this a bedtime nap. This isn't always easy. If your child is happy with this, then by all means carry on, but if they are unhappy and seem like they're desperate to go back to bed, abandon this tactic.
- Get your child outside in broad spectrum daylight in the late afternoon, to try to help their circadian signalling.
- Try to keep your child in the dark when they wake up, and use some early rising tools to help.
- Try a scheduled awakening (see page 233).

Very frequent night-waking

If you have a child waking in the night beyond the young toddler period, this can be very difficult and tiring. Most people accept that babies wake in the night, but most parents do not expect to still be regularly woken in the night for an older child. Yet, it is remarkably common.

Start by ruling out obvious reasons for them waking up:

- Check your red flags (mouth-breathing, snoring, strange limb movements, night sweating) – see chapter 3
- Discomfort (itching, cramps, wind, constipation, bedwetting) – see chapters 4 and 6
- Illness, teething, allergy, pain, fever
- Nightmares, night terrors, anxiety – see chapter 6
- Big changes in their world
- Something in their room that is scary or exciting

Next, try some quick wins. These may or may not improve your nights, but they are all gentle, risk-free and could possibly reduce at least some of the night wakes passively:

- Clean up their diet – more whole foods, less processed food, more fruit and vegetables and more water.
- More exercise – if you can, and if your child is able.
- Love bombing – filling your child's love tank, preferably by tapping into their love language, can be a game changer.
- One-to-one time – this doesn't need to be an unmanageable length of time. Just 10 minutes can make a big difference.
- Calm down any drama at bedtime – revisit chapter 3 to see if there are any changes you could make to bedtime.
- Use a social story to explain how bedtime will go – see chapter 10 for an example.

Then, decide how you plan to handle the night wakes:

- Passive approach – make it easier for both of you when your child wakes in the night.
- Easy fixes – just work on bedtime, and hope that this translates into nighttime improvements as well.
- Active nighttime changes – you may want to follow through with a strategy to help improve your nights. Be warned though; this may mean less sleep in the short term.

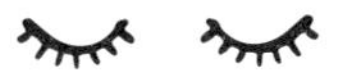

Passive approach
You might choose this approach if you haven't the capacity to make big changes at night. You might also not have the headspace or will, or this might simply fit better with your style of parenting. These approaches focus on maximising everyone's sleep, and minimising stress. For example, you might decide to buy a bigger bed to facilitate easier and more comfortable bedsharing. Or you might take your child's mattress out of their cot and put it on the floor next to a single mattress for yourself, so you can easily attend to them in the night. Perhaps this means putting a camp bed or mattress in your room, so that your child can snuggle up near you, without waking you. It might also include strategies such as nightlights to reduce fear of the dark, or meditation tracks to reduce anxiety. At its heart, the passive approach is about positively embracing nighttimes for what they are. It's not about giving up, but more about acceptance.

Easy fixes
Easy fixes might be for you if the sleep situation you're facing is relatively specific or simple, or you lack the capacity for big changes. Sometimes, it's also a good idea to try these before you embark on nighttime changes. These approaches include making adjustments to timings, and changing bedtime. You might make changes to the environment, such as improving the black-out blinds, increasing exercise to capitalise on your child's physical fatigue, and working on sleep hygiene. Or the bedtime changes might relate to bedtime boundaries and limits, restructuring the length, order, or person involved. You might incorporate a social story or comfort object. This approach would also include making some changes to daytime naps if applicable for your child. You could, of course, also incorporate some or all of the passive approaches as well.

Active nighttime changes
Finally, you may need or want to make some changes to your nights. Again, you can also utilise some or all of the strategies within the passive and easy fix approaches. Perhaps you feel this is appropriate because your nights are so difficult, or because your child is struggling to manage their day with their nighttime sleep situation as it is. This approach is likely to involve you doing something different overnight. This still does

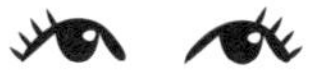

not need to involve you being non-responsive, but it may involve less sleep, as you might need to support your child in the night in a different location, or a different bed, or during night-weaning for instance. Making a change in the night is likely to lead to a temporary reduction in the amount of sleep, as it may be harder, and take longer to settle your child. Review the options and different sleep tools you can use in chapter 10 to decide which strategy might be best for your family.

The trouble with troubleshooting

One final thought: as you finish this chapter, I hope you feel that you have some areas to work on. The trouble with troubleshooting is that, through necessity, I cannot possibly cover every situation. You will almost certainly have to find the 'best fit'. This book covers sleep in a very broad sense. There are many areas that might not feel immediately obviously applicable in your situation, but the more open-minded you can be about what might work, the more chance you have of making some improvements. The idea is that there may not be just one single improvement you can make, but by chipping away at numerous areas, you will probably be able to feel better, and sleep better. By tackling sleep in this bitesize way, it is also more manageable and less stressful. I wish you luck.

CONCLUSION

Sleep issues in the toddler to tween age group can feel lonely, frustrating and daunting. I hope it is clear that you are far from alone. Maybe one day people will talk openly about how normal it is for little people to need bigger people to help them. Perhaps one day this book will be faintly amusing and quaint, because everyone has known for decades about supporting children holistically and responsively with sleep. I hope so. But, until then, I hope it brings you comfort. I hope it brings you a sense of solidarity. I hope you feel validated, heard, understood and seen.

This is not your fault, and it is also not your child's fault. It's so easy to travel down Blame Lane, but a huge part of the release from sleep grief and anxiety is to accept that some things are the way they are. Not because you screwed up, and not because you're unlucky, and not because your child is a 'bad sleeper'. Just because. Letting go of the need to blame and feel blamed is freeing and cathartic, and even this process in itself will make you feel less fatigued.

I also hope you now realise just how many areas of your child's life affect sleep and, conversely, how much sleep affects many areas of their life. We are not neat and tidy, with our issues packed up in little compartments. As humans, we are complex and sometimes messy. Sleep is sometimes the cause, and sometimes the symptom. Unpacking this can take a little bit of cunning.

It may feel overwhelming and frustrating, but by digging into the issues, you can uncover new ways to get to know your child, connect with them and support them. You can turn your frustration into a fearless

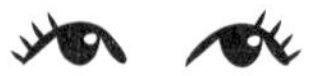

embrace of your child's uniqueness. Through knowledge, patience and sometimes detective work, you can find out why sleep has become your nemesis, and begin to turn the sleep ship around.

Finally, I hope it is clear that sleep in the toddler to tween age group is not as simple as it might seem. It's not simply a case of applying sleep techniques that work for babies and making a more 'grown up' version. Older children have different sleep dramas, different sleep needs, and different factors affecting sleep. They also express themselves differently, react differently and need a different approach.

However you choose to approach your child's sleep – whether you are comforted by more understanding, uncover areas to improve, or make some big changes – I hope you now have some tools to equip you for the journey.

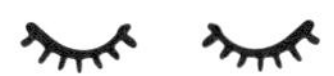

ACKNOWLEDGEMENTS

This book has been a joy to write. It's been churning around in my brain for years, and now that it's written I feel both relieved that it's out in the world (hopefully helping thousands of families), but also a little bereft! I've genuinely never enjoyed writing a book as much as this one. I hope you can feel the support reaching out to you from within its pages – that's what I was imagining as I wrote, sometimes deep into the night.

When I started to try to get my thoughts down in an articulate way, I realised how many areas of sleep usually come up when I'm supporting an older child's family. It's really not just about sleep – otherwise this book would be 10 percent of the size that it is! I realised how many resources I usually point to, and how many experts I refer out to. I wanted this to be a complete resource for families, so I just kept on writing.

Just like when I work with families and refer out, I wanted to include the voices and expertise of the sorts of professionals that sometimes need to be involved. I'm enormously grateful and humbled by the willingness of so many people around the world to be involved with a project like this. The book would not be the resource that I hope it is without you all. You all have my eternal gratitude.

Thank you as ever to my extended family – my parents for raising me kindly, to the extent that I now think of them more as friends, my patient husband who had the grace to not even bat an eyelid when I announced that I was writing another book, and our girls – who demonstrate their brilliance every day. I take a tiny bit of credit for how fantastic they are...

Finally, thank you to the team at Pinter & Martin for your enthusiasm for this book. Your patience and flexibility, as well as commitment to this project, has been heart-warming.

REFERENCES

Introduction

1. Hirshkowitz M., Whiton K., Albert S.M., et al. (2015). National Sleep Foundation's updated sleep duration recommendations: final report. *Sleep Health.* 1(4):233–243.
2. Airhihenbuwa, C.O., Iwelunmor, J.I., Ezepue, C.J., Williams, N.J., & Jean-Louis, G. (2016). I sleep, because we sleep: a synthesis on the role of culture in sleep behavior research. *Sleep medicine*, *18*, 67-73.
3. Cao, J., Herman, A.B., West, G.B., Poe, G., & Savage, V.M. (2020). Unraveling why we sleep: Quantitative analysis reveals abrupt transition from neural reorganization to repair in early development. *Science Advances*, *6*(38), eaba0398.
4. Reynaud, E., Forhan, A., Heude, B., Charles, M.A., Plancoulaine, S., Annesi-Maesano, I., ... & de Lauzon-Guillain, B. (2018). Night-waking and behavior in preschoolers: a developmental trajectory approach. *Sleep medicine*, *43*, 90-95.
5. Kahn, M., Sheppes, G., & Sadeh, A. (2013). Sleep and emotions: bidirectional links and underlying mechanisms. *International Journal of Psychophysiology*, *89*(2), 218-228.
6. Fang, H., Tu, S., Sheng, J., & Shao, A. (2019). Depression in sleep disturbance: A review on a bidirectional relationship, mechanisms and treatment. *Journal of cellular and molecular medicine*, *23*(4), 2324-2332.
7. Gao, Q., Kou, T., Zhuang, B., Ren, Y., Dong, X., & Wang, Q. (2018). The association between vitamin D deficiency and sleep disorders: a systematic review and meta-analysis. *Nutrients*, *10*(10), 1395.

Chapter 1: How sleep works

1. Bathory, E., & Tomopoulos, S. (2017). Sleep regulation, physiology and development, sleep duration and patterns, and sleep hygiene in infants, toddlers, and preschool-age children. *Current problems in pediatric and adolescent health care*, *47*(2), 29-42.
2. Kim, P., Oster, H., Lehnert, H., Schmid, S.M., Salamat, N., Barclay, J.L., ... & Rawashdeh, O. (2019). Coupling the circadian clock to homeostasis: The role of period in timing physiology. *Endocrine reviews*, *40*(1), 66-95.
3. Quante, M., Mariani, S., Weng, J., Marinac, C.R., Kaplan, E.R., Rueschman, M., ... & Wang, R. (2019). Zeitgebers and their association with rest-activity patterns. *Chronobiology international*,*36*(2), 203-213.
4. Walker, M. (2017). *Why we sleep: The new science of sleep and dreams*. Penguin UK.
5. McMahon, W.R., Ftouni, S., Drummond, S.P., Maruff, P., Lockley, S.W., Rajaratnam, S.M., & Anderson, C. (2018). The wake maintenance zone shows task dependent changes in cognitive function following one night without sleep. *Sleep*, *41*(10), zsy148.
6. Scholle, S., Beyer, U., Bernhard, M., Eichholz, S., Erler, T., Graneß, P., ... & Koch, G. (2011). Normative values of polysomnographic parameters in childhood and adolescence: quantitative sleep parameters. *Sleep medicine*, *12*(6), 542-549.
7. Currie, A., & Cappuccio, F.P. (2007). Sleep in children and adolescents: A worrying scenario: Can we understand the sleep deprivation–obesity epidemic? *Nutrition, Metabolism and Cardiovascular Diseases*, *17*(3), 230-232.
8. Kopasz, M., Loessl, B., Hornyak, M., Riemann, D., Nissen, C., Piosczyk, H., & Voderholzer, U. (2010). Sleep and memory in healthy children and adolescents – a critical review. *Sleep medicine reviews*, *14*(3), 167-177.

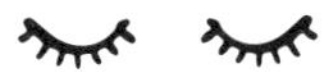

9. Maski, K.P., & Kothare, S.V. (2013). Sleep deprivation and neurobehavioral functioning in children. *International Journal of Psychophysiology, 89*(2), 259-264.
10. Beebe, D.W., Rose, D., & Amin, R. (2010). Attention, learning, and arousal of experimentally sleep-restricted adolescents in a simulated classroom. *Journal of Adolescent Health, 47*(5), 523-525.

Chapter 2: Self-soothing

1. Caballero, A., Granberg, R., & Tseng, K.Y. (2016). Mechanisms contributing to prefrontal cortex maturation during adolescence. *Neuroscience & Biobehavioral Reviews, 70*, 4-12.
2. Anders, T.F. (1979). Night-waking in infants during the first year of life. *Pediatrics, 63*(6), 860-864.
3. Bigelow, K.M., & Morris, E.K. (2001). John B. Watson's advice on child rearing: Some historical context. *Behavioral Development Bulletin, 10*(1), 26.
4. Woodhouse, S.S., Scott, J.R., Hepworth, A.D., & Cassidy, J. (2020). Secure base provision: A new approach to examining links between maternal caregiving and infant attachment. *Child Development, 91*(1), e249-e265.
5. Adshead, G. (2018). Security of mind: 20 years of attachment theory and its relevance to psychiatry. *The British Journal of Psychiatry, 213*(3), 511-513.
6. Bowlby, J. (1960). Separation anxiety: A critical review of the literature. *Journal of Child Psychology and Psychiatry, 1*(4), 251-269.

Chapter 3: Supporting sleep without sleep-training

1. McMahon, W.R., Ftouni, S., Drummond, S.P., Maruff, P., Lockley, S.W., Rajaratnam, S.M., & Anderson, C. (2018). The wake maintenance zone shows task dependent changes in cognitive function following one night without sleep. *Sleep, 41*(10), zsy148.
2. Brazelton, T.B. (1978). Introduction. Organization and Stability of Newborn Behavior: A Commentary on the Brazelton Neonatal Behavior Assessment Scale. *Monographs of the Society for Research in Child Development, 43*, 1-13.
3. Kuypers, L. (2011). *The zones of regulation*. San Jose: Think Social Publishing.
4. Keyhanmehr, A.S., Movahhed, M., Sahranavard, S., Gachkar, L., Hamdieh, M., & Nikfarjad, H. (2018). The effect of aromatherapy with rosa damascena essential oil on sleep quality in children. *Research Journal of Pharmacognosy, 5*(1), 41-46.
5. Shahidi, B., Khajenoori, F., Najarzadegan, M.R., Mameneh, M., Sheikh, S., Babakhanian, M., ... & Ghazanfarpour, M. (2019). A Systematic Review of the Effectiveness of Aromatherapy Massage on Sleep in Children and Infants. *International Journal of Pediatrics, 8*(5), 11233-11241.
6. France, K.G., McLay, L.K., Hunter, J.E., & France, M.L. (2018). Empirical research evaluating the effects of non-traditional approaches to enhancing sleep in typical and clinical children and young people. *Sleep Medicine Reviews, 39*, 69-81.
7. Motaghi, M., Borji, M., & Moradi, M. (2017). The effect of orange essence aromatherapy on anxiety in school-age children with diabetes. *Biomedical and Pharmacology Journal, 10*(1), 159-164.
8. Thompson, S.B. (2014). Yawning, fatigue, and cortisol: expanding the Thompson Cortisol Hypothesis. *Medical hypotheses, 83*(4), 494-496.
9. Dominguez-Ortega, G., Borrelli, O., Meyer, R., Dziubak, R., De Koker, C., Godwin, H., ... & Fox, A.T. (2014). Extraintestinal manifestations in children with gastrointestinal food allergy. *Journal of Pediatric Gastroenterology and Nutrition, 59*(2), 210-214.
10. Jenkins, T.A., Nguyen, J.C., Polglaze, K.E., & Bertrand, P.P. (2016). Influence of tryptophan and serotonin on mood and cognition with a possible role of the gut-brain axis. *Nutrients, 8*(1), 56.

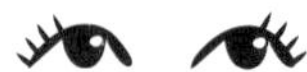

11. Huiberts, L.M., & Smolders, K.C. (2020). Effects of vitamin D on mood and sleep in the healthy population: interpretations from the serotonergic pathway. *Sleep Medicine Reviews*, 101379.
12. Mol, S.E. & Bus, A.G. (2011). To read or not to read: a meta-analysis of print exposure from infancy to early adulthood. *Psychological Bulletin*, 137, 267.
13. Shahaeian, A., Wang, C., Tucker-Drob, E., Geiger, V., Bus, A.G. & Harrison, L.J. (2018). Early Shared Reading, Socioeconomic Status, and Children's Cognitive and School Competencies: Six Years of Longitudinal Evidence. *Scientific Studies of Reading*, 22, 485-502.
14. Webb, S. & Rodgers, M.P.H. (2009). Vocabulary Demands of Television Programs. *Language Learning*, 59, 335-366.
15. Clague, L. & Levy, R. (2013). Bookbuzz: evidence of best practice. www.booktrust.org.uk/globalassets/resources/research/bookbuzz-2012-13-final-report.pdf
16. Kirsch, I., De Jong, J., Lafontaine, D., McQueen, J., Mendelovits, J. & Monsieur, C. (2003). Reading for change: Performance and engagement across countries: Results of PISA 2000.
17. Gariepy, G., Danna, S., Gobiņa, I., Rasmussen, M., de Matos, M.G., Tynjälä, J., ... & Brooks, F. (2020). How are adolescents sleeping? Adolescent sleep patterns and sociodemographic differences in 24 European and North American countries. *Journal of Adolescent Health*, *66*(6), S81-S88.
18. Eliasson, A.H., & Lettieri, C.J. (2017). Differences in sleep habits, study time, and academic performance between US-born and foreign-born college students. *Sleep and Breathing*, *21*(2), 529-533.
19. Williamson, A.A., Rubens, S.L., Patrick, K.E., Moore, M., & Mindell, J.A. (2017). Differences in sleep patterns and problems by race in a clinical sample of black and white preschoolers. *Journal of Clinical Sleep Medicine*, *13*(11), 1281-1288.
20. Zreik, G., Asraf, K., Tikotzky, L., & Haimov, I. (2020). Sleep ecology and sleep patterns among infants and toddlers: a cross-cultural comparison between the Arab and Jewish societies in Israel. *Sleep Medicine*, *75*, 117-127.
21. Takahashi, M., Wang, G., Adachi, M., Jiang, F., Jiang, Y., Saito, M., & Nakamura, K. (2018). Differences in sleep problems between Japanese and Chinese preschoolers: a cross-cultural comparison within the Asian region. *Sleep medicine*, *48*, 42-48.

Chapter 4: Lifestyle factors

1. Mendelson, M., Borowik, A., Michallet, A.S., Perrin, C., Monneret, D., Faure, P., ... & Flore, P. (2016). Sleep quality, sleep duration and physical activity in obese adolescents: effects of exercise training. *Pediatric Obesity*, *11*(1), 26-32.
2. Williams, S.M., Farmer, V.L., Taylor, B.J., & Taylor, R.W. (2014). Do more active children sleep more? A repeated cross-sectional analysis using accelerometry. *PloS one*, *9*(4), e93117.
3. Schwarzenberg, S., Georgioff, M., *et al* (2018). Advocacy for Improving Nutrition in the First 1000 Days to Support Childhood Development and Adult Health. *Pediatrics*, 141 (2), e20173716
4. Emmett, P.M., Jones, L.R. (2015). Diet, growth, and obesity development throughout childhood in the Avon Longitudinal Study of Parents and Children. *Nutr Rev*. 73 Suppl 3(Suppl 3):175-206. doi: 10.1093/nutrit/nuv054. PMID: 26395342; PMCID: PMC4586450.
5. Cordain, L., Eaton, S.B., Sebastian, A., Mann, N., Lindeberg, S., Watkins, B.A., et al. (2005). Origins and evolution of the Western diet: health implications for the 21st century. *The American Journal of Clinical Nutrition*, 81: 341-354.
6. David, L., Maurice, C., *et al* (2013) Diet rapidly and reproducibly alters the human gut microbiome. *Nature*, 505(7484):559-563.

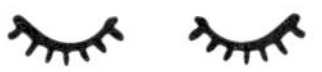

7. Valdes Ana, M., Walter, Jens, Segal, Eran, Spector, Tim D. (2018). Role of the gut microbiota in nutrition and health. *BMJ*; 361 :k2179
8. McDonald, D., Hyde, E., Debelius, J.W., Morton, J.T., Gonzalez, A., Ackermann, G., ... & Goldasich, L.D. (2018). American Gut: an open platform for citizen science microbiome research. *Msystems*, *3*(3), e00031-18.
9. Taylor, C.M., Wernimont, S.M., Northstone, K. and Emmett, P.M. (2015). Picky/fussy eating in children: Review of definitions, assessment, prevalence and dietary intakes. *Appetite*, 95, 349-359
10. Taylor, C.M. and Emmett, P.M. (2019). Picky eating in children: causes and consequences. *Proceedings of the Nutrition Society*, 78, 161-169
11. https://www.ellynsatterinstitute.org/
12. Coulthard, H., & Sealy, A. (2017). Play with your food! Sensory play is associated with tasting of fruits and vegetables in preschool children. *Appetite*, *113*, 84-90.
13. Brekke Stangeland, E. (2017). The impact of language skills and social competence on play behaviour in toddlers. *European Early Childhood Education Research Journal*, *25*(1), 106-121.
14. Storli, R., & Hansen Sandseter, E.B. (2019). Children's play, well-being and involvement: how children play indoors and outdoors in Norwegian early childhood education and care institutions. *International Journal of Play*, *8*(1), 65-78.
15. Badura, P., Geckova, A.M., Sigmundova, D., van Dijk, J.P., & Reijneveld, S.A. (2015). When children play, they feel better: organized activity participation and health in adolescents. *BMC public health*, *15*(1), 1090.
16. Flowers, E.P., Timperio, A., Hesketh, K.D., & Veitch, J. (2019). Examining the features of parks that children visit during three stages of childhood. *International journal of environmental research and public health*, *16*(9), 1658.
17. Mavoa, J., Carter, M., & Gibbs, M. (2018). Children and Minecraft: A survey of children's digital play. *New media & society*, *20*(9), 3283-3303.
18. Rich, A. (1976). *Of woman born: Motherhood as experience and institution* (1st ed.). New York: Norton.
19. Ruddick, S. (1989). *Maternal thinking: Toward a politics of peace.* Boston: Beacon Press.
20. Winnicott, D., 1953. Transitional Objects and Transitional Phenomena—A Study of the First Not-Me Possession. *International Journal of Psycho-Analysis*, 34, pp.88-97.

Chapter 5: Little kids, big feelings

1. Chess, S., Thomas, A., & Birch, H. (1959). Characteristics of the individual child's behavioral responses to the environment. *American Journal of Orthopsychiatry*, *29*(4), 791.
2. Rutter, M., Birch, H.G., Thomas, A., & Chess, S. (1964). Temperamental characteristics in infancy and the later development of behavioural disorders. *The British Journal of Psychiatry*, *110*(468), 651-661.
3. Schore, A. (2003) *Affect Regulation and the Repair of the Self.* New York: W.W. Norton & Co.
4. Siegel, D. & Hartzell, M. (2014) *Parenting from the Inside Out.* London: Scribe Publications.
5. Raphael Leff, J. (2008) *Parent-Infant Psychodynamics: Wild Things, Mirrors & Ghosts.* London: Whurr Publishers.
6. Cooper, A. & Redfern, S. (2016) *Reflective Parenting: A Guide to Understanding What's going on in your child's mind.* London: Routledge.
7. Siegel, D. Payne Bryson, T. (2011) *The Whole Brain Child. 12 Proven Strategies to Nurture your Child's Developing Mind.* London: Robinson.
8. Bion, W.R. (1962). *Learning from experience.* London: Karnac.

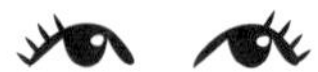

9. Green, R.W. (2016) *Raising Human Beings. Creating a Collaborative Partnership with your Child.* New York: Scribner.
10. Markham, L. (2012) *Peaceful Parent, Happy Kids. How to Stop Yelling and Start Connecting.* New York: Penguin Books Ltd.
11. Rothenberg, W.A., Weinstein, A., Dandes, E.A., & Jent, J.F. (2019). Improving child emotion regulation: effects of parent–child interaction-therapy and emotion socialization strategies. *Journal of Child and Family Studies, 28*(3), 720-731.
12. Gottman, J.M., & DeClaire, J. (1997). *The heart of parenting: How to raise an emotionally intelligent child.* Simon & Schuster.
13. Singer, P. (2011). *The expanding circle: Ethics, evolution, and moral progress.* Princeton University Press.
14. Neldner, K., Crimston, D., Wilks, M., Redshaw, J., & Nielsen, M. (2018). The developmental origins of moral concern: An examination of moral boundary decision making throughout childhood. *PloS one, 13*(5), e0197819.
15. Dweck, C. (2012). *Mindset: Changing the way you think to fulfil your potential.* Hachette UK.
16. Cope, E., Bailey, R., Parnell, D., & Kirk, B. (2018). What young children identify as the outcomes of their participation in sport and physical activity. *Health Behavior and policy review, 5*(1), 103-113.

Chapter 6: Things that bump, walk, leak and yell in the night

1. Simon, S.L., & Byars, K.C. (2016). Behavioral Treatments for Non-Rapid Eye Movement Parasomnias in Children. *Current Sleep Medicine Reports, 2*(3), 152-157.
2. Provini, F., Tinuper, P., Bisulli, F., & Lugaresi, E. (2011). Arousal disorders. *Sleep medicine, 12,* S22-S26.
3. McDonald, A., & Joseph, D. (2019). Paediatric neurodisability and sleep disorders: clinical pathways and management strategies. *BMJ Paediatrics open, 3*(1).
4. Gogo, E., Van Sluijs, R.M., Cheung, T., Gaskell, C., Jones, L., Alwan, N.A., & Hill, C.M. (2019). Objectively confirmed prevalence of sleep-related rhythmic movement disorder in pre-school children. *Sleep medicine, 53,* 16-21.
5. Stallman, H.M., Kohler, M.J., Biggs, S.N., Lushington, K., & Kennedy, D. (2017). Childhood sleepwalking and its relationship to daytime and sleep related behaviors. *Sleep and Hypnosis (Online), 19*(3), 61-69.
6. Provini, F., Tinuper, P., Bisulli, F., & Lugaresi, E. (2011). Arousal disorders. *Sleep medicine,* 12, S22-S26.
7. Nevéus, T. (2017). Pathogenesis of enuresis: Towards a new understanding. *International Journal of Urology, 24*(3), 174-182.
8. Borg, B., Kamperis, K., Olsen, L.H., & Rittig, S. (2018). Evidence of reduced bladder capacity during nighttime in children with monosymptomatic nocturnal enuresis. *Journal of Pediatric Urology, 14*(2), 160-e1.
9. Joinson, C., Sullivan, S., von Gontard, A., & Heron, J. (2016). Stressful events in early childhood and developmental trajectories of bedwetting at school age. *Journal of Pediatric Psychology, 41*(9), 1002-1010.
10. Dominguez-Ortega, G., Borrelli, O., Meyer, R., Dziubak, R., De Koker, C., Godwin, H., ... & Fox, A.T. (2014). Extraintestinal manifestations in children with gastrointestinal food allergy. *Journal of pediatric gastroenterology and nutrition, 59*(2), 210-214.
11. Tsai, J.D., Chen, H.J., Ku, M.S., Chen, S.M., Hsu, C.C., Tung, M.C., ... & Sheu, J.N. (2017). Association between allergic disease, sleep-disordered breathing, and childhood nocturnal enuresis: a population-based case-control study. *Pediatric Nephrology, 32*(12), 2293-2301.
12. Kato, T., Blanchet, P.J., Montplaisir, J.Y., & Lavigne, G.J. (2003). Sleep Bruxism and Other 24. Disorders with Orofacial Activity during Sleep. *Sleep and movement*

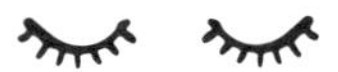

disorders, 273.
13. Machado, E., Dal-Fabbro, C., Cunali, P.A., & Kaizer, O.B. (2014). Prevalence of sleep bruxism in children: a systematic review. *Dental press journal of orthodontics*, *19*(6), 54-61.
14. Sharon, D., Walters, A.S., & Simakajornboon, N. (2019). Restless Legs Syndrome and Periodic Limb Movement Disorder in Children. *Journal of Child Science*, *9*(01), e38-e49.
15. Primhak, R., & Kingshott, R. (2012). Sleep physiology and sleep-disordered breathing: the essentials. *Archives of Disease in Childhood*, *97*(1), 54-58.
16. Harrison, R., Edmiston, R., & Mitchell, C. (2017). Recognising paediatric obstructive sleep apnoea in primary care: diagnosis and management. *British Journal of General Practice*, *67*(659), 282-283.
17. Reckley, L.K., Song, S.A., Chang, E.T., Cable, B.B., Certal, V., & Camacho, M. (2016). Adenoidectomy can improve obstructive sleep apnoea in young children: systematic review and meta-analysis. *The Journal of Laryngology & Otology*, *130*(11), 990-994.
18. So, H.K., Li, A.M., Au, C.T., Zhang, J., Lau, J., Fok, T.F., & Wing, Y.K. (2012). Night sweats in children: prevalence and associated factors. *Archives of Disease in Childhood*, *97*(5), 470-473.
19. Miller, G.F., Coffield, E., Leroy, Z., & Wallin, R. (2016). Prevalence and costs of five chronic conditions in children. *The Journal of School Nursing*, *32*(5), 357-364.
20. Martire, L.M., & Helgeson, V.S. (2017). Close relationships and the management of chronic illness: Associations and interventions. *American Psychologist*, *72*(6), 601.
21. Knight, L.K., & Depue, B.E. (2019). New frontiers in anxiety research: The translational potential of the bed nucleus of the stria terminalis. *Frontiers in Psychiatry*, *10*, 510.

Chapter 7: Big changes, big deals
1. Polanczyk, G.V., Salum, G.A., Sugaya, L.S., Caye, A., & Rohde, L.A. (2015). Annual research review: A meta□analysis of the worldwide prevalence of mental disorders in children and adolescents. *Journal of Child Psychology and Psychiatry*, *56*(3), 345-365.
2. Koopman□Verhoeff, M.E., Serdarevic, F., Kocevska, D., Bodrij, F.F., Mileva□Seitz, V.R., Reiss, I., ... & Luijk, M.P. (2019). Preschool family irregularity and the development of sleep problems in childhood: a longitudinal study. *Journal of Child Psychology and Psychiatry*, *60*(8), 857-865.
3. Golberstein, E., Gonzales, G., & Meara, E. (2016). *Economic conditions and children's mental health* (No. w22459). National Bureau of Economic Research.
4. Fosco, G.M., & Lydon□Staley, D.M. (2019). Implications of Family Cohesion and Conflict for Adolescent Mood and Well□Being: Examining Within□and Between□ Family Processes on a Daily Timescale. *Family Process*.
5. Eyre, O., Hughes, R.A., Thapar, A.K., Leibenluft, E., Stringaris, A., Davey Smith, G., ... & Thapar, A. (2019). Childhood neurodevelopmental difficulties and risk of adolescent depression: the role of irritability. *Journal of Child Psychology and Psychiatry*, *60*(8), 866-874.
6. Wlodarczyk, O., Pawils, S., Metzner, F., Kriston, L., Klasen, F., Ravens-Sieberer, U., & BELLA Study Group. (2017). Risk and protective factors for mental health problems in preschool-aged children: cross-sectional results of the BELLA preschool study. *Child and Adolescent Psychiatry and Mental Health*, *11*(1), 12.
7. Wamser-Nanney, R., & Chesher, R.E. (2018). Presence of Sleep Disturbances Among Child Trauma Survivors: Comparison of Caregiver and Child Reports. *Journal of Child & Adolescent Trauma*, *11*(4), 391-399.

8. Lai, B.S., La Greca, A.M., Colgan, C.A., Herge, W., Chan, S., Medzhitova, J., ... & Auslander, B. (2020). Sleep problems and posttraumatic stress: children exposed to a natural disaster. *Journal of Pediatric Psychology*, *45*(9), 1016-1026.
9. Dimov, S., Mundy, L.K., Bayer, J.K., Jacka, F.N., Canterford, L., & Patton, G.C. (2019). Diet quality and mental health problems in late childhood. *Nutritional neuroscience*, 1-9.
10. Fosco, G.M., Mak, H.W., Ramos, A., LoBraico, E., & Lippold, M. (2019). Exploring the promise of assessing dynamic characteristics of the family for predicting adolescent risk outcomes. *Journal of Child Psychology and Psychiatry*, *60*(8), 848-856.
11. Bennett, S.D., Cuijpers, P., Ebert, D.D., McKenzie Smith, M., Coughtrey, A.E., Heyman, I., ... & Shafran, R. (2019). Practitioner Review: Unguided and guided self□help interventions for common mental health disorders in children and adolescents: a systematic review and meta□analysis. *Journal of Child Psychology and Psychiatry*, *60*(8), 828-847.
12. Schofield, G. and Beek, M., 2018. *Attachment handbook for foster care and adoption*. Coram BAAF.
13. Bowlby, J., 1973. Attachment and loss: Volume II: Separation, anxiety and anger. In *Attachment and Loss: Volume II: Separation, Anxiety and Anger* (pp. 1-429). London: The Hogarth Press and the Institute of Psycho-analysis.
14. Bowlby, J., 1988. A secure base: Clinical applications of attachment theory (collected papers). *London: Tavistock*, pp.134-155.
15. Bowlby, J., 1969. Attachment and loss v. 3 (Vol. 1). *Random House*.
16. Ainsworth, M.D.S., Bell, S.M. and Stayton, D.J., 1971. Attachment and exploratory behavior of one year olds. *The origins of human social relations*, pp.17-52.
17. Ainsworth, M.D., Blehar, M., Waters, E. and Wall, S., 1978. Patterns of attachment.
18. Schofield, G. and Beek, M., 2014. *Promoting attachment and resilience: A guide for foster carers and adopters on using the Secure Base model*. BAAF.
19. Furman, W., & Buhrmester, D.(2009). Methods and measures: The network of relationships inventory: Behavioral systems version. *International Journal of Behavioral Development*, *33*, pp.470-478.
20. Killick, S. and Boffey, M., 2012. Building relationships through storytelling. *England: The Fostering Network Wales*, pp.12-48.
21. Perry, B. (2003). Effects of Traumatic Events on Children. Booklet. Child Trauma Academy.
22. Van Der Kolk, B. (2015). *The Body Keeps The Score*. Penguin Books. Kindle Edition.
23. Levine Ph.d., Peter A.; Kline, Maggie. (2010). *Trauma Through a Child's Eyes: Awakening the Ordinary Miracle of Healing* (p.4). North Atlantic Books. Kindle Edition.
24. Bhreathnach, É. (2018). International Association for the Study of Attachment Plenary Paper. *Sensory Information, Sensory Integration and Strategic Functioning*. Florence.
25. Van Gulden. H. (2010). *Learning the Dance of Attachment*. Lulu.com
26. Minnis, H. (2020). *What's Behind The Trauma*. 'ACEs, Attachment, and Trauma: new advances in understanding and treatment' – 2020 Emanuel Miller Memorial Lecture and National Conference. ACAMH. London. 13 March 2020.
27. Crittenden, P. (2015) *Raising Parents: Attachment, Representation and Treatment*. Willan Publishing.
28. Siegel, Daniel J.; Bryson, Tina Payne. *The Power of Showing Up (Mindful Parenting)* Scribe Publications Pty Ltd. Kindle Edition.
29. Bhreathnach, É. (2018). International Association for the Study of Attachment Plenary Paper. *Sensory Information, Sensory Integration and Strategic Functioning*.

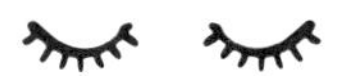

Florence.
30. Bhreathnach, É. (2020). *The Scared Gang.* (Boxset 3rd Edition). Aldertree Press. Available from www.sensoryattachmentintervention.com
31. Karst, P. (2018). *The Invisible String.* Little, Brown Young Readers US.
32. Atkinson, M.; Hooper, S. (2015). *Once Upon A Touch...Story Massage for Children.* Singing Dragon.
33. Quayle, S. (2014) *The Mouse's House: Children's Reflexology for Bedtime or Anytime.* Singing Dragon.

Chapter 8: Children with disability and complex needs

1. Brockmann, P.E., Damiani, F., Nunez, F., Moya, A., Pincheira, E., Paul, M.A., & Lizama, M. (2016). Sleep-disordered breathing in children with Down syndrome: Usefulness of home polysomnography. *International Journal of Pediatric Otorhinolaryngology, 83*, 47-50.
2. Rossignol, D.A., & Frye, R.E. (2011). Melatonin in autism spectrum disorders: a systematic review and meta□analysis. *Developmental Medicine & Child Neurology, 53*(9), 783-792.
3. Cuesta, S.O., & Delrio-Hortega, I.M. (2016). Use of Melatonin in Children and Adolescents with Primary Sleep Disorders and Sleep Disorders Associated to Autism Spectrum Disorder and Attention Deficit-Hyperactivity. *Journal of Pediatric Care, 2*(1).
4. Bruni, O., Alonso-Alconada, D., Besag, F., Biran, V., Braam, W., Cortese, S., ... & Curatolo, P. (2015). Current role of melatonin in pediatric neurology: Clinical recommendations. *European Journal of Paediatric Neurology, 2*(19), 122-133.

Chapter 9: All about naps

1. Staton, S., Rankin, P.S., Harding, M., Smith, S.S., Westwood, E., LeBourgeois, M.K., & Thorpe, K.J. (2020). Many naps, one nap, none: A systematic review and meta-analysis of napping patterns in children 0–12 years. *Sleep Medicine Reviews, 50*, 101247.
2. Thorpe, K., Staton, S., Sawyer, E., Pattinson, C., Haden, C., & Smith, S. (2015). Napping, development and health from 0 to 5 years: a systematic review. *Archives of Disease in Childhood, 100*(7), 615-622.
3. Reichert, C.F., Maire, M., Gabel, V., Viola, A.U., Götz, T., Scheffler, K., ... & Salmon, E. (2017). Cognitive brain responses during circadian wake-promotion: evidence for sleep-pressure-dependent hypothalamic activations. *Scientific reports, 7*(1), 1-9.
4. Staton, S., Rankin, P.S., Harding, M., Smith, S.S., Westwood, E., LeBourgeois, M.K., & Thorpe, K.J. (2019). Many naps, one nap, none: A systematic review and meta-analysis of napping patterns in children 0-12 years. *Sleep Medicine Reviews*, 101247.
5. Spencer, R.M., Campanella, C., de Jong, D.M., Desrochers, P., Root, H., Cremone, A., & Kurdziel, L.B. (2016). Sleep and behavior of preschool children under typical and nap-promoted conditions. *Sleep health, 2*(1), 35-41.

Chapter 10: All about nights

1. Galland, B.C., Taylor, B.J., Elder, D.E., & Herbison, P. (2012). Normal sleep patterns in infants and children: a systematic review of observational studies. *Sleep Medicine Reviews, 16*(3), 213-222.
2. Hoyniak, C.P., Bates, J.E., Staples, A.D., Rudasill, K.M., Molfese, D.L., & Molfese, V.J. (2019). Child sleep and socioeconomic context in the development of cognitive abilities in early childhood. *Child Development, 90*(5), 1718-1737.
3. Rickert, V.I., & Johnson, C.M. (1988). Reducing nocturnal awakening and crying episodes in infants and young children: A comparison between scheduled

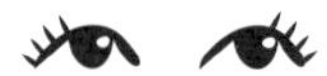

awakenings and systematic ignoring. *Pediatrics, 81*(2), 203-212.
4. Galland, B.C., & Mitchell, E.A. (2010). Helping children sleep. *Archives of Disease in Childhood, 95*(10), 850-853.
5. Taylor, D.J., & Roane, B.M. (2010). Treatment of insomnia in adults and children: a practice□friendly review of research. *Journal of Clinical Psychology, 66*(11), 1137-1147.

Chapter 11: Night feeding

1. Brown, A. (2018). What do women lose if they are prevented from meeting their breastfeeding goals?. *Clinical Lactation, 9*(4), 200-207.
2. Dettwyler, K.A. (2004). When to wean: biological versus cultural perspectives. *Clinical Obstetrics and Gynecology, 47*(3), 712-723.
3. Brockway, M., & Venturato, L. (2016). Breastfeeding beyond infancy: a concept analysis. *Journal of Advanced Nursing, 72*(9), 2003-2015.
4. Thompson, A.J., Topping, A.E., & Jones, L.L. (2020). 'Surely you're not still breastfeeding': a qualitative exploration of women's experiences of breastfeeding beyond infancy in the UK. *BMJ Open, 10*(5), e035199.
5. Gupta, A., Suri, S., Dadhich, J.P., Trejos, M., & Nalubanga, B. (2019). The world breastfeeding trends initiative: implementation of the global strategy for infant and young child feeding in 84 countries. *Journal of Public Health Policy, 40*(1), 35-65.
6. Scott, J., Davey, K., Ahwong, E., Devenish, G., Ha, D., & Do, L. (2016). A comparison by milk feeding method of the nutrient intake of a cohort of Australian toddlers. *Nutrients, 8*(8), 501.
7. Ramamurthy, M.B., Sekartini, R., Ruangdaraganon, N., Huynh, D.H.T., Sadeh, A., & Mindell, J.A. (2012). Effect of current breastfeeding on sleep patterns in infants from Asia□Pacific region. *Journal of Paediatrics and Child Health, 48*(8), 669-674.
8. Yip, S.H., Romano, N., Gustafson, P., Hodson, D.J., Williams, E.J., Kokay, I.C., ... & Bunn, S.J. (2019). Elevated prolactin during pregnancy drives a phenotypic switch in mouse hypothalamic dopaminergic neurons. *Cell Reports, 26*(7), 1787-1799.
9. Hassoun, D. (2018). Natural Family Planning methods and Barrier: CNGOF Contraception Guidelines. *Gynecologie, obstetrique, fertilite & senologie, 46*(12), 873-882.
10. Gust, K., Caccese, C., Larosa, A., & Nguyen, T.V. (2020). Neuroendocrine Effects of Lactation and Hormone-Gene-Environment Interactions. *Molecular Neurobiology*, 1-11.
11. Pomeranz, J.L., Palafox, M.J.R., & Harris, J.L. (2018). Toddler drinks, formulas, and milks: Labeling practices and policy implications. *Preventive Medicine, 109*, 11-16.
12. Harris, J.L., & Pomeranz, J.L. (2020). Infant formula and toddler milk marketing: opportunities to address harmful practices and improve young children's diets. *Nutrition Reviews.*
13. Milanaik, R., Fruitman, K., Teperman, C., & Sidhu, S. (2019). Bottles at Bedtime: Prevalence of the Use of Milk/Formula in the Bottle as a Sleep Aid in Toddlers Aged 13–35 Months.
14. Pritchard, N. (2019). A practical approach to the assessment of faltering growth in the infant and toddler. *Paediatrics and Child Health, 29*(9), 407-410.
15. Harrison, M., Dewey, K., & National Academies of Sciences, Engineering, and Medicine. (2020). Existing Recommendations on How to Feed. *Feeding Infants and Children from Birth to 24 Months: Summarizing Existing Guidance.*
16. Boone, K.M., Geraghty, S.R., & Keim, S.A. (2016). Feeding at the breast and expressed milk feeding: Associations with otitis media and diarrhea in infants. *The Journal of Pediatrics, 174*, 118-125.
17. Kashyap, N., Katlam, T., Avinash, A., Kumar, B., Kulshrestha, R., & Das, P. (2019). Middle ear infection in children and its association with dental caries. *Medicine and*

Pharmacy Reports, *92*(3), 271.

18. Chen, X., Xia, B., & Ge, L. (2015). Effects of breast-feeding duration, bottle-feeding duration and non-nutritive sucking habits on the occlusal characteristics of primary dentition. *BMC Pediatrics*, *15*(1), 46.

Chapter 12: Troubleshooting

1. Jones, S. E., Lane, J. M., Wood, A. R., van Hees, V. T., Tyrrell, J., Beaumont, R. N., ... & Weedon, M. N. (2019). Genome-wide association analyses of chronotype in 697,828 individuals provides insights into circadian rhythms. *Nature communications*, 10(1), 1-11.
2. Clara, M. I., & Gomes, A. A. (2020). An epidemiological study of sleep– wake timings in school children from 4 to 11 years old: Insights on the sleep phase shift and implications for the school starting times' debate. *Sleep medicine*, 66, 51-60.
3. Fontanellaz-Castiglione, C. E., Markovic, A., & Tarokh, L. (2020). Sleep and the adolescent brain. *Current opinion in physiology*, 15, 167-171.

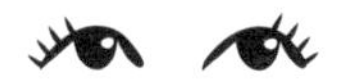

INDEX

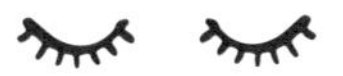

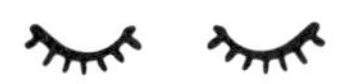

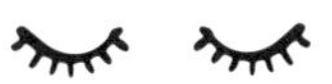